MANAGING THE INTERNAL MARKET

edited by
Ian Tilley

P·C·P
Paul Chapman
Publishing Ltd

For Helen

Paul Chapman Publishing Ltd
144 Liverpool Road
London
N1 1LA

British Library Cataloguing in Publication Data

Managing the Internal Market
  I. Tilley, Ian
  658.8

ISBN 1 85396 195 7

Typeset by Hewer Text Composition Services, Edinburgh
Printed and bound by Athenaeum Press Ltd, Newcastle upon Tyne, U.K.

A B C D E F G H 9 8 7 6 5 4 3

Contents

List of figures and tables

Glossary of Abbreviations

DGH   District general hospital
DGM   District general manager
DHA   District health authority
DMU   Directly managed unit
DoH   Department of Health
ECR   Extra-contractual referral
FHSA   Family health services authority
GP   General practitioner
GPFH   GP Fundholder/holding
NHS   National Health Service
NHSME   NHS Management Executive
NHST   NHS Trust
RAWP   Resource allocation working party
RHA   Regional health authority
RM   Resource management
RMI   Resource management initiative
UGM   Unit general manager

Notes on contributors

John Appleby is the Manager of the Central Policy Unit of the National Association of Health Authorities and Trusts. His previous publications include *Financing Health Care in the 1990s* (with Ray Robinson) and *A Review of Capital and Capital Charges: Cutting through the Confusion*. He is also currently the economics correspondent for the *British Medical Journal* and has worked as a health economist and information specialist since 1981.

Juan Baeza studied social administration at Goldsmiths' College and is at present a research assistant on the NHS Organizational Change Project of the Business School, University of Greenwich.

Liz Cairncross was formerly Senior Research Fellow at the Centre for Corporate Strategy and Change at the Warwick Business School. Her research interests and practical experience span the areas of health and housing, particularly as they relate to user involvement and consultation.

Shah Ebrahim is Professor of Health Care of the Elderly at the London Hospital Medical College. He has written *Essentials of Health Care of the Elderly* (with G. L. Bennett) and has coedited (with J. George) *Health Care for Older Women*. Currently he is on secondment to the DoH working on health-care policy for elderly people prior to becoming the Professor of Clinical Epidimiology at the Royal Free Hospital School of Medicine.

Ewan Ferlie is the Associate Director of the Centre for Corporate Strategy and Change at the Warwick Business School. He has collaborated on *Shaping Strategic Change* (with Andrew Pettigrew and Lorna McKee). Dr Ferlie's research interests encompass the introduction of quasi markets in health care and the role of the new health authorities and Trusts.

Nigel Fisher is a Consultant Psychiatrist at Springfield University Hospital and Honorary Senior Lecturer at St George's Hospital Medical School. He has an interest in monitoring developments in the provision of psychiatric services. His research interests include the epidemiological aspects of homelessness, medical ethics, and the physical health of long-stay psychiatric patients.

Simon Frostick is a Senior Lecturer in Orthopaedic and Accident Surgery at the University of Nottingham and Honorary Consultant at Queen's Medical Centre, Nottingham. He has edited *Medical Audit: Rationale and Practicalities* (with P. J. Radford and W. A. Wallace) and 'Medical audit in orthopaedics' in *Current Opinion in Orthopaedics* (August 1992). The development of medical audit and its relation to resource management is one of his particular research interests.

David Hunter is Professor of Health Policy and Management and Director of the Nuffield Institute for Health Services Studies at the University of Leeds. His past publications include *Coping with Uncertainty: Policy and Politics in the NHS* (with S. Harrison and C. Pollitt), *The Dynamics of British Health Policy* (with S. Harrison, G. Marnoch and C. Pollitt), 'The reluctant managers: clinicians and budgets in the NHS' in *Financial Accountability and Management* (1988) and 'Managing medicine: A response to the "crisis"' in *Social Science and Medicine* (1991). As well as holding the post of Deputy Director of the School of Public Health at the University of Leeds, Professor Hunter is a non-executive member of Leeds Health Authority.

Michael Kerin is the Chief Executive of Greenwich and Bexley Joint Commissioning for Health which was established by Bexley and Greenwich Health Authorities and Greenwich and Bexley Family Health Services Authority.

Susan Kerrison is a Research Fellow in medical audit at Brunel University's Health Economics Research Group. She has written 'Organisational aspects of the audit process', *British Medical Journal* (1992) (with T. Packwood and M. Buxton). She has also completed an in-depth case study of the introduction of medical audit at four hospitals.

Valerie Little is the Head of Commissioning for Sandwell Health Authority. She has 15 years' experience of working in NHS planning and information at both Regional and District level. At present she holds a visiting lectureship at the Health Services Management Centre of the University of Birmingham.

David MacKerrell is a Principal Lecturer in Accounting at the Business School, University of Greenwich, and involved in the School's NHS Organizational Change Project. He has had wide experience of accounting for management information at controller/director level, chiefly in multinational service industry groups.

Alan Maynard is the Director of the Centre for Health Economics at the University of York. He has edited *Public–Private Mix for Health* (with G. McLachlan) and *Competition in Health Care* (with A. J. Culyer and J. Posnett). He has been a member of the Health Services Research Committee of the Medical Research Council since 1986 and a former member of the Economic and Social Research Council. He is also at present a non-executive member of York NHS Trust Hospital.

Julian Nettel is the Divisional Manager of King's Healthcare and also Executive-in-Residence at the University of Ottawa, Ontario, Master in Health Administration Program.

Louis Opit is Professor of Community Medicine at the Centre for Health Services Studies (CHSS) at the University of Kent at Canterbury. His publications include *Commissioning of General Surgery for the West and East Kent Consortia, Elderly Care Planning Model, Wessex Regional Health Authority*, and *Needs-Based Community Care Purchasing for the Elderly: Handbook to Accompany Wessex Interactive Computer Model*, all put out by the CHSS.

Andrew Pettigrew is Professor of Organizational Behaviour and Director of the Centre for Corporate Strategy and Change, the Warwick Business School. He has published extensively including *The Politics of Organisational Decision-Making, The Awakening Giant, Managing Change for Competitive Success* (with R. Whipp) and *Shaping Strategic Change* (with E. Ferlie and L. McKee). Professor Pettigrew is President of the British Academy of Management.

Raymond Pietroni is a GP in Camberwell, London. He is also Chairman of the South London Umbrella Group of GPs which represents their views on the commissioning process.

Wendy Ranade is a Senior Lecturer in Government at the University of Northumbria in Newcastle and Vice-Chair of Newcastle Health Authority. She has written *To market, to market. . .* (with John Appleby) and *A Future for the NHS?*.

Ray Robinson is Deputy Director of the King's Fund Institute. He has written *Competition and Health Care* (with C. Propper and J. Le Grand) and *Economics of Social Problems*. Previously he was Reader in Economics at the University of Sussex and he has produced many articles and books on the economics of social policy.

David Salt has studied at the London School of Economics and the University of North London before taking up his present post of research assistant on the NHS Organizational Change Project at the Business School, University of Greenwich.

Roger Seifert is a Senior Lecturer in Industrial Relations at the Centre for Industrial Relations, Keele University. He has published *Industrial Relations in the NHS* and *Teacher Militancy*. He is currently leading a research project into industrial relations in hospitals.

Paula Smith is a research officer on the Monitoring Managed Competition Project of the National Association of Health Authorities and Trusts. Formerly she held the position of Research/Information Assistant with the National Association for the Care and Resettlement of Offenders.

Peter Spurgeon is the Director of the Health Services Management Centre at the University of Birmingham. His publications include editing *The Changing Face of the NHS in the 1990s* (with P. Bennett and J. Weiman), *Current Developments in Health Psychology* and *Implementing Change in the NHS* (with F. Barwell). Professor Spurgeon is working closely with both purchaser and provider organizations and is particularly interested in the new skills required to implement the current Reforms in the NHS.

Stephanie Stanwick is the Workforce Planning and Education Manager at the Nursing Directorate of South East Thames Regional Health Authority (SETRHA). Her area of research is skill-mix nursing and she also works with SETRHA's Corporate Business Teams which are responsible for monitoring the commissioning process.

Robin Stott is a Consultant Physician and the Medical Director at the Guy's and Lewisham NHS Trust. He has written on a range of topics from patient involvement in care to the nuclear arms race and its health-care implications. His long-term interests are mainly focused on how those working in curative care might advance standards of health in general.

Ian Tilley is the Project Director of the NHS Organizational Change Project and Reader at the Business School, University of Greenwich. His publications include *The Students' Companion to the Accounting Framework* (with J.K. Henderson and R.L. Mathews) and *Capital, Income and Decision Making* (edited with Peter Jubb). His research interests are in public-sector management, the management of change and the organizational aspects of financial control systems.

Stuart Turner is a Senior Lecturer in Psychiatry at University College, London, and the Lead Consultant for Mental Health Services in Bloomsbury and Islington Health Authority. He has published on various mental health aspects of stress, trauma and disaster. He is co-director of the Traumatic Stress Clinic at the Middlesex Hospital.

Angus Wallace is Professor of Orthopaedic and Accident Surgery and Head of the Department at the University of Nottingham. He is a joint editor of *Medical Audit: Rationale and Practicalities* (with S.P. Frostick and P.J. Radford). His specialty is shoulder surgery and he has a particular interest in the provision of orthopaedic care to the community.

Foreword

The wide range of contributors to *Managing the Internal Market* provide a timely opportunity to take stock of the NHS Reforms. Written from different perspectives, they reflect not only on the experience of the changes which have been made to the NHS itself, but also on the wider changing environment in which they are taking effect.

An understanding of this changing environment is vital to any appreciation of where we are now and where we should be going in terms of the NHS internal market. The Reforms were conceived by a government with a large majority in its third term, led by Mrs Thatcher. *Working for Patients* was launched in January 1989 by Secretary of State Kenneth Clarke, who had no qualms about a policy characterised by broad direction, bold brush strokes and banner headlines such as 'Money will follow the patient'. This approach caught the imagination of many who, like Mr Clarke, believed that the NHS needed just such a liberating shock to its system to wean it from its caution, conservatism and adherence to perceived Spanish practices.

In four years, the world has moved on in terms of national politics and economics, personalities and, above all, the understanding which can be gained from the operation so far of the internal market in the NHS.

The liberation is apparent in many places: the role of GP Fundholders (GPFHs – see the 'Glossary of abbreviations'), the greater influence of GPs generally, the potential speed of decision-making in NHSTs and the greater flexibility of working practices from many different disciplines.

Many other changes are under way where the effects will not be clear for some time: mergers of DHAs and FHSAs into larger commissioning authorities and, from April 1993, different relationships with local authority social services departments over care in the community.

The Reforms have also thrown up a number of specific issues which must be examined honestly and openly. These include the long term relationship of GP Fundholding and DHA/FHSA purchasing and the sheer cost of administering the contract-based internal market – a 'bureaucratic overhead' which few managers would attempt to deny. The role of the consumer in influencing market decisions must also be addressed.

In parallel with the structural and cultural changes is evidence of significant change in clinical practice as the market forces have added further impetus to the proportion of work carried out on a day basis, via minimally invasive techniques or drug therapies. These changes contributed significantly to the public perception of an NHS in crisis late in the financial year 1992/93, as many providers had consumed the money provided by DHA purchasers via block contracts, often with significant increases in the number of patients treated, and were able only to treat GPFHs' patients for non-urgent conditions in the last months of the year.

This situation emphasised the potential capacity of the NHS in much of the United Kingdom to meet more of the demand for health care than can be currently funded. It also accentuated the continuing inadequacy of information systems to support an undertaking as complex as the NHS internal market. Although there is evidence of progress, this remains a dangerously vulnerable aspect of the Reformed NHS.

The question which must be addressed during the coming year is the extent to which a market in health should be regulated. This book provides much evidence and analysis which should contribute to that debate, as should its advocacy of a continuing role for research and development, whether that be in health needs assessment or in organisational models.

Pamela Charlwood
Regional General Manager,
South Western Regional Health Authority and former Director,
Institute of Health Services Management

Preface

This collection considers the management and operation of the main NHS purchaser and provider institutions operating in the internal market in the acute sector into the second year of contracting. Newly commissioned academic overviews of the implementation process and scholarly studies of particular key issues are presented in Part 1 along with extensive practitioner accounts in Part 2 from NHS management and the medical and nursing professions of their experiences of the implementation of 'managed competition' and the interpretations they placed on these experiences. This blending of levels, approaches and perspectives within the confines of one book is designed to produce a distinctive and worthwhile addition to the literature on 'managed competition' and associated health Reforms.

The NHS is probably the most publicly valued part of either the public sector or welfare state. The hospitals and other Units of the NHS acute sector are ultimately much concerned with such difficult issues as pain, suffering, disease and death. How a society deals with such matters defines something of its nature. The policy intent behind the NHS market, and related measures, is designed to alter fundamentally the organization and management of the Service. It cannot avoid having some effect on these burdensome, often unspoken, issues of life and death that lie at the heart of all health services. Differing perceptions of this effect are in part responsible for the intense controversy accompanying the Government's health Reforms, none more so than with the focus of this book, the quasi market in hospital services.

All this is likely to mean that *Managing the Internal Market* and the account it offers of the functioning of the key institutions of this NHS market will appeal to general readers. Beyond this, the main specialist readerships it is aimed at are:

(1) NHS managers and those from the many clinical professions who, officially or otherwise, find themselves undertaking a managerial function alongside their other duties;
(2) students training to enter NHS management or these clinical professions;

(3) students undertaking courses with a social-policy or management-of-change dimension of varying proportions for which the Health Service Reforms are included as a major and significant instance.

When the contributors agreed to write for this book, they were asked to produce a chapter that stood on its own as well as being part of a collection. This has necessitated a degree of repetition between some of the chapters. Further, the endnotes to Chapters 2–19 were added by me as editor and are therefore my responsibility, not that of the individual contributors. The parts of the book written by me in my editorial role – this preface, the Introduction and Chapters 1 and 20 – contain no endnotes as, in this case, links with other chapters are best shown directly in the text itself.

The chapters are not of equal length. Some of the academic contributions of Part 1 are considerably longer than the practitioner accounts of Part 2. But the longest chapters, Chapters 12 and 14, are in Part 2. Furthermore, these two chapters were based on interviews with a DHA commissioner and senior manager in a large provider Unit, respectively. This was done as an accessible way of starting to consider some of the key managerial issues faced by many occupants of these two key roles in the NHS market.

My thanks go to Juan Baeza for help in making initial contact with potential contributors and for providing some early references on 'managed competition', and who, with David Salt, assisted me with the interviews that formed the basis of Chapters 12 and 14. I would also like to thank David Salt who, armed with lengthy lists, hunted down literature which I have used, directly or otherwise, in my editorial role. My thanks also go to Ginnie Malone and more recently Fraser Nicolaides, and their colleagues at the Riverside House Library, University of Greenwich, for helping David secure these references. I also wish to record my appreciation of the assistance David Fenton provided at the time of the establishment of a research project at the University into the Government's health Reforms, of which this book is a by-product. I thank Sue Proudfoot and Mary Spence for continuing that assistance.

Special appreciation goes to contributors for writing effectively to their briefs; without their efforts this book would not exist. I particularly want to thank my publisher and editor, Paul Chapman, for helping me conscientiously and effectively throughout, despite some delays my end. I am grateful for word processing and other help from Helen Tilley and Trish Fazackerley. I most want to thank Helen and Jonathan Tilley for their invaluable and loving support during the editing stages of this book.

Ian Tilley
Business School
University of Greenwich

Introduction:

The Main Institutions of the Internal Market

What briefly does the internal market involve? The purpose of this introduction is to offer a thumbnail sketch of the key institutions of the NHS market in the acute sector for those whose existing knowledge of this area is limited. Readers with this institutional background could well skip this introduction.

At this stage it is sufficient to depict the internal market as separating the hospital service into *purchasers* – the district health authorities (DHAs – refer to the 'Glossary of abbreviations' for a list of all commonly used acronyms in this book), GPFHs and private-sector buyers. The DHAs have still unfamiliar responsibilities to assess their residents' health needs, plan provison and write contracts to secure that provision. The health-care *providers* – the NHSTs, DMUs and private-sector contractors – agree to supply health care in accordance with agreements drawn up between themselves and purchasers. This is shown diagrammatically in Figure 1.

Thus far the internal market in acute services has some recognizable qualities of a market-place as the term is commonly used. However, on closer inspection 'managed competition', as it now tends to be called in NHS documents, is a market like no other in either the way it functions or the controversy it continues to evoke. Some of the special qualities of this NHS market, the subject matter of the entire book, emerge, even at this stage, as the nature of its key participating institutions is briefly reviewed. In fact, the introduction works its way systematically through the institutions mentioned in Figure 1.

THE DISTRICT HEALTH AUTHORITIES

The first types of purchasing institution in Figure 1, the DHAs, obtain health-care services for their local residents. With the change from the RAWP (resource allocation working party) to the new weighted capitation formula, funding is based strictly on the resident population, weighted for age, sex and marital status (Perrin 1992: 223). Non-residents can only be treated individually on an extra-contractual referral (ECR) basis.

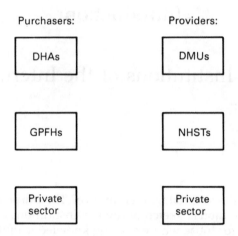

Figure 1   The purchaser/provider split created by the Reforms: the main
institutions of acute contracting

The health services provided are of either a 'core' or 'non-core' variety. The
former, which includes accident and emergency services, must be provided
locally. The latter, being of the elective kind, may involve waiting lists and the
like. In theory at least, all this elective work could be contracted to providers,
inside or outside the DHA area.

The District's responsibilities are for both hospital and community services. As Chapter 12 indicates, the DHAs are likely to be involved in
a reduced share of hospital commissioning, the extent of the reduction
depending on how much acute-services contracting moves to GPFHs over
the next few years. Whatever happens to their hospital commissioning,
DHAs will certainly be heavily involved in community contracting. Already
there have been mergers and other types of joint purchasing agreements
between DHAs. Increasingly FHSAs are joining these larger purchasing
institutions.

However, for the first 2 years of commissioning in the acute sector, from
1991 to 1993, DHAs have been the dominant hospital purchaser. Services
have chiefly been purchased from providers with block agreements which
specify the number of completed episodes to be supplied in a particular
broad specialty at a given average price. In future, other conditions to do
with quality, access, waiting times, complaints procedures and the like are
more and more likely to be specified as well as price. Increasingly providers
are thinking in terms of more refined agreements (cost-and-volume contracts
with triggers at one or more volume levels, or per-case contracts) which

they see as 'sharing the risks' between themselves and the purchaser more equitably. A lack of provider knowledge of detailed specialty cost behaviour as work loads alter is just one obstacle currently limiting moves away from block agreements.

THE GENERAL PRACTITIONER FUNDHOLDERS

DHAs are a pre-Reform institution whose remit has been greatly altered. GPFHs are the second and newly created type of purchasing institution in Figure 1, in the same way that NHSTs are the new supplying institution for the Reformed NHS. What GPFH and NHST share in common is a 'far greater degree of managerial and financial autonomy' than DHAs and DMUs (Whynes 1991: 14). GPFHs are a major extension and development of the GP's role as patient advocate and gatekeeper with respect to hospital provision. Initially intended for large practices – large in terms of patient list size – the size criterion has been reduced as the scheme has taken off. GPs apply to their RHA and, if they are successful, Region gives them a practice budget which is deducted from the DHA's funding. It is designed to cover some additional practice staff costs and drug costs with the lion's share for acute-service contracting by the GPFH for particular types of elective surgery, out-patient clinics and ancillary services such as X-ray and pathology on behalf of their patients.

GPFHs are able to vire or move funds between the different areas in which they can contract and, if they have a budget surplus, this can be used for practice improvements and additional contracting in the following year. Some practices have made large 'windfall gains' in this way which have proved controversial, given that they can be ploughed back into the practice owned not by the NHS but by the GP partners. Two even more controversial features of GP Fundholding are, first, the alleged special treatment their patients receive from hospitals to the disadvantage of other GPs' patients, thus forming the basis of the criticism that GPFH is creating a 'two-tier' NHS, and, second, the fact that the GPFHs are not effectively accountable, in any institutional sense, for their actions within the internal market. The FHSAs have only rather limited powers in terms of clinical accountability. The RHAs provide practice budgets for GPFHs but cannot, as yet, audit either the effectiveness of their use of such budgets or its wider implications for other GPs and other patients.

THE PRIVATE-SECTOR PURCHASERS AND PROVIDERS

The last type of both provider and purchaser listed in Figure 1 is the private sector. Private hospitals tend to be concentrated around providing certain types of elective surgery; consequently, they are 'a significant supplier' (Birch 1985: 281) of such procedures, in particular some types of plastic surgery, orthopaedic and gynaecological procedures – terminations of pregnancy (TOPs), *in vitro* fertilization (IVF), and elective hysterectomies. Since the

Reforms, private hospitals (and private beds in NHS hospitals) have been used, quite extensively in some cases, to clear waiting lists, in addition to private hospitals and laboratories receiving NHS work in areas such as pathology and radiography. As is made clear in Chapter 18, DHAs contract mainly with privately owned residential and nursing homes.

In their purchasing, the private sector might place its patient in a private bed in an NHS hospital for a procedure it cannot undertake, for example neurosurgical procedures requiring postoperative intensive care. Private hospitals and private laboratories also contract for support services from the NHS.

THE DIRECTLY MANAGED UNITS

Considered institutionally the main NHS suppliers, the DMUs and newly established NHSTs, share quite a lot in common. An important exception to this is the purchaser/provider split which is likely to be more complex, even fraught, for DMUs – compared to NHSTs – when each seeks a DHA contract. This is because the management of the DMU report to and are appraised annually by District. Another potential way the divide could become blurred is the DHA relying on the local DMUs' doctors for technical advice. However, the DHA might just as easily rely on an NHST's doctors, if there is a Trust nearby. Chapters 12 and 14 present two quite different ways of dividing providers from purchasers, only one of which seemed to produce a rapid and fairly clear separation of the two roles.

This said, there are a large number of commonalities between DMUs and NHSTs in their management and operation which emerge from looking at Figure 2. This figure presents a diagrammatic representation of information and financial flows between institutions. It is particularly important to remember that the focus of Figure 2 is the provider, be it NHST or DMU, and its main institutional linkages. Thus, other links, for example between GPs, RHAs and FHSAs, are ignored.

What does Figure 2 reveal? The main funding circuit is DoH → RHA → DHA and then from the DHA and GPFHs in the form of contracts with providers. There can be monies flowing from the DoH and RHA for various initiatives although, as the centre devolves more decision-making, especially to its NHSTs, even if to be carried out within Departmental guidelines, these monies and initiatives will probably reduce. Thus, training, research and so on will become more locally based decisions, with all the attendant opportunities for innovation, and dangers too, that this implies. As mentioned above, there are financial flows between the private sector and providers. Further, funding moves between the educational institutions such as the medical, nursing and paramedical schools (for physiotherapists, radiographers, speech, occupational and art therapists) and the provider.

In relation to the information flows in Figure 2, large numbers of instructions and circulars pass from the centre to the health authorities and providers and flow back in the form of routine and specially gathered reports and returns, regular and *ad hoc* meetings and other communications. In terms of information flows between the DHA and providers, these include help from the providers, consultants and doctors in specifying precisely what will be sought in the way of contracts and needs assessment of the resident population. This was noted at the start of this section as was its contribution to a certain blurring of the purchaser/provider split, certainly for DMUs but also for NHSTs, at least in the early years.

One feature of the internal market, and the Reforms generally, is an enhanced status for GPs. This is discussed not only in Chapter 13 but also in several other chapters in Part 2. Clearly, even with the relatively small volume of purchasing by GPFHs in today's NHS, they have, at least, improved communications with and their influence on hospitals. If only because of their feared volatility in placing contracts, feared not only by DHAs but by providers, Trusts as much as DMUs, GPFHs command a new respect in the hospital world.

But non-GPFHs are likely to be courted as well, firstly because they might always apply to become Fundholders, and secondly because they are likely to have a degree of influence, in some cases major influence, with the DHA and the acute contracts it places. In fact, when this influence becomes sufficiently institutionalized and strong, one has effectively moved from the

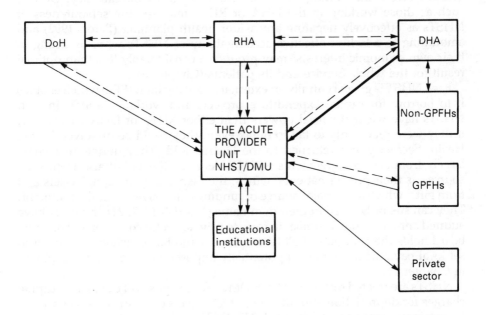

Figure 2 The acute provider and its relation to other institutions.
– – – – Information flow; ——— financial flow

Government's version of the purchaser/provider divide to that advocated by the Labour Party (1992: 15) which wants not only to abolish GPFHs and NHSTs, the newly introduced institutions of the Conservatives' Reforms, but also to 'create a central role for GPs in the process of setting and monitoring service agreements. Health authorities will be responsible for establishing panels of GPs to specify the level of services and standards that should be developed through service agreements for their locality.'

THE NATIONAL HEALTH SERVICE TRUSTS

To complete my brief review of the main institutions in the NHS market, I will consider the special features of NHSTs, the newly established providing institutions which, with the 'third wave' of Trusts in 1993, are likely to be the dominant provider of hospital services.

The first and crucial difference is that Trusts are established as 'self-contained financial entities' (Perrin 1992: 228). Not only are the DMU's assets transferred to the Trust but also the Trust board is managerially responsible for the affairs of the Trust. Its only accountability is direct to the Secretary of State thus bypassing RHA and DHA planning and funding, including capital funding, procedures. How this is regarded is likely to be significantly affected by where one is located. Trust managers might even describe this as a welcome liberation from the 'stifling' effects of health authority bureaucracy. Others, such as those working in the DHA or RHA, may see the separateness of NHSTs as effectively negating any wider health planning (Paton 1992) and amounting to a lack of effective accountability of NHSTs who, by acting in their own economic interests, may produce a considerably less than optimal result for the whole Service and its patients (Chapter 8).

Each NHST is given centrally an external financing limit (EFL) which enables it to borrow for capital expenditure projects and working capital. In fact, NHSTs have wider financial powers than either RHAs or DHAs. However, if they were repeatedly to fail to break even, they could be dissolved by the Health Secretary and returned to the District fold. They derive an income largely from service agreements with DHAs and GPFHs but also from such sources as their private patients' wings, the disposition of capital assets and from gifts, which are a major source of funding expensive medical equipment. They can sue or be sued in their own name (Morrish 1992: 21) and must have audited annual accounts similar in form to private-sector companies. The Trust board holds the contracts of all its employees and has considerable power to set local pay and conditions, a potentially important change that is explored in Chapter 11.

NHSTs are treated differently from DMUs for purposes of calculating capital charges for depreciation and interest (which affects contract prices) as well as for retained surpluses (Perrin 1992: 233–6). They can advertise their services, although this power has not yet been extensively used. As with GPFHs on the commissioning side, NHSTs are the Government's preferred organizational and legal form for the supply of acute services. They are expected to be entrepreneurial in approach and thence be at the forefront in deploying private-sector innovations in NHS Units – for example, in marketing, business information systems and human resource management. Clearly central to this is the expectation that NHSTs are actively to seek new business, both new contracts outside their NHS District and from the private sector in those specialties and other services where they have excess capacity available now or expected in the future. Gynaecology, orthopaedics (see Chapter 16 below), radiology and biochemistry are the most likely candidates.

OTHER INSTITUTIONS

Foremost here must be the RHAs which, like the DHAs, are losing many of their planning and monitoring functions, especially as more NHSTs and GPFHs arise. They still, however, receive funding from the DoH which is redistributed to DHAs after top slicing to cover their own administration and support services costs (Regional stores, training and development, etc.). Thus there is a considerable degree of compulsion in terms of receiving these services from Region, something increasingly resented by DHAs and DMUs, given the NHSTs' freedom from DHAs. Further, as other functions are devolved downwards to DHAs and DMUs, having to buy Regional services could appear to be an anachronism from a bygone age. The current management fashion, both in the private (Moss Kanter 1990) and public sectors is to favour the contracting out of support services and is certainly against being required to take them from 'head office' at a price, quantity and quality over which the 'purchaser' has little or no influence. Additionally, RHAs fund their Regional specialties and medical and nurse education costs and the extra costs of teaching hospitals in the form of SIFTR (Service Increment for Teaching and Research).

As Chapter 12 makes clear, no other NHS institution is in a situation of greater role uncertainty today than the RHAs. DHAs and DMUs are likely to bemoan their costliness and see them as out of touch, yet the Regions still influence crucial resource flows to DHAs and DMUs. Whether they will be abolished and their functions taken over by an enlarged NHSME; or handed over to NHSTs and the DHAs (the latter are themselves enlarging through mergers with other DHAs and FHSAs and may end up as something like the old Areas); or simply reduced in size; or even given new powers, most critically explicit regulatory powers over all purchasers and providers, including GPFHs and NHSTs; is unclear. The Government itself still appears somewhat undecided about the vital regulatory dimension to the Reforms.

The last institution to be covered in this section is the community health council (CHC) which is independent of the institutions mentioned above and has a somewhat vague role of commenting on the performance and operation of NHS institutions in its own geographical area and of giving advice on proposed changes in local provision, for example site rationalizations like those mentioned in Chapter 8. They could, potentially, be an effective voice for local residents and many do attempt that role. However, whilst their status within the emerging new system remains unclear, this is a difficult role to discharge. Given the new requirements on the DHA for strategic planning and needs assessment, and, as Chapter 6 points out, the real legitimacy problems of DHAs in these roles, the CHCs could be given a much more definitive role and clearer powers by the policy-makers.

CONCLUSION

Having provided an institutional thumbnail sketch of the main players in the NHS acute-sector market, what then is the nature and scope of this book on the management and operation of these institutions in the market? Answering that is the task of the next chapter.

REFERENCES

Birch, S. (1985) Tread carefully: private waters, *Health and Social Service Journal*, 6 June, 710–11.
Labour Party (1992) *Your Good Health: A White Paper for a Labour Government*. London: Labour Party.
Morrish, A. (1992) What are Trusts allowed to do?, *Health Services Management*, April, 21–3.
Moss Kanter, R. (1990) *When the Giants Learn to Dance: Mastering the Challenges of Strategy, Management and Careers in the 1990s*. London: Unwin.
Paton, C. (1992) *Competition and Planning in the National Health Service: The danger of Unplanned Markets*. London: Chapman & Hall.
Perrin, J. (1992) The National Health Service, in D. Henley *et al.* (eds.) *Public Sector Accounting and Financial Control*. London: Chapman & Hall, 215–47.
Whynes, D. (1991) When the future is in futures, *Health Service Journal*, 4 April, 14–15.

1
Approaching the Internal Market:
The Nature and Scope of the Book

Ian Tilley

This book brings together both health academics and practitioners to consider the stage currently reached in the creation of an internal market in acute health-care services within the implementation of the overall change programme provided for in the Government's health Reforms (in particular, DoH 1989a, 1990a, 1991, 1992). The present chapter introduces this collection and defines the nature and scope of the book.

THE TASKS OF THE CURRENT CHAPTER

During the so-called period of 'steady state' in 1991–2 when the Department of Health (DoH) required purchasers and providers in the market to focus on establishing the institutional framework for the Reforms rather than alter existing referral patterns, Le Grand (1991: 1266) spoke, not unexpectedly, of there being 'much yet to be discovered'. A year later Harrison *et al.* (1992: 118) were talking of there still only being 'the most preliminary and fragmentary' information about how this health-care market operates, even in what senses it might meaningfully be called a market.

However, the existence of this market and the Reform programme posed important questions for managers, health-care professionals and employees generally, policy-makers, and all of us as potential or actual users of the services NHS hospitals provide. These questions and their urgency spawned 'voluminous conjecture', a large ephemeral literature which is only slowly now yielding to a new phase of a more grounded, considered understanding of the operations of this market of which, hopefully, *Managing the Internal Market* will play its part.

It differs from many other accounts, particularly in the way it provides a forum in which different professionals can speak at a variety of levels, perspectives and angles. Their accounts were chiefly written as the first year of contracting drew to a close up to around the first half of the second year, 1992–3. Clearly it is early days in terms of being able to observe the NHS market. Furthermore it would be quite unrealistic to claim comprehensiveness and typicality for all aspects of the contributors' accounts.

Thus, *Managing the Internal Market* is a work of the second, more considered phase in the understanding of the dynamics of the quasi market in health and the Reforms generally. The sheer size of the Health Service, its importance in British society, and the political consensus that surrounds the separation of health purchasers and providers, if not the form this separation takes under the current Conservative Government's health policy, guarantees that this area will continue to be studied in the long term.

The current chapter has the following tasks:

(1) To establish something of the importance accorded the internal market.

(2) To remind readers how controversial this quasi market is in an overall programme of change whose hallmark is its contentiousness both inside the Health Service and beyond.

(3) To examine briefly the preparedness of the NHS purchaser and provider institutions for the implementation of the internal market within the overall health policy. The reasons for this discussion are, first, that it is not really commented upon elsewhere in the collection and, second, that success and failure in this area will influence the entire implementation process.

(4) To consider the scope of the collection, what the book includes and, particularly important at this stage, what is excluded from its brief.

(5) To outline the broad approach that informs the collection and, leading on from that, the structure of the book.

THE IMPORTANCE OF THE INTERNAL MARKET

Change programmes, especially in health, tend to evoke colourful epithets which are not only indicative of the political, occupational (for NHS employees) and other allegiances of those uttering them but are also likely to emerge in stark terms. Thus, the accounts given about the effects of planned changes like the introduction of the internal market into the acute sector are likely to say either that nothing has really altered or the opposite: everything is now different. Such polarized, dichotomous reactions are perhaps less true in change situations outside of the NHS where those living with large-scale change are likely to forget 'about the many continuities with the pre-change situation' (Pettigrew 1985).

Relatively early examples of health commentators stressing this discontinuity when talking about the internal market include Culyer *et al.* (1990: 2): 'The means by which the objectives embodied in the Reforms are to be achieved is the creation of a competitive market on the supply side where providers, public and private, compete for budgets of publicly financed purchasers'. Likewise Millar (1990: 1597): 'Contracts are the glue that will hold the whole system together after April 1991.' Both portray this market as the prime mover 'driving' the whole package of change. Several years on it is easy enough to find interpreters of the Reforms speaking of the 'new contract culture' (Ham *et al.* 1992: 24) or even now to find commentators talking of 'the revolution begun with *Working for Patients*' (Health Service Journal 1992a: 14).

Others are much more cautious, referring to the importance of the 'subsequent linguistic softening' in which the term internal market has become officially metamorphosed into 'managed competition' (Ashburner *et al*. 1991: 4) or the Reforms are referred to as a 'potentially massive change' (Appleby 1992: xi). But some recent surveys – the one reported in Chapter 7 below and/or in Agnew (1992), say – speak even in Year Two of the market as still having little or no real effect.

What can be concluded at this stage? First, the perceptions of commentators and the conversations with NHS personnel will, as often as not, reveal polarized opinions in which the internal market is portrayed either as the driving force or having no real influence at all. Second, although perceptions are doubtless important, the impact of 'managed competition' or the Reforms overall appears to be complex and varied depending on such factors as location and type of Unit. Most of the chapters in this book offer opinions and evidence about this and Chapters 7 and 8 research the question directly.

THE CONTROVERSIAL NATURE OF THE INTERNAL MARKET

One thing that is clear, however, is that the NHS internal market, quasi market or 'managed competition' is the most controversial aspect of current health policy which is itself perhaps the most debated policy for health since the creation of the Health Service. In fact, 'the management and organization of the British Health Service has seldom been off the front pages of national and local newspapers' (Cox 1991: 109). The first large-scale redundancies by the new Trusts were announced at the Guy's and Lewisham (Davies 1992: 12) and Bradford NHS Trusts. As Chapter 15 indicates, the media focus was particularly intense on the former NHST given its 'flagship' prominence.

The NHS market is vaunted by some as the core to instilling a new vigour, efficiency and business-like quality to Britain's biggest enterprise, the NHS. A few political commentators would see it as stopping short of its potential. For example, Butler (1989: 336–7) called early for contract management for NHS hospitals but its formal introduction at least has not yet been considered. Far more common is for critics to disparage the internal market and the whole policy as, first, denying and ignoring underfunding in the NHS and misdirecting attention into the Service's alleged 'inefficiency' when it was, till the changes, one of the cheapest and most efficient health services in the industrialized world; second, as attacking quality of patient care in a market only oriented to prices and economic matters whereas patient care ought to be the first and foremost goal of the NHS around which policy-makers, managers, clinicians and other NHS employees unite; and, third, as the prelude to the direct privatization of the service (Socialist Health Association 1988: 9; Cook 1991) or a more indirect process of privatization, given the public importance and popularity accorded the NHS:

The [White Paper] proposals introduce a structure which will facilitate subsequent privatization. The market will have been segmented, the assets evaluated, product lines developed, and an information system capable of being used as a billing system will be in place. Whilst the present ministers may protest that privatization is not their aim, future ministers are unlikely to feel so constrained. As some self-governing hospitals grow and flourish, it is highly likely that they will wish to become fully independent of the National Health Service and what Minister of the new right could deny them that freedom?

(Roberts 1990: 113)

Others speak of increased secrecy, and harsh treatment for 'whistle blowers' (MSF 1992: 1), especially in NHSTs operating in the internal market, and of 'an accountants' paradise' (Gerrard 1991: 24) with escalating administrative costs generally, given the complexity and uncertainty introduced by 'managed competition'. Other commentators stress the element of progression from compulsory competitive tendering (refer Key 1988 and Asher 1987) of laundry, cleaning and catering services in the 1980s to contracting all clinical services in the 1990s (Bach 1989); alternatively this is regarded as a 'different order of magnitude and significance' (Perrin 1992: 225). Some have 'regretted the lack of any pilot testing of the changes' (Charlwood 1991); others still speak of the Reforms as 'a dangerous experiment' (Hunter and Webster 1992: 26). The DoH (1990b: 21) suggested the Reforms would not change such issues as research funding in the NHS; recently Peter Woodford, Chief Scientist at the DoH, said 'Research and development are in danger of being squeezed out by the need of providers to obtain contracts' and it would require the intervention of NHSME to resolve this problem (Health Service Journal 1992b). This raises the wider question of the paradox of a market with a powerful centre, the DoH, which can intervene in that market. Finally, Snell (1991: 18–19) recently reported that 'A circular from the DoH, offering advice on decontamination of equipment contaminated with Hepatitis B and HIV, has been sent to DMUs for action, but the NHSTs for information only.' This example again raises the question of the role of the centre but also questions of accountability of NHSTs. One could also extend this to GPFHs. Such issues arise in Chapters 12 and 13.

PREPAREDNESS FOR THE INTERNAL MARKET

In management-of-change programmes, even and perhaps especially those on the scale of the Government's Reforms of the NHS hospital service, ensuring adequate preparations for the changes is a first and essential step. This is not meant in some absolute or static sense. The conception of what and how to reorganize is constantly evolving so it would be unhelpful to criticize the health policy-makers and DoH officals for not planning everything ahead of starting the implementation process. None the less, if the actual preparations are too far down the other end of the spectrum, the complications this creates are likely to dog the change process throughout.

An assessment of the degree of preparedness within the NHS to implement 'managed competition' and, in particular, how purchasers and providers are coping in the early years of what is the rapid implementation of large-scale change in a very big organization needs to be undertaken somewhere in the collection. As I commissioned no contributor to write directly on this theme, the assessment, albeit a brief one, will be conducted in this first chapter which is supplemented by some material in later chapters, especially Chapters 12 and 14.

The assessment offered here will simply consist of a short response to the following three questions:

(1) Why did the policy-makers decide on a relatively fast implementation of the NHS market and related Reforms of the hospital service?
(2) What problems has this created for providers?
(3) What difficulties has this created for purchasers?

Why a rapid implementation?

The Thatcher Government which initiated the health Reforms produced a health version of 'the change model' it had deployed in the Civil Service, education and in the public sector generally: one aspect of this is what March and Olsen (1989: 64) call 'intentional transformation through process of radical shock': 'Major structural changes in institutions are made in the hope that such changes will destabalise political arrangements and force a permanent realignment of the existing system.'

The Health Service was adjudged by the policy-makers as a very large organization with a track record for trenchant resistance to significant change stretching back to its inception. Furthermore, the resistors had unparalleled effectiveness within a public sector that was perceived by the Government as generally resisting changes to its own organization and management. In the case of the NHS this 'pre-eminence' largely stemmed from the role played by doctors and consultants in such resistance with their ability to appeal to science, medical ethics and successes due mainly to the advent of many new cures, 'wonder drugs' and treatments, which still dazzle so many of us.

The separation of purchaser – mainly the DHAs and GPFHs – from provider – chiefly DMUs and NHSTs – depended so much on the 'availability of relevant, accurate and timely' (Smith 1990: 110) information about prices, work loads, quality standards and so on. Some (e.g. Kelly 1991: 28) called this a 'Herculean task'. Others were much less sympathetic. For instance, the Labour Party (1992: 4) spoke of 'the tragedy' of pushing up the historically low administrative costs of the NHS compared with health services elsewhere as the internal market imposed 'extra transaction costs' and created an 'elaborate new paperchase of contracts and invoices' which, in an allegedly underfunded NHS, could only mean fewer financial resources being available to treat patients.

One academic commenting on the degree of preparedness for change says:

NHS managers find the rules of their game [i.e. instructions and circulars from

the DoH] change rapidly, and seem to be devised 'off the cuff' by the DoH
. . . like the governments of Eastern Europe, [the Department] has introduced
a market before setting up the policies and organisations needed to make the
market work.

(Cumella 1991: 22)

What needs to be assessed is how fair these strident voices of criticism
are being. On the one hand, the introduction of the internal market and
associated Reforms was clearly a top-down process and therefore it is
incumbent upon the politicians and DoH officials to have made adequate
plans and communicated the Reform process. On the other hand, no major
change process can or should be fully planned prior to implementation.
Later chapters will present more of the detail needed to reach a balanced
assessment. All that can be done here is to highlight something of the
different situations providers and purchasers find themselves in, given a
speedy implementation process which was designed to minimize the fierce
internal opposition expected and rapidly demonstrate the benefits of 'the new
world'.

The preparedness of providers

As will soon become apparent, the available literature concentrates on the
providers and problems around their readiness for the changes because
the centre itself was much more concerned with the health-care suppliers.
None the less, this literature seems more preoccupied with weaknesses
in the suppliers' preparations than their strengths. These were said to
include:

(1) *The lack of senior managers in the NHS appropriately trained in commercial
     management* (Perrin 1992: 227) and capable of effectively leading NHSTs.
     For instance, in their recent study Marriott and Mellett (1991b: 23)
     found a definite gap existing between managers' financial skills and
     those which will be needed to operate efficiently the novel procedures
     in the Reformed NHS. Despite efforts to reduce such gaps, they
     appear to extend to all managerial competences whose importance
     has been enhanced with the introduction of 'managed competition':
     marketing, contracting, personnel management along with finance and
     IT skills.

(2) *The rudimentary nature of the budgetary and accounting systems vital to the
     financial control, planning, pricing and billing requirements of the internal
     health market.* In a recent survey 74% of chief executives in charge
     of NHSTs 'felt their IT systems were holding back implementation'
     (Agnew 1992: 8). Professor John Perrin (1992: 247), a leading expert
     in NHS accounting and finance has said that, in time, these problems
     will be solved but this will be costly. Other observers (e.g. Mayston
     1992: 47) have reached the same conclusions.
        RMI, which began the upgrading of hospital information systems

before the Reforms, has become the model (Appleby 1992: 25) and has been extended and become integral to the current Reform process. The Chartered Institute of Public Finance and Accountancy (CIPFA) is developing 'guides to good practice' in significant problem areas (Wise 1991: 25) and NHS accounting research, so long neglected, is now the most researched part of public-sector accounting (Lapsley 1991: 12). Despite all this, it would be wrong to assume that private-sector management accounting with its attendant organizational values – the model for much of the Reform process – is without fundamental criticism on its home ground, far less in the NHS (Johnson and Kaplan 1987; Bromwich and Bhimani 1989; Ward 1992).

(3) Linked to (2) above but a significant difficulty for NHS managers, especially in provider Units, is *the minimal knowledge of the details of cost behaviour of the treatments, procedures and the like being sold to purchasers and thence no really firm basis on which to make sound pricing decisions.* An essential premise behind the internal market is that there will be reliable comparative cost data (Perrin 1988: 141) and prices based upon them. The intended net result is supposed to be a new structure of incentives rewarding the efficient Unit and, within it, individual departments, 'firms' of doctors and clinical directorates, and forcing inefficient Units and their component parts to change if they want to survive. There are many barriers to the internal market in NHS hospitals operating like a purely competitive market, but with a dearth of timely and relevant information about costs and prices, it is very difficult to see how, in practice, the internal market can ground its efficiency claims until this situation significantly alters. At present I am aware of no NHS Unit of any size that has full and adequate information of cost behaviour.

The view of the academic accountants is to urge a cautious approach until the problem eases: 'The DoH would be ill-advised to remove the current restrictions to a freer market [so-called steady state] before health-care costing and consequently pricing is improved' (Ellwood 1991: 28). Yet the DoH did remove the restrictions shortly after this comment was made and, although it is a matter of judgement, it is hard to see even now there being enough information to move easily out of 'steady state'.

One of the overheads that the NHS accountants must include in their contract prices is capital charging, making an explicit charge for the use of the capital assets used as part of the level playing field that the Government's policy-makers wanted. Quite apart from whether such an approach is fair – to the London teaching hospitals, say, with their vast capital costs – the preparations in this area have been criticized: 'The calculations which underpin the whole system [of capital charging] have proved so awry throughout the country that the DoH has effectively written off the first twelve months as a mere paper exercise. Year One has been renamed Year Zero' (Moore 1992: 27).

Specialty costing, which still forms the basis of many service agreements, was something that was emerging under Körner (Ellwood 1990: 26). Quite realistically the early advice from the centre was to keep costing simple and seek short cuts (NHSME 1991a, 1991b) and to use block contracts but, as Chapter 12 makes clear, these are not without their problems either. In fact, some of the leading figures on NHS accounting and finance have concluded that 'specialty costs offer little if any contribution to the contracting process' (Prowle *et al.* 1989: 51). The reality is that some Units do not even generate their own specialty costs but simply adapt DoH national average specialty costs (Perrin 1992: 246).

The difficulties around management information are generating responses such as new concepts (e.g. Carter 1991), training packages (Marriott and Mellett 1991a) and a contracts database with a billion-plus words (Appleby 1991: 36).

The preparedness of purchasers

There is no doubt that the problems for purchasers, particularly DHAs which are required to undertake needs assessments and so forth, are at least as great as those faced by providers. The centre has been slow to generate the required advice and support as, till recently, its attention has been much more on provider difficulties.

I will briefly consider the preparedness of purchasers under two headings.

(1)   GPs and their information systems
The internal market poses obvious challenges in terms of both the managerial skills and information systems for GPFHs. None the less, I will consider only the latter which has implications for all GPs as the non-GPFHs too are likely to be much more effective champions of their patients' interests if they possess adequate information systems.

The imposition of the GP contract prior to the main health Reforms did induce considerable change relating to the provision of business information. Over 90% of GPs in a survey reported changes of an adminstrative nature arising from the GP contract but from a very uneven baseline indeed:

> On the whole prior to the implementation of the new contract there was a wide disparity in the records kept by doctors with regard to both practice activities and accounting records. The most efficient practices kept information on all aspects of the practice, they also monitored their income and expenditure and produced budgets. But it would appear that some practices kept hardly any records at all, for example 7.6 per cent did not keep a petty cash book and a similar number did not keep an age/sex register of patients.
>
> (Greenfield *et al.* 1991: 31)

Moving from all GPs to the GPFHs, how were they chosen? Although it has been lowered, size in terms of patient list was a publicly stated criterion for selection. It is also important in terms of which GPs are likely to apply as the 'start-up and running costs of the accounting and administrative systems and computing needed for each Fundholding practice are substantial' (Perrin 1992: 229). Another commentator reached similar conclusions in terms of which applications for GPFH status were successful in the early days of the scheme: 'In the event, judgemental criteria centring upon high motivation plus managerial and computer capacity were used in selecting practices. Beyond this, the rules under which the scheme would operate had to be created as it went along' (Robinson and Scheuer 1992: 19).

Smith captures something of the degree of change required of GPs just in the business information field as they become GPFHs:

> The introduction of budgets would of course require formal pricing of all services used by general practice. Each practice would require information on the use of resources, and financial planning models to monitor performance against budgets. Again, such systems are available, although their implementation in general practice would impose considerable costs, particularly in terms of requirements for additional managerial expertise.
>
> (Smith 1990: 131)

None the less, it seems that the emergence of GPFHs has been less problematic in terms of preparedness than is the case for NHS hospitals in their provider role. Perhaps this is significantly related to the fact that most of the early GPFHs were the strongest in terms of their existing information systems and so forth. What this will mean as the criteria soften and larger numbers of GPFHs emerge is unclear. It will largely depend on how successfully what was found to be good practice in the early days can be more widely diffused.

(2) The DHAs and their new responsibilities

In this section the concern is simply how well prepared were DHAs for their new roles and duties? Once again information is critical, and both the quantity and quality needs to increase greatly (Ives 1991: 22).

I will only consider two areas where preparations have been important:

(1) *Those arising from administering their side of the contracting system.* As was established above, the providers too have a great need to upgrade information systems. The most distinctive feature of weighted capitation, the new funding formula, is that DHAs are only responsible for, and paid with respect to, their resident populations. DHAs must be able to: identify residents and non-residents; establish and monitor contracts with all their suppliers in both the hospital and community sectors; collect their funding; and disburse contract payments (Perrin 1992: 223), including ECRs which could be to providers anywhere in the UK.

(2) *Making an audit of their resident population's health needs.* This underlies the whole planning and contracting process and yet, in the second year of contracting, it was still being said that a centre, preoccupied with NHSTs and perhaps GPFHs – the two elements in the equation and perhaps the most favoured ones – had provided 'little guidance about how health needs should be assessed' (Pollock 1992: 26). Clearly this was a quite 'radical change' in approach but, as Chapter 12 makes

clear, DHA commissioners, even supported by a Director of Public Health, lack the knowledge or legitimacy to make such choices on their own about health needs or the appropriate treatments to deal with those needs. Until the Department undertakes or sponsors the many difficult, costly and often hotly debated assessments of procedures and treatments plus national studies of health needs, DHA purchasers can only really make marginal changes to existing patterns, thereby holding up this crucial aspect of the Reforms and altering contracting patterns towards the primary/community area and away from secondary, hospital-based care (DoH 1991).

As May (1992: 23) has observed, there is a real danger that commissioners will fill this lacuna with 'magic formulae' such as will occur from an over-reliance on such measures as quality-adjusted life years (QALYs). In fact, what the internal market with its requirements for the assessments of health needs and the efficacy of various treatments has revealed is that current NHS information systems are geared to activity and financial matters. The required reorientation purchasers urgently need can only occur over the long term. This gap between the current reality and what is required might be expected to stimulate a vigorous response (Fitchett 1991: 24) yet current progress is less than encouraging: 'A shortage of resources, skills, expertise and information to develop a good population needs assessment impedes service development and is compounded by a crisis in funding in many provider units, and will inevitably rebound on purchasers' (Pollock 1992: 27).

In sum, what can be concluded about the readiness of purchasers and providers to implement the Reforms, including the quasi health market? First, the nature and pace of the change programme have both been political decisions. Second, in the context of a speedy introduction of the market, both the policy-makers and DoH could not do everything and had to make difficult choices on what area they would stress. Thus, despite the problems providers face, they have received much more attention than purchasers, certainly DHA purchasers with their new and important responsibilities for needs assessment and the like, the real emergence of which have been delayed as a consequence.

The next task for this first chapter of *Managing the Internal Market* is to consider the book's ambit, what falls within its scope and what will be regarded as outside its confines.

THE SCOPE OF THE COLLECTION

A useful starting point is in what setting contributors consider the internal market. All chapters focus on 'managed competition' but within the context of the overall Reform programme. To consider the internal market in isolation is in no sense feasible or worthwhile. Thus, the purpose of the collection is to examine 'managed competition' functioning within the package of NHS

Reforms. The spotlight is firmly placed on this quasi health market, its modes of management and operation at the key institutional levels and into the beginning of the second year of the implementation.

Few would challenge the important role that health care has played in creating our modern world nor that changes in the methods of funding and health-care delivery will continue to play a significant role. The current health agenda in the UK (DoH 1991) and elsewhere points in three basic directions:

(1) towards a greater emphasis on preventive, promotive – and even complementary – approaches as opposed to 'curative', high-tech medical interventions in a hospital setting;
(2) consequently, more stress on primary and community-based health provisioning and less on the acute, hospital-centred provision;
(3) concern about the funding of the health budget, cost containment and possibly changing roles for managers and the various clinically based professionals in health-care delivery.

In Britain today this third direction, the economic and managerial dimension, has not only received more attention than the other two – which more directly define the medical domain – but also it is likely to affect how they develop.

Managing the Internal Market reflects this situation and thus is concerned with the Government's health Reforms and the quasi health market in the acute sector, currently the main legislative and policy expression of the economic and managerial dimension actually affecting the present health scene when the contributors wrote their chapters. Furthermore, to keep the collection at a suitable size, the focus is on the health Reforms in England even though similar changes are occurring elsewhere in the UK.

Care in the community (Griffiths 1988; DoH 1989b, 1990a), officially launched in April 1993, involves, among other things, the creation of a "social-care market" for the elderly, the mentally ill, and mentally and physically handicapped. Though the NHS is involved, local government social service departments are the lead agency and hold the funding. Thus, these developments effectively fall outside the scope of this book. Consistent with what has already been said about the acute-sector stress of this book, the community side of health-care commissioning receives strictly limited attention, only being mentioned in discussing important changes likely to occur in the DHA purchasing role (Chapter 6) and, on the provider side, where medical specialties either already straddle the complex and often confusing acute/community divide (Chapter 17) or fear that the internal market will push them in this direction (Chapter 18).

At the centre of the changes in the acute sphere is the division between purchasing and supplying functions. However, as it is a necessary, but 'not wholly sufficient' (Appleby 1992: 152–3), step in creating the quasi health market and, as all the major political parties accept the divide but both Labour and the Liberal Democrats are vociferous in their disapproval of the internal market, most of the analysis must involve a detailed consideration of the institutional setting within which the internal market operates. In other words, a careful look at the management and ways of functioning of the new institutions that have been created, the NHSTs and GPFHs, and the pre-existing ones, the DHAs and FHSAs, that have seen their remits radically redefined or, as was pointed out in the introduction, the RHAs and the community health councils (CHCs) who have yet to see their remits clearly specified.

To focus the book effectively on the management and operation of these institutions requires that much be de-emphasized, even ignored. Thus, the 'first step' of the health Reforms, the imposition of a new GP contract in the face of British Medical Association and doctor opposition is only briefly touched on in Chapter 13. Indicative prescribing budgets (DoH 1990c) to limit costs and prevent over-prescribing are entirely omitted. FHSAs are considered in Chapter 12 as merger partners for DHA purchasers but not, for instance, with respect to the adequacy of their regulatory powers over GPs. Similarly GPFHs appear to be emerging as important purchasers and other GPs are, in a variety of ways, beginning to influence the services offered by hospitals, the ways their clinicians work and the contracts placed by DHAs. These are important concerns in this book and are indeed referred to by many of the contributors. Other functions of GPs, important though they might be from a different angle, do not enter this collection.

Likewise, the effects of the reduction in the membership of health authorities (DoH 1990a, Schedule 1), and the elimination of local authority and trade union membership from such bodies are not considered here, although a research team at the Centre for Corporate Strategy and Change, Warwick University, has, for some time, been undertaking important research on these and related matters (see, for instance, Pettigrew *et al*. 1991).

Similarly, Opportunity 2000 (NHSME 1992), a recent attempt to boost the proportion of women managers in the public sector, including the NHS, is not included in *Managing the Internal Market* as it is far too early to be able to grasp how this might affect the management and functioning of main institutions of the internal market. Project 2000 (UKCC 1986), the upgrading of nurse education making it more college based, is similarly not covered as it is far too early in its implementation to draw from it any lessons in terms of 'managed competition'. Likewise, the training of medics and paramedics is not included. None the less, it is a central feature of this book to stress the multidisciplinary nature of the operation and management of the NHS. In this sense professional training and, for example, the still small amount that is included in such education about the Reforms and the management function in the Service will have an influence on the implementation of the Reforms including the NHS market.

Finally, audit arrangements for NHSTs (DoH 1990a) and the details of how interest on capital and depreciation are charged (Perrin 1992; Prowle *et al*. 1989; HFM/CIPFA 1991; DoH 1990d, 1990e) are not covered in this book and only appear to the extent they affect contracting strategies (for example, in Chapter 12). The nature and impact of tax relief on private medical insurance for older people is not covered, although Chapter 18 considers the daunting question of financing health care of the elderly in the face of a rapidly ageing British population.

What then will the collection concentrate upon? To reiterate, the central focus is the management and operation of the main providers and purchasers in the quasi market in acute health care into Year Two of contracting as 'steady state' begins to disappear.

THE BROAD APPROACH AND STRUCTURE OF THE BOOK

Having defined the scope of *Managing the Internal Market*, what can be said about the conception behind the book as a whole? This helped decide such matters as which contributors to seek out to write chapters and what sort of brief to negotiate with them and thence what gives the book its unity and distinctiveness. Having clarified the conception that informs the book, its structure can be presented.

The book's underlying conception

If the concern is with the management and functioning of the key institutions in the internal market in acute services, a key managerial issue is about the management of change: implementing this quasi market and related measures at different levels in the NHS. An adequate account of the NHS health market needs to consider both macro issues, including the funding and policy initiatives from government, and the dynamics at the more micro level within and between different institutions and levels in the NHS, and the interaction between macro and micro levels.

Furthermore, the management-of-change task needs to involve the recognition that:

- The NHS is a very large, multiprofessional organization.
- The different professions possess different and changing power in hospitals and other parts of the acute service. Practitioner perspectives on internal market implementation, that is the views held by professional groupings about this implementation, will have an effect on outcomes.

   When thinking about power and change, what is crucial is what Pettigrew (1985) calls 'power in possession'. For example, one plausible implication that might be generally imputed about RMI (Packwood *et al.* 1991) is that it is likely nurse managers' budgets, and thence their power organizationally, will be subsumed within a larger multiprofessional budget covering an entire specialty or group of specialties, and usually headed by a consultant as clinical director. This could indeed be what happens in a particular instance but, even if it is, how concretely this is brought about, how the consultant and nurse manager relate to one another, and how each, and their associated professional groupings, define the situation – the differing practitioner perspectives – will all affect how this power in possession works in particular cases.

- If power and influence in the NHS are complex and often diffused so too is the managerial role, be it about internal market implementation or anything else. There are, of course, those officially designated as

NHS managers, be their backgrounds purely administrative or clinical. Additionally, at every level in the NHS there are large numbers of clinicians with *de facto* managerial roles as an aspect of their jobs.

- Beyond this, the detailed technical knowledge and widespread social prestige accorded doctors especially will limit and make complex the exercising of the managerial role in the Health Service. This makes the policy decision to replace 'consensus management' involving the major NHS groupings by one general manager at each level (Griffiths 1983) a knotty one indeed, and may well speak against the effectiveness of forcing a general manager on reluctant clinicians.

Another factor of note for policy-makers and change managers alike is that such clinicians deal with sick people who are frequently suffering pain and some of whom will die. How people relate to such issues is complex inside the hospital itself (Menzies Lyth 1988: 46 ff.) or beyond it (Ariès 1983). What it means is that, first, health care in a quasi market or not is a 'social good' like no other. For instance, the present Government education reforms seem to be proceeding more rapidly than their counterpart in health despite many similarities in policy intent and solution. This stems from the relatively greater power of doctors compared with teachers and, ultimately, because the former deal with illness, pain and death on a daily basis, whereas education deals with things of a different order.

The approach summarized and its implications for this book

What then are the requirements of a readings book on 'managed competition' implementation that responds to the above considerations?

(1) It needs to offer broadly based macro accounts (much of Part 1) and, where possible, offer detailed research into key questions (Chapters 7, 8, 9 and 11).

(2) The macro accounts in Part 1 require elaboration and grounding in more detailed work on the management and operation of key institutions in the market (Part 2). The aim is to discover something of their interests, strategies and resources – financial, information and symbolic resources. Furthermore, this more micro work needs to reflect the multiprofessional nature of these institutions, especially what is introduced by the medical and nursing professions in the provider Units, the DMUs and NHSTs. The aim is to uncover something of both the different professional perspectives held with respect to the NHS market and generalizations based on the experience to date of different groups in that market.

Although Parts 1 and 2 were organized to respond to the above requirements, they do unavoidably fall short of them to a significant degree. Let's illustrate this just in relation to the practitioner accounts of Part 2. First, of the areas and perspectives actually covered, considerable research is required to develop these and judge how typical they are of the functions and views they outline.

Second, clearly Part 2 is incomplete and, although one book can do no more, the omissions could be of significance in gaining a comprehensive picture. For instance, it could be interesting to compare accounts offered by a Director of Public Health in his or her role of supporting the commissioning process with what is said on purchasing in Chapters 6 and 12. It would also be worthwhile to see more medical specialties represented than was possible in Part 2 and to know much more about the NHS's largest occupational group, the nurses, in the different acute settings in which they work and their experiences in such areas as contracting and budgets. Other clinicians (radiographers, phamaceutical chemists, dieticians) and non-clinicians (porters, clerical workers) would complete this part of the picture. Certainly a greater variety of accounts of DHAs, GPs and hospitals in more diverse circumstances would add much of real importance.

Nevertheless, to some extent some of these incompletenesses can be worked with even within the confines of this one book. For example, the need to understand DHAs, GPs and hospitals in a wider range of situations can be partly covered by considering the micro accounts of Part 2 in relation to the more widely cast work of Part 1. Thus, Chapters 14 and 15 on hospital management could be read in relation to Chapters 7 and 8.

The other response is to acknowledge frankly that much more research is required and justified for such an important organization as the NHS and its acute wing. This is especially the case as the NHS is currently at an important phase in its organization history, the implementation of the internal market and associated changes. This major need for extensive further organizational research and development is directly considered in Chapter 20.

One thing is clear: it is not possible for any one book to fully deliver all the requirements indicated above to produce a comprehensive account of the NHS acute-sector market.

The basic structure of the book

The purpose of this subsection is to move beyond the already explained macro/practitioner accounts split of Parts 1 and 2 and to think briefly about the more detailed contours of the book.

Chapters 2–5 present four different types of overview. They are preceded, first, by the Introduction, a brief review of the main purchaser and provider institutions of the acute-sector internal market intended to assist readers whose prior knowledge of the NHS market and associated Reforms is rather limited, and, second, this chapter (Chapter 1) which, although also broadly cast, is not an overview of some part of the management or operation of the internal market or ways of understanding that market. Its main task is simply to provide guidelines readers may find useful in approaching the collection itself.

Chapter 2 offers a broad overview and assessment of the historical development of the Reforms, particularly the internal market, and includes coverage of such matters as the crucial doctor–manager relationship and the place of RMI in that. Chapter 3 discusses different types of health markets with varying degrees of regulation. Chapter 4 is a useful compendium of the key economic issues involved. Finally, Chapter 5 looks at the vexed and important questions of how to conceptualize the internal market which has some market-like qualities but is none the less a market like no other.

From the foundations provided by the overviews of Chapters 2–5, Part 1 moves on to consider a series of issues crucial to the broad brush strokes used in Part 1. Chapter 6 is a comprehensive account and assessment of the new role of DHA purchasing by an academic specialist in public health with practical experience in assisting DHA commissioners in that role. Chapter 7 presents those results obtained to date of significance for understanding the operation of the internal market obtained from a National Association of Health Authorities and Trusts (NAHAT) large-scale survey commissioned by the King's Fund into the overall Reform process. Chapter 8 focuses on hospital strategies and the ways in which they are affected by the NHS market. Chapter 9 draws on Brunel University research into the place of quality in contracting. Chapter 10 considers the vagaries of NHS management accounting, a function much enhanced by 'managed competition'. Somewhat provocatively and certainly interestingly the contributor presents this as offering a series of new opportunities for provider managements operating in the market. Part 1 closes with Chapter 11 offering as comprehensive an account as is currently possible of the new industrial relations possibilities open to NHSTs in the quasi market.

Part 2 starts with the new purchasing function: Chapter 12 is an extended interview with a DHA commissioner about his new role in the market and Chapter 13 considers the enhanced role of GPs under 'managed competition', be they GPFHs or not, and from the standpoint of a GP who is critical of much that has flowed from the internal market and the Reform process.

Chapters 14 and 15 are about providers and the altered role of the hospital management and are written by a professional manager and doctor/manager, respectively. Chapter 14, like Chapter 12, is in the form of an extended interview and examines how 'external changes' including the internal market have wrought internal change to a large inner London hospital. Chapter 15 focus on Trust status and something of the experiences to date of the 'flagship Trust', the Guy's and Lewisham NHS Trust.

Chapters 16–18 focus on three medical specialties and Chapter 19 on nursing, all in relation to 'managed competition'. In Chapter 16 two orthopaedic surgeons in a large hospital in the Midlands consider the threats and opportunities for their specialty, one commonly tipped to be an income generator if excess capacity is available, although more general surgery is by no means always cast in such a role. Chapters 17 and 18 consider the two 'Cinderella specialties' some early commentators imagined might face difficulties in a 'competitive situation'. Chapter 17 is written by two psychiatrists and Chapter 18 by a consultant in health care of the elderly. Both are London based; the psychiatrists seem less concerned than might be predicted by the advent of the NHS market, which is probably due to some extent to the statutory backing behind some of their services and also because psychiatry straddles both the acute and community sectors; when organized within an NHST, the psychiatric consultants not infrequently opt to join a

Trust. The author of Chapter 18 is much more critical of the market and overall Reforms as, like the psychiatric contributors, this consultant in health care of the elderly sees the likelihood of his specialty being pushed firmly out of the acute sector as the internal market bites. Unlike the psychiatrists, however, he bitterly laments this, perhaps because the internal market emerged at an earlier stage in the institutionalization of health care of the elderly as a distinct specialty than was the case with psychiatry, and therefore seems likely to destroy much that has been so recently created. Chapter 19 considers some of the implications, especially the effects on industrial relations, of 'managed competition' for nurses, and in that sense links well with Chapter 11 which surveys the overall industrial relations picture.

Chapter 20 lists and briefly enumerates some themes that I see as underlying much of the collection. These are briefly explained and one is explored in more depth to provide support for the idea of an enhanced, more varied and novel approach to organizational research and development, something that is supported in a variety of other ways as well. Given that the effects of the internal market and the health Reforms generally are greatly under-researched, this is a fitting way to close the book.

REFERENCES

Agnew, T. (1992) Managers' verdict: internal market does not work, *Health Service Journal*, 5 November, 8.

Appleby, J. (1991) Compact for Contracts, *Health Service Journal*, 25 April, 36.

Appleby, J. (1992) *Financial Health Care in the 1990s*. Buckingham: Open University Press.

Ariès, P. (1983) *The Hour of our Death*. Harmondsworth: Penguin.

Ashburner, L. *et al.* (1991) Organisational restructuring and the new Health Authorities: continuity or change? Papers presented to the British Academy of Management Conference, University of Bath, September.

Asher, K. (1987) *The Politics of Privatization: Contracting Out Public Services*. Basingstoke: Macmillan.

Bach, S. (1989) Trading for health services: lessons from the competitive tendering experience, *Journal of Management in Medicine*, 160–6.

Birch, S. (1985) Tread Carefully: Private Waters, *Health and Social Service Journal*, 6 June, 710–1.

Bromwich, M. and Bhimani, A. (1989) *Management Accounting: Evolution not Revolution*. London: Chartered Institute of Management Accountants.

Butler, E. (1989) Contract management of hospitals – Canadian lessons for the UK, *Journal of Management in Medicine*, 335–44.

Carter, N. (1991) *Case-Mix Analysis for Contracting and Pricing: A View from a Unit General Manager*. London: Heathcare Financial Management Association/Chartered Institute of Public Finance and Accountancy.

Charlwood, P. (1991) Finding funds for health, *Health Service Journal*, 6 June.

Cook, R. (1991) Cook releases health action plan for first 100 days. Press release, 23 September. London: House of Commons.

Cox, D. (1991) Health Service management – a sociological view: Griffiths and the non-negotiated order of the hospital, in J. Gabe *et al.* (ed.) *The Sociology of the Health Service*. London: Routledge, 89–114.

Culyer, A.J. *et al.* (eds.) (1990) Reforming health care: an introduction to the economic issues, in *Competition in Health Care: Reforming the NHS*. London: Macmillan, 1–11.

Cumella, S. (1991) To market, to market . . ., *Health Service Journal* (14 November), 22–3.

Davies, P. (1992) A different guise?, *Health Service Journal*, 12 March, 12.

DoH (Department of Health) (1989a) *Working for Patients.* London: HMSO.

DoH (Department of Health) (1989b) *Caring for People: Community Care in the Next Decade.* London: HMSO.

DoH (Department of Health) (1990a) *National Health Service and Community Care Act 1990.* London: HMSO.

DoH (Department of Health) (1990b) *Funding and Contracts for Hospital Services. Working for Patients Working Paper 2.* London: DoH.

DoH (Department of Health) (1990c) *Indicative Prescribing Budgets for General Medical Practitioners. Working for Patients Working Paper 4.* London: DoH.

DoH (Department of Health) (1990d) *Capital Charges. Working for Patients Working Paper 5.* London: DoH.

DoH (Department of Health) (1990e) *Capital Charges: Funding Issues. Working for Patients Working Paper 9.* London: DoH.

DoH (Department of Health) (1991) *The Health of the Nation: A Consultative Document for Health in England.* London: HMSO.

DoH (Department of Health) (1992) *The Patient's Charter: Raising the Standard.* London: HMSO.

Easton, J. (1991) Service to the community, *British Journal of Healthcare Computing,* (July), 30–1.

Ellwood, S. (1990) Competition in health care, *Management Accounting* [UK], (April), 24–8.

Ellwood, S. (1991) Costing and pricing healthcare, *Management Accounting* [UK] (November), 26–8.

Fitchett, M. (1991) M25 Syndrome, *Health Service Journal,* (5 December), 24–5.

Gerrard, N. (1991) Figuring out the future, *Health Service Journal,* 11 July, 24.

Greenfield, S. *et al.* (1991) *The Impact of 'Working for Patients' and the 1990 Contract on General Practitioners' administrative systems.* London: Certified Accountant Publications.

Griffiths, R. (1983) *NHS Management Inquiry Report.* London: Department of Health and Social Security.

Griffiths, R. (1988) *Community Care: An Agenda for Action.* London: HMSO.

Ham, C. *et al.* (1992) Contract culture, *Health Service Journal,* 7 May, 22–4.

Harrison, S. *et al.* (1992) *Just Managing: Power and Culture in the National Health Service.* London: Macmillan.

Health Service Journal (1992a) Is gin the tonic? *Health Service Journal,* 16 April, 14.

Health Service Journal (1992b) Reforms 'threat to research', *Health Service Journal,* 12 November, 6.

HFM/CIPFA (Healthcare Financial Management Association/Chartered Institute of Public Finance and Accountancy) (1991) *Introductory Guide to NHS Finance.* London: Healthcare Financial Management.

Hunter, D. and Webster, C. (1992) Here we go again, *Health Service Journal,* 5 March, 26–7.

Ives, S. (1991) Your flexible friend, *British Journal of Healthcare Computing* (June), 22–5.

Johnson, H. T. and Kaplan R. S. (1987). *The Rise and Fall of Management Accounting.* Boston, Mass.: Harvard Business School Press.

Kelly, M. (1991) The need to know, *British Journal of Healthcare Computing* (February), 28–9.

Key, T. (1988) Contracting out ancillary services, in R. Maxwell (ed.) *Reshaping the NHS.* Oxford: Policy Journals, 65–81.

Labour Party (1992) *Your Good Health: A White Paper for a Labour Government.* London: Labour Party.

Lapsley, I. (1991) Accounting Research in the National Health Service, *Financial Accountability & Management* (Spring), 1–14.

Le Grand, J. (1991) Quasi-markets and social policy, *Economic Journal*, September, 1,256–67.

March, J. G. and Olsen J. P. (1989) *Rediscovering Institutions: The Organisational Basis of Politics*. New York: Free Press.

Marriott, N. and Mellett, H. (1991a) Bridging the skills gap, *Certified Accountant* (October), 34–5.

Marriott, N. and Mellett, H. (1991b) *The financial awareness of managers in the Reformed NHS*. Occasional Paper No. 10. London: Chartered Association of Certified Accountants.

May, A. (1992) Perfect purchasing, *Health Service Journal* (16 July), 22–4.

Mayston, D. (1992) Internal markets, capital and the economics of information, *Public Money & Management* (January–March), 47–53.

Menzies Lyth, I. (ed.) (1988) The functioning of social systems as a defence against anxiety: a report on a study of the nursing service of a general hospital, in *Containing Anxiety in Institutions: Selected Essays, Volume 1*. London: Free Association Books.

Millar, B. (1990) Contracts are about real money changing hands, *Health Service Journal*, 25 October, 1597.

Moore, W. (1992) Zero plus one equals zero, *Health Service Journal* (30 January), 27–8.

MSF (Manufacturing, Science, Finance) (1992) Sacked whistle blower: support grows, *MSF*, vol. 5, no. 3, p. 1.

NHSME (National Health Service Management Executive) (1991a). *Purchasing for Health: 16 May 1991 Conference Report*. London: DoH.

NHSME (1991b). *Purchasing Intelligence October 1991*. London: DoH.

NHSME (1992) *Women in the NHS: An Action Guide to the Opportunity 2000 Campaign*. London: HMSO.

Packwood, T. *et al.* (1991) *Hospitals in Transition: The Resource Management Experiment*. Milton Keynes: Open University Press.

Perrin, J. (1988) *Resource Management in the NHS*. London: Chapman & Hall.

Perrin, J. (1992) The National Health Service, in D. Henley *et al.* (eds.) *Public Sector Accounting and Financial Control*. London: Chapman & Hall.

Pettigrew, A. M. (1985) *The Awakening Giant: Continuity and Change in Imperial Chemical Industries*. Oxford: Basil Blackwell.

Pettigrew, A. *et al.* (1991) *Authorities in the NHS: The Leadership Role of the New Health Authories: An Agenda for Research and Development*. Coventry: Centre for Corporate Strategy and Change, University of Warwick.

Pollock, A. (1992) Split decisions, *Health Service Journal* (8 October), 26–7.

Prowle, M. *et al.* (1989) *Working for Patients – The Financial Agenda*. London: Certified Accountant Publications.

Roberts, J. A. (1990) The marketeers and the National Health Service, in I. Taylor (ed.) *The Social Effects of Free Market Policies: An International Text*. Hemel Hempstead: Harvester Wheatsheaf.

Robinson, R. and Scheuer, M. A. (1992) Fishing for Fundholders, *Health Service Journal* (13 January), 18–20.

Smith, P. (1990) Information systems and the White Paper proposals, in A. J. Culyer *et al* (eds) *Competition in Health Care*. London: Macmillan, 110–37.

Snell, J. (1991) Riding the wave, *Nursing Times*, 25 September, 18–19.

Socialist Health Association (1988) *Their Hands in our Safe: A Critique of Ring-Wing Proposals on Financing the NHS*. London: SHL.

UKCC (United Kingdom Central Council for Nursing, Midwifery and Health Visiting) (1986) *Project 2000: A New Preparation for Practice*. London: UKCC.

Ward, K. (1992) *Strategic Management Accounting*. London: Butterworth/Chartered Institute of Management Accountants.

Wise, J. (1991) *Extra Contractual Referral Price Tariffs: An Analysis of Orthopaedic Prices*. London: Chartered Institute of Public Finance and Accountancy.

Part 1

THE MACRO PICTURE

2

The Internal Market: The Shifting Agenda

David J. Hunter

A central feature of the NHS Reforms has been their concern with means rather than ends. It is the *process* of change which has absorbed the attention of policy-makers and managers rather than the *direction* or *outcomes* desired from that change. Consequently, the purpose of the Reforms has been of a shifting nature and generally unclear. The reasons for this are complex. This chapter seeks to identify the key elements in the development of the Reforms, in particular the move to an internal market, to offer explanations for them and to assess the implications of the shift in thinking about the notion of an internal market from its initial conception.

BACKGROUND TO THE NHS REFORMS

The notion of an internal market in the NHS has its origins in the ideas of a number of analysts and health economists but perhaps its most influential architect is Alain Enthoven, Professor of Public and Private Management at Stanford University, California. Enthoven has articulated the concept of a managed market in the US health-care system for a number of years. He applied his ideas to the British NHS in a pamphlet (Enthoven 1985). At that time there was no hint of a major review of the NHS. This was not announced until 1988. The two came together by happy coincidence rather than by conscious design.

The NHS Review itself proved to be a somewhat confused affair with various agendas in existence, not all of them consistent with each other. Ostensibly the result of a funding 'crisis' in the Service, the Review had little to say about finance. Rather, its starting point was the importance of better management and of using existing resources more effectively. In this respect the Review proposals (DoH 1989) were consistent with, and built upon, the Griffiths management changes introduced in 1983 (Harrison *et al.* 1990). But the Review went further in the direction of introducing market principles into the NHS based on elements of competition among provider Units which would be separate from the planning and purchase of care. In this respect the Reforms had more in common with the Government's own political ideology and abiding faith in the virtues of competition and in ending public-sector monopolies. It is conceivable that the Government would have gone further but was constrained from doing so because of the NHS's popularity with the general public.

It was doubtless sensitivity to the likelihood of a negative public reaction to the proposals which resulted in some ambivalence on the part of the Government over how it should best present its Reforms. There is no doubt that the Government's position shifted in the run-up to, and subsequently in the course of, the first year of the Reforms which were introduced in April 1991. The lead-up to the Reforms was significant since there was a 2-year period between the appearance of the White Paper and the start of the implementation process. Most of this time was taken up with the NHS and Community Care Bill in order to allow it to reach the statute-book in 1990 and become an Act. Perhaps predictably during this time ministers were more bullish about the Reforms especially when so many groups were opposed to them, including the majority of the public. The then Secretary of State for Health, Kenneth Clarke, who was charged with the task of getting acceptance for the Reforms, had his own particular style of presentation and of securing commitment. Essentially it was to go on the attack and not give an inch to his adversaries. Clarke's view was that achieving change in an organization as inherently conservative as the NHS was only achievable by attacking in a highly confrontational manner rather than trying to secure commitment through consensus. Change would only be diluted if there was any attempt at appeasement. It would be resisted and therefore there was no course other than one which sought to destabilize the status quo. For this reason he resisted calls for pilots and experiments to test the changes. To respond to these would be to play into the hands of those opposed to the changes.

Prior to the start of the implementation of the proposals there was much macho rhetoric in evidence concerning the desirability of competition and market principles. For instance, it was Clarke's firm belief, as he told the Social Services Committee in March 1989, that the forces of competition would keep costs to a minimum (Davies 1989). However, in the course of discussion and the development of more detailed proposals as the Bill passed through Parliament, much of the more colourful language became progressively played down. A principal reason for the shift was the change of minister. William Waldegrave succeeded Clarke in November 1990, and while he did not slow down the moves towards a market system – for example, the introduction of first-wave NHSTs and GPFHs maintained its momentum – he did tone down the use of the language of business, competition and the market-place. Indeed, on this score he quite deliberately sought to distance himself from the rather more combative style of his predecessor.

Moreover, while Waldegrave maintained the Government's commitment to the principles of the Reforms and commenced to implement them largely in the spirit intended by Kenneth Clarke, he also sought to put his own distinctive stamp on developments. These took the form of (a) putting more emphasis on the role of purchasing or commissioning in the new-style NHS, and (b) developing an explicit strategy for health which resulted in the consultative document *The Health of the Nation* which appeared in 1991. A White Paper outlining the Government's health strategy awaits publication. The two developments initiated by Waldegrave are closely linked. Neither followed directly from the Reforms themselves, which were almost exclusively concerned with introducing supply-side changes without really attending to the question of what the changes were actually for. It also seems likely that Clarke's chief interest lay in the machinery of the provider-side changes and not in the strategic needs assessment role of the purchasing health authorities. This is not to say that attention would not have been given to this role in time, but under Waldegrave there was a perceptible shift in this direction.[1] Whether intended or not, this had the effect of distracting attention from the market-type changes and of giving the NHSME a major stream of work around what the role of purchasing for health gain should entail. The Welsh had already shown the way in this area and the NHSME/DoH therefore had a model to look at and adapt. In the process, the centre became distanced from the controversial proposals surrounding the setting-up of NHSTs, GPFH practices and the other paraphernalia of an internal market and became preoccupied, at least in public, with establishing a strategic framework in which these changes were intended to improve the nation's health.

AN INTERNAL MARKET IN THE NHS

Enthoven's proposal for an internal market within the NHS is sketched out in five brief pages in his 1985 pamphlet. Under his scheme, each DHA would receive a RAWP-based per capita revenue and capital allowance. Each DHA would continue to be responsible for the provision of comprehensive care for its own resident population but not for people from other areas without appropriate compensation. The DHA would be paid for emergency services to outsiders at a standard cost. It would be paid for non-emergency services to outsiders at negotiated prices. It would control referrals to providers outside the District and it would pay for them at negotiated prices. Enthoven saw the development of DHAs along these lines being akin to health maintenance organizations in the USA. In addition, Enthoven proposed that wages and working conditions would be negotiated locally, although he conceded that this was merely a desirable rather than an essential part of the model. Hospital consultants and other doctors would contract with Districts and Districts would be free to enter into all sorts of contractual arrangements, including short-term contracts and contracts with incentive payments with increased productivity.

Under Enthoven's scheme, each District would have a balance sheet and an income statement. It would be free to borrow at government long-term interest rates up to some agreed limit on debt. A District owning valuable property could sell it, keep the proceeds and add the interest receipts to its revenues. In addition, each District would be in a position to buy and/or sell services or assets from other Districts or the private sector. A District would therefore resemble a nationalized company. In these circumstances, formerly poor Districts would be able to buy services for their residents from outside the District. They might eventually provide more services themselves although they might find that they could do better buying services from outside their own boundaries. In such a model, Districts would have much more freedom to manage as their authorities thought best.

For Enthoven, such a scheme provided managers with many more incentives and the freedom to be able to use resources more efficiently. They could buy services from producers who offered good value. They could use the possibility of buying outside as bargaining leverage to get better performance from their own providers. They could sell off assets such as valuable land in order to redeploy their capital most effectively. Unlike the normal bureaucratic model, they would not get more money by doing a poor job with what they had. Managers would be assured that they could retain all the savings made and use them on the highest priority needs in their districts as defined by them. An internal market model would force the development of proper costing systems and would create much more efficiency and cost sensitivity in those DHAs that were selling as well as buying services from neighbouring authorities. For Enthoven, the change in the internal economic structure of the NHS would be quite fundamental. However, it would be almost invisible to most patients and therefore could be deemed politically attractive.

For the model to work effectively Enthoven listed a number of essential prerequisites. These included:

- incentives to make cost-effective decisions;
- suitably trained managers who could analyse alternatives and make efficient choices;
- a culture of buying and selling health-care services;
- reasonably good cost information;
- a supply of information on how to improve efficiency;
- medical decision-making which would need to be free of the conflict of interest that existed.

Enthoven remained concerned that the model had imperfections in so far as it did not contain powerful incentives for District managers to make their decisions in the best interests of patients in the face of political pressures to do otherwise. In his view, it would still be the case that managers might give in to pressures to favour inside suppliers in the interests of keeping peace in the family. There might also be pressures on Districts to use their own personnel rather than declare them redundant and spend the money elsewhere. Pressures might also come from consultants anxious to develop a full range of services in the District for the sake of autonomy, control, prestige and so on. Enthoven believed the central problem of the NHS was an ability to remain quite insensitive to the best needs of the population for appropriate health care. Unless there was reliance upon consumer choice[2] to motivate efficient and responsive performance, it was all too easy for monopolies to determine what they wanted to do so that services became profession led rather than user driven.

Drawing on Enthoven's ideas, the NHS White Paper (DoH 1989) set out what an internal market would entail within the NHS. Essentially, it involves the separation of two functions: the provision of hospital and community health services, entailing the ownership of health-care institutions and the employment of direct-care staff, and the purchase (or commissioning) of care, that is, the allocation of funds to providing institutions through contracts so as to ensure that the needs of a population are met. Figure 2.1 is an attempt to illustrate the intended dynamics of the internal market within the NHS. It is evident that the proposed market might consist of up to four different types of institution competing for the resources of a particular DHA or GPFH. Arrangements between a DHA and private-sector hospitals, NHSTs or DMUs owned by a different DHA will be contractual, as will arrangements between GPFHs and all institutions. In the case of DMU, the relationship will be a management budget, a quasi contract with similar provisions to commercial contracts, since the intention is that DHAs should not be so closely involved in the management of hospitals as was the case prior to 1991. The separation of purchasing and provision is the basis of the market.

The proposed system rests heavily on the assumption that DHAs and GPFHs will be prepared to commit resources prospectively to meet the anticipated health needs of their population of patients, retaining only a relatively small proportion of funds for contingencies. For some 'core' services, such as accident and emergency, or immediate medical and surgical admissions, contracts will necessarily be let locally, although not necessarily within the DHA's boundaries. The precise definition of what constitutes a core service is for local determination. Other services, that is, where patients and their GPs have time to choose when and where to seek hospital treatment, may be the subject of a contract with hospitals in any location. Contracts will need to specify the type of patient or procedure involved, the standards to which treatment will be given (implying a quality-control mechanism) and a basis of price. Most contracts will also be expected to specify the number of cases or level of service over which they will apply.

All of this sounds fine in theory but is not so readily realized in practice. While it is impossible to comment definitively on the impact of the internal market after the first year of operation, it is possible to speculate on what might happen on the basis of the experience of the past 12 months or so. Before doing so, however, it is important to point out that in many respects the first year of the Reforms was an unusual one. In the event, it proved to be a general election year which resulted in the NHS Reforms having an extremely high political profile which the Government was anxious to manage closely. As a result, far from the changes leading to more devolution and decentralization – the essence of an internal market arrangement – the changes paradoxically led to more central control in the NHS than has existed at any time in the Service's history. Not only were the Trusts directly accountable to the centre rather than to local health authority control but the centre kept very close reins on what was happening within the Service at all levels in order that no political embarrassment should occur prior to the general election which took place in April 1992. It was also the case that the government was prepared to invest quite large sums of additional money in the NHS to lubricate pressure

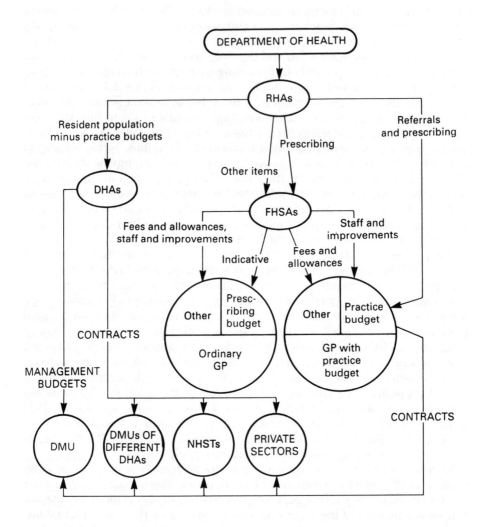

Figure 2.1 Proposed main funding flows in the English NHS by 1992/3. *Source*: Harrison *et al.* (1990)

points and to enable the initial changes to occur more smoothly than might otherwise have been the case.

Any assessment of the Reforms must therefore take into account the fact that their alleged success might have been achieved by the injection of new money rather than by the Reforms themselves. In any event, it is impossible to say after 1 year whether or not an internal market is working effectively or having a beneficial impact on the health of local populations. Such changes will take many years to determine. Moreover, the first year of the Reforms for the reasons cited above was one of 'steady state' and endeavouring to achieve 'a smooth take-off'. As a consequence, the operation of the contractual system was restricted to placing block contracts with provider Units for existing services. In short, the operation of a market in health care has taken the form of largely maintaining the status quo rather than seeking to disturb it in any fundamental way. The attempt to change the profile of service delivery and to purchase for health gain has been more apparent than real. The high-flown rhetoric and ambitious claims for purchasing have not been matched so far by the actions of purchasing authorities on the ground. However, the NHSME in an assessment of the first 6 months of the new NHS claimed that the changes were 'leading to improvements in the quality of care, greater responsiveness to individuals and even better value for money from the growing NHS budget' (NHSME 1991: 2). Of course many of the claimed improvements in the number of patients treated or the reduction of waiting lists might well have occurred anyway regardless of the Reforms.

SOME CONCERNS WITH AN INTERNAL MARKET

Observers have expressed concern that an internal market and the emergence of competition in health care will result in greater inequities and a reduction in the accessibility of some services. For example, the House of Commons Social Services Committee in a report published in 1989 noted that evidence from the USA suggested that markets are good for hospitals but bad for patients unless closely monitored (Social Services Committee 1989). There is little experience in the UK of placing Health Service contracts or of monitoring them on any scale.[3] There is particular ignorance when it comes to quality and outcome measures and their application. For the Committee, the principal fears about an internal market were: that patients may have less immediate access to hospital treatment if they have to travel far for specialized treatment; the potential problems of providing specialist treatment for patients with more than one specialist need; the potential financial and other difficulties for patients having to travel longer distances for treatment; potential problems of communication between GPs and specialists; and the considerable cost consequences of going over to a system of trading in health services, including the possibility that some hospitals which are 'inefficient' would have to close.

The Committee went on to conclude that in a 'simple' internal market – where DHAs were purchasers and all hospitals were DHA owned and competing for contracts from the parent DHA and neighbouring authorities – then the Government's proposals would represent an improvement on the present system. But the Committee was concerned that the Government's plans were not for such a simple internal market but for the furtherance of competition in all aspects of Health Service provision as articulated to the Committee by the then Secretary of State, Kenneth Clarke. Consequently, the proposal to establish NHSTs to compete with DMUs and to establish GPFH practices to compete with DHAs as purchasers of health care would give rise to the potential for considerable 'gaming'. The Committee was not convinced that such a system would be able to achieve the Government's objective of improving services for all patients in all areas.

The Committee was also concerned that the plans to establish an internal market were to begin to operate in advance of the availability of accurate data for the costing of treatments and other procedures. While a market can operate without true costings and hospitals can make broad-brush assumptions about costs in order to set their prices, such an approach is not likely to succeed in eliminating the efficiency trap in which hospitals find themselves. Without accurate information the market would be a distorted one. Resources could go to where prices are lowest rather than to where costs are lowest. Finally, the Committee was concerned that some of the fundamental consequences of introducing a market in health care remained to be worked out. These related to how services could be better planned by DHAs; how access to care could be guaranteed and patient choice extended; and to the monitoring and regulation of the quality of services that would need to be put in place. It is not clear, 1 year on, whether these concerns have been adequately addressed by the Government or by local health authorities.

Striking the right balance between competition and regulation will not be easy, as the evidence from the USA shows. Constraining the competitive spirit by introducing too many safeguards may prove to be self-defeating. Equally, allowing competition to operate in an unregulated fashion is likely to produce results which are inconsistent with the aim of providing accessible and comprehensive services.

MANAGING CLINICAL ACTIVITY

If the NHS Reforms are to succeed then this will involve major adaptation in the relationship between the medical profession and managers. Various attempts have been made over the last 40 years or so to achieve a closer integration between medical decisions and political and management decisions. But they have achieved only partial success. The Griffiths NHS Management Inquiry Report in 1983 stressed that 'closer involvement of doctors is critical . . . to effective management at local level' (Griffiths 1983).[4] The NHS Reforms introduced in 1991 seek to redefine the relationship between doctors and managers in a number of ways:

- extending and accelerating the RMI;
- monitoring pay flexibility and greater flexibility over conditions of service;
- medical audit for all doctors;
- introducing changes in consultants' contracts, job descriptions and appointments;
- reforming the system of distinction awards.

If the support of the medical profession is not forthcoming or is lost in the course of implementing the Reforms then it is unlikely that they will prove to be effective. If untrammelled clinical freedom is not a serious option then neither is overtly aggressive management. Working *with* the medical profession to secure the required shift in clinical culture is, as the Government appears to recognize, the only sure way forward. In the confrontational phase, post-White Paper, when Kenneth Clarke was Secretary of State for Health, it seemed that the Government's strategy was one of going on the attack in respect of forcing changes through and imposing them upon the medical profession. As was noted earlier, this combative strategy gave way to a more conciliatory one when Waldegrave succeeded Clarke as Health Secretary.

Perhaps RMI has been the most important in respect of the attempt to shift the culture of medicine more towards one which acknowledges the importance of management within the medical domain. Much useful progress has been made in respect of the initiative since its introduction in 1986. On the other hand, progress has been slow and clearly cannot be rushed. As the architect of the initiative, Ian Mills, emphasized at the time, 'the resource management programme is principally about changing attitudes and encouraging closer teamwork in managing resources among patient care professionals and between such professionals and other managers'.

Research evidence shows that it is taking time to win over many clinicians to the principles of RM and to allay fears about an erosion of clinical autonomy (Pollitt *et al.* 1988). Rushing the roll-out of RM, when all the evidence suggests that there is a need for careful nurturing of the initiative in order to ensure that its fragility does not lead to its collapse, suggests proceeding with some caution. From the limited evidence available to date, four lessons may be drawn from this early experience. First, the support and commitment of doctors is crucial to the success of RM. Second, investment in the necessary information systems is essential. Third, incentives for doctors to encourage them to support RM are necessary. It is not simply a matter of financial incentives but of incentives which enable doctors to see improved results in their work and to raise the quality of care. Finally, the achievement of these changes cannot be rushed. A long haul is unavoidable and to attempt to short-circuit it runs the risk of jeopardizing the entire initiative (Packwood *et al.* 1991).

It seems likely that doctors will remain suspicious of RM if they perceive it as a tool to be used by managers to cut costs and focus on the narrow financial aspects of clinical work. The painstaking progress made in the RMI pilot sites could be lost as doctors become concerned that managers who have become politicized are operating according to directives from the centre rather than to signals coming up from front-line professionals. The initial RMI was informed by a rather different philosophy which put the emphasis on improved effectiveness and more efficacious interventions whereby those providing services on the ground were able to influence the decision-making at higher levels and take part in genuinely devolved management arrangements to improve health-care provision. In the rush to implement the NHS Reforms it is important not to lose the valuable gains there have been since the introduction of the RMI. If there is not unity of view, or at least an approximation of one, between doctors and managers then it will be doctors who win at the end of the day by simply 'gaming' the system. Evidence from the USA is available to support the view that introducing an overtly aggressive management style into the clinical field may be counterproductive and ultimately self-defeating (Ham and Hunter 1988). Doctors are adept at finding ways around controls over their work which they believe to be unacceptable. In the USA it has been shown that as fast as regulations and review protocols are written, physicians learn to circumvent them, resenting the intrusion into their clinical autonomy.

TOWARDS AN INTERIM ASSESSMENT

At the core of the Government's NHS Reforms is the creation of an internal market to promote competition among service providers with a view to improving the efficiency and effectiveness of service delivery and to making it more responsive to user preferences. The key components of the internal market are the separation of purchaser/provider responsibilities; the creation of NHSTs which are intended to compete with each other, with DMUs and providers in the private sector; and GPFH practices which can be expected to compete with DHAs and FHSAs in the purchase of services for their patients.

The NHS has been launched on a huge experiment and no one knows what the likely outcome will be, least of all the Government. Indeed, ministers have gone on record as saying that a measure of the success of the Reforms will be that in 5 years' time the NHS will look very different from how it looks now. It is not so much what the differences will be that interests ministers at this stage but rather the fact that there will be differences. In short, it is the process of reform that is at issue rather than the direction, purpose and anticipated outcomes from it. The Government's own position in regard to the changes has shifted over the years since the White Paper's appearance in 1989.

In the first phase there was much talk of competition and markets in health care as providing incentives to change which no other reforms in the Health Service had been able to achieve so effectively. However, tough talk about competition began to give way in the face of mounting public and professional hostility to the Reforms to a new language which did not contain words like 'markets' and 'competition'. It was quite noticeable that with the change in Secretary of State a marked shift in the vocabulary describing the Reforms was discernible. William Waldegrave sought to play down all talk of markets and competition and tried to shift the debate on to new ground, in particular by articulating the need for a strategy for health that would provide a framework to guide all the activities for purchasers and providers at local level. However, the shift in language did not constrain him from announcing a second wave of NHSTs in April 1992 or from increasing the number of GPFH practices. While the public language used to describe the Reforms may have changed, the momentum to secure the changes sought in the NHS and Community Care Act 1990 (DoH 1990) went ahead as planned.

With the general election which took place in April 1992 over and a new

Secretary of State installed in the DoH it remains to be seen how far the rhetoric surrounding the Reforms will continue as it has been shaped over the last year or so or whether it will change again. The view at the time of writing is that there will be no major departure from the position delineated by the Department and by the new Secretary of State's predecessor. As noted earlier, the stress on 'steady state' and on not unleashing the Reforms has made it difficult to assess their impact. Not a lot has actually changed on the ground. Purchasers have more or less been maintaining a position of 'more of the same' rather than seeking to begin to disturb the historical patterns of care and commitments which authorities have maintained and added to over the years.

The presumption must be that the Government will now ease the pressure on health authorities and providers not to rock the boat and will gradually take the brakes off, thereby allowing the internal market to operate with more freedom than has been allowed hitherto. The dilemma for ministers, however, remains one of finding the optimal balance between freedom on the one hand and control on the other. If all they achieve are complex and bureaucratic billing and regulatory arrangements then the chances are that this will only serve to stultify the very innovation that is being encouraged. Since such an outcome would negate the whole thrust of the Reforms for improved efficiency, it seems unlikely that ministers will be enthusiastic to go too far down this road. On the other hand, the political risks of taking the brakes off completely and allowing the internal market total freedom is that there is great potential for profound political embarrassment in respect of the market inevitably throwing up winners and losers. It is not clear how far ministers are prepared to endure the political pain that could result from allowing the internal market to operate freely. While not letting go risks making a mockery of the Reforms, allowing too much freedom risks setting in train a sequence of events which may prove difficult, if not impossible, to control in practice.

This was one reason why the Social Services Committee in its 1989 report on the NHS advocated that the idea of the internal market be studied further. The Committee recommended that to test its practicability limited experiments should be arranged. Moreover, it took the view that if the concept of the internal market was to be taken further it would require to be very carefully planned, monitored and assessed to ensure that too high a price was not paid for its benefits. The Committee was emphatic in its view that an internal market 'should not be introduced nationally before a thorough piloting has been done'. It pointed out that

> markets in health care are complex. Introducing competition into the NHS, along with the other changes, will undoubtedly change the incentive structure which currently operates. To begin with, the incentives might not be sufficiently strong to bring about price competition rather than collaboration and the setting up of cartels. Alternatively, competition may become so severe that 'unfair methods' are used with undesirable results. By changing the incentive structure in the NHS, a very wide range of predictable and unpredictable consequences are likely to result.
> (Social Services Committee 1989: 5)

At this stage in the unfolding of the Reforms we are on the threshold of a dilemma. Nobody yet knows whether the changes that will emerge from the Reforms are desirable and can be managed effectively or whether they will prove to be undesirable and in practice be impossible to manage. Either way, the degree of predictability in mapping the future is minimal. This was always going to be the case from the moment the White Paper (DoH 1989) appeared. In some ways, the Government is correct in concluding that there will always be opposition to change and that the forces in favour of change will always be weaker than those pressing for maintaining the status quo. If one is serious about change, one may be forced to ignore a certain level of opposition and protest. Revolutions are not made through consensus. This is fair enough provided that the groups required to implement the changes successfully are not so alienated from the change process that they seek to sabotage the Reforms or take them off in directions that are not intended.[5] As was pointed out earlier, the Reforms offer ample opportunity to 'game' the system and divert the Reforms from their ostensible aims.

If the NHS has been founded on a set of principles that preach the virtues of collective provision and allocation of resources made available by governments for health then at the very least it seems important that such principles are preserved in any attempts to reform health-care provision. The danger otherwise is that fragmentation will occur and the system as a whole will cease to function in a coherent or integrated manner. At the end of the day, the question is whether an internal or provider market will prove more or less successful at bringing about improvements in health-care provision and in the status of people's health or whether central planning and direction remain necessary to bring about change in health status. Of particular relevance here is the whole area of community services for the so-called priority groups. Many would argue that they have not done particularly well out of the former central planning arrangements. Arguably they risk doing even less well under an internal market system which might be inclined to favour acute services and address the needs of the so-called 'worried well' rather than needs of the chronically sick.[6] Moreover, it is conceivable that central planning failed not because the model was flawed but because no one was seriously committed to it. On the other hand, the appeal of GPFH to observers like Glennerster is precisely that 'it shifts the balance of power and finance from the top of the service to the bottom. It puts purchasing power and choice nearer the patient, informed by his or her doctor' (Glennerster 1992).

How successful an internal market will be in addressing such concerns remains to be seen. The Government is not insensitive to the issues raised in this final section which is one reason why the language used to describe the Reforms has shifted over the past couple of years or so from a vigorous defence of the market-place in health care and the notion of competition to a position where the Reforms are deemed in reality to be about better management and the better use of existing resources. Whether or not this is a tenable position will be determined by the ability of the Reforms to deliver a better health service. The difficulty here lies in the definition of a 'better' health service. Is it simply increased patient throughput and shorter waiting lists? Or is it better health which may be quite a different matter?

NOTES

1 See p.191 for another account of the lack of emphasis on purchasing in the earlier days of the Reforms.
2 See p.263 for an argument against the feasibility of consumer choice as a reality in the case of health care of the elderly.
3 Refer to Chapter 9 for further discussion on the problems of monitoring quality in health care.
4 See pp.223–4 for further information on doctors as managers, as the system has evolved in one provider Unit.
5 Cf. p.271 where the argument is put that for the Reforms to work there must be a feeling of common ownership of the changes by all staff charged with carrying through the initiatives.
6 See Chapters 16, 17 and 18 for varying views on how well specialties (in acute and other sectors) and their client groups are faring under the internal market plus pp.193–5 and pp.214–5 for a manager's view of the winners and losers.

REFERENCES

Davies, P. (1989) White Paper show – with no support act, *Health Services Journal*, 23 February, 223.
DoH (Department of Health) (1989) *Working for Patients*. London: HMSO.
DoH (Department of Health) (1990) *The National Health Service and Community Care Act 1990*. London: HMSO.
Enthoven, A. (1985) *Reflections on the Management of the NHS*. London: Nuffield Provincial Hospitals Trust.
Glennerster, H. (1992) GP fundholding: promising and far-reaching – but with problems, *Times Higher Educational Supplement Health Summary*, ix, no. III, March, 6.
Griffiths, R. (1983) *NHS Management Inquiry Report*. London: Department of Health and Social Security.
Ham, C. and Hunter, D.J. (1988) *Managing Clinical Activity in the NHS. Briefing Paper No. 8*. London: King's Fund Institute.
Harrison, S. *et al.* (1990) *The Dynamics of British Health Policy*. London: Unwin Hyman.
NHSME (National Health Service Management Executive) (1991) *NHS Reforms: The First Six Months*. London: NHSME.
Packwood, T. *et al.* (1991) *Hospitals in Transition: The Resource Management Experience*. Milton Keynes: Open University Press.
Pollitt, C. *et al.* (1988) The reluctant managers: clinicians and budgets in the NHS, *Financial Accountability and Management*, 231–3.
Social Services Committee (1989) *Resourcing the NHS: The Government's Plan for the Future of the NHS*. Eight Report, Session 1988–89. London: HMSO.

3

Regulation or Free Market for the NHS?: A Case for Coexistence

Peter Spurgeon

BACKGROUND TO THE 'IMPLIED MARKET'

It is important to understand the cultural assumptions underlying the NHS Reforms in as much as they constitute an implied internal market in health care. Over the past decade the UK Government has pursued a consistent and vigorous policy towards the whole of the public sector. The philosophical motivation behind this policy would seem to be a desire to control total public expenditure and, if possible, substitute alternative forms of resourcing as a replacement for public input. There are some fundamental and pervasive values at work here, most notably:

(1) Increased accountability – at both institutional and personal levels, public organizations have been made more directly accountable for how public money is used.
(2) Multiple providers – slowly but steadily additional and alternative providers have been encouraged to enter the previous monopoly of public provision.
(3) Differential service levels – no longer is the universality of service provision paramount, thus allowing a range of service types and levels to emerge.
(4) Consumer choice – great emphasis has been given to the idea that consumers should exercise a direct choice over what services they receive and where they are provided, both within public provision and incorporating alternative providers.

In summary, then, these values express the concept of market forces with a range of providers offering different levels of service and the public exercising choice in terms of cost and quality of provision.

The basic operational reforms in the health sector that underpin this market philosophy may be identified as:

(1) the separation of purchaser and provider roles with contracts or service agreements as the basis of the purchaser–provider relationship;

(2) the establishment of NHSTs as organizations responsible for the provision of health care;

(3) the creation of GP Fundholding enabling GPs to purchase some services directly on behalf of their patients.

Some ambiguities in these structures have become obvious fairly quickly. For example, would the capacity of some GPFHs to exert direct pressure on hospitals to secure access or treatment for their patients result in a two-tier Health Service with patients on Fundholder lists being placed in an advantageous position above other ordinary GP patients? Similarly, do NHSTs somehow sit just outside the normal NHS structures and represent a Trojan horse towards privatization (whatever the concept of privatization means to different individuals)?

Both of these issues have received rather sensational press coverage and can almost certainly be resolved quite readily should they become serious problems. Perhaps more serious was the sense of ambiguity existing within the relationship between purchasers (DHAs) and providers (Units). For the most part the latter group remained DMUs meaning that, although they were solely concerned with the provision of health care and were receiving contracts from the purchaser, they were also ultimately still responsible to the old DHA (the main purchaser). Indeed, UGMs in charge of DMUs still have a direct line-management relationship to the DGMs with the latter being responsible to the RHAs for the performance of the Units in their Districts. Thus, those placing contracts were also responsible for the staff delivering on those contracts.

It can be argued that the Reforms are, in fact, predicated on a model where all providers are NHSTs. The return of a Conservative Government in April 1992 suggests that there will be steady progress towards this position.[1] In the interim, different health authorities took up varying positions on a dimension of degree of separation. The more extreme positions saw purchasers largely disown the Units, encouraging them to manage their own affairs and to proceed towards Trust status as soon as possible. This 'hands-off' approach was true to the spirit of purchaser/provider but it did create some sense of schizophrenia in the purchaser general managers who remained accountable for Unit performance. The contracts placed between purchaser and provider tended to reflect the philosophical stance taken in that some contracts emphasized the split by identifying elements like penalty clauses and referring to 'soliciting alternative providers'. Indeed some health authorities set explicit targets of identifying alternative suppliers and thereby started to create the competitive environment. Other contracts were written in a cooperative spirit and largely built around what the provider could deliver.

The notion of placing and withdrawing contracts is the weapon of the purchaser and is of course also the essence of the 'implied market'. Nichol (1991) describes the key features of the market-oriented Reforms as:

(1) the ability of the purchaser to represent consumer choice by setting standards and targets free of the conflict of interest that existed when they were also responsible for the supply of health care;

(2) the right of purchasers to place contracts as and where they feel the interests of this population will be best served.

He specifically uses the phrase 'good performance is rewarded, poor performance is penalised'. Here we see the 'implied market' come into focus: there will be winners and there will be losers as a consequence of the operation of market forces.

However, judgements about the functioning of the internal market or indeed the degree to which it needs to be managed or regulated may be premature. The Government has argued strongly that it is far too early to evaluate the outcome of the market at work. In pursuit of a 'smooth take-off' legislation has tended to retard the action of potential market forces. Ham (1992) has suggested that progress on the principal competitive elements underpinning the market has been slow. He argues that purchasers have been preoccupied with developing managerial arrangements for the purchasing process and for links with DMUs. At a more macro level there has been a focus on mergers of Districts,[2] the development of purchasing consortia and relationships with the new-style FHSAs. Equally GPFHs have been surrounded by guidelines to avoid controversial and politically sensitive issues. Finally, contracts during the first year were largely block contracts and, on central advice, based upon historical patterns of service. The consequence was pretty much 'steady state' and contained hardly any radical departures from traditional service patterns.

It may be too early for evaluative statements and some uncertainties still exist but the outcome of the 1992 general election would suggest the retention of the purchaser–provider separation with a provider base consisting largely of Trusts. The 'implied market' may well become a reality and there are some initial facets that might be used to consider how this market in health care is to be managed. However, before looking at these specific factors it may be useful to understand some general properties of markets.

THE NATURE OF MARKETS

Health-care systems of various types, and in a number of countries, are currently under scrutiny as to how total expenditure on health might be restrained. Implicit in this concept of constraint is, of course, the less palatable notion of rationing the provision of health care. It is only fair to acknowledge that rationing of health-care provision has always existed implicitly even in centralist, planned, publicly funded systems. However, as rationing becomes a pressing requirement and more explicit, governments may wish to withdraw from obvious direct involvement. Instead the market can be allowed to operate and through its own interplay of forces resolve conflicts of resource shortfall. This movement towards market mechanisms is somewhat ironic since many existing for-profit systems are experiencing problems both in terms of cost containment and the equity achieved in levels of provision. Public health systems, by and large, have been more successful in controlling aggregate expenditure (OECD 1990).

This perception of market forces as the arbiter or allocator of resources is a rather extreme view of the process of competition. It is perhaps only in conditions of virtually perfect competition that the market will be efficient in an allocative sense. There are in fact a whole range of market structures with varying degrees of rules and regulation. A key aspect in determining the appropriateness or efficiency of a particular market form is the nature of the goods or services in question. With regard to health care as a good, there are some important discrepancies in its characteristics as far as the theory of competition is concerned. Perhaps the most notable is the concept of information asymmetry (Arrow 1963) where the doctor (supplier) and patient (customer) are markedly different in their capacities to determine the precise nature of health need or to determine the effectiveness of any proposed provision.[3] A high degree of competition would normally see a similarly high level of transactions, with some degree of trial and error within the purchaser behaviour. This is manifestly not the case with health care.

The inability of for-profit systems to contain costs, coupled with the higher specific costs of hospitals in a competitive environment (based upon their high-tech, high-quality competitive image), does not seem to augur well for a movement towards a market-based health-care system. However, we need to ask just what form of market is envisaged for health care in the UK.

Mullen (1990) has offered some valuable insight and clarification as to what might be meant by the term 'internal market' and its operation. The origin of the internal market is usually attributed to Enthoven (1985). His original writing was directed particularly at dealing with the issue of the flow of patients in and out of their District of residence. Enthoven actually said that each DHA would continue to be responsible to provide, and pay for, comprehensive care for its own resident population, but not for other people without compensation. However, a much more patient-led system with GPs shopping around for the best access or lowest price seemed to become common parlance. Mullen then describes two types of 'internal market'.

Type I: the health authority receives funding for its population and has specific responsibility for the health care provided to that population. It may in varying degrees provide and purchase. It is implied that residents of the home health authority may be treated only by 'approved' or 'contracted' providers.

Type II: the health authority again receives funding for its population and may again be a direct provider of services. However, residents can seek treatment anywhere and their home authority is obliged to reimburse the provider.

Reality appears to be largely Type I with resources for home residents allocated to the DHA who have a responsibility to purchase health care but may also provide through the continued existence of DMUs. But there are also Type II elements in the emerging new UK system, specifically the provision of emergency services and the ability of GPs to refer patients anywhere.[4] Both sets of costs must be met irrespective of whether or not a contract exists. This is a very important distinction since the Type I aspect represents a more regulated managed-market structure, whilst the lesser Type II aspects provide a forum for the competitive aspects of the market to function. It is this relative balance that has led to the use of the term 'implied internal market' here and for others to describe the internal market in health-care as more rhetoric than reality.

Debate about the internal market, especially by those opposed to the concept, has tended to focus rather unfairly on a more extreme, highly competitive version of a market. The previous discussion makes it clear that this emphasis may be misplaced. The implications of a more constrained market and indeed the intention of the advocates of competition in health care may be less controversial and more viable. For example, as von Otter (1991) suggests, the competitive influence in health-care provision is aimed at securing:

(1) greater internal efficiency of provider organizations;
(2) greater responsiveness of service provision to patients' preferences;
(3) increased managerial effectiveness.

These then are the more reasonable, more laudable goals of the internal market. The question to be asked is how far will the Reforms underpinning the internal market enable these objectives to be delivered? How far might an excessive, over-zealous form of competition inhibit the attainment of these objectives? What degree of market management might be required to balance and stabilize these effects? As previously mentioned, it is too early to be properly evaluative. However, some genuine aspects such as purchasing, contracting and GPFH are in place. It is possible to examine what has happened so far and what this may mean for managing the internal market.

IMPACT OF THE INTERNAL MARKET

Purchasing role

Despite a number of attempts at reform over the past decade it is probably fair to say that the NHS has not been notably responsive to attempts to change its operation. The majority of initiatives seem to have resulted in little more than structurally superficial changes. This very powerful resistance was largely based upon the fact that the professional view of appropriateness of services remained paramount. Medical staff and managers have effectively blocked most previous initiatives and remained the determinants of which services shall be delivered and developed, and also how they will be provided. The NHS has been a provider-dominated organization. The apparent unresponsiveness of the Service was not a conscious or antagonistic rejection but more the outcome of a set of predisposing factors. An excessive demand for an 'apparently free service' delivered by highly trained specialists with relatively limited alternative supply options combined to create a very one-sided situation. As Ham (1991) says, 'the setting-up of the purchaser role provides a significant opportunity to exercise a counterbalancing force to this provider power'.

The notion that the DHA will purchase health services as required by its resident population according to the 'needs' of that population raises a host of technical and ethical problems in the implementation of the purchaser role. Unfortunately, the concept of need is far less precise than it would at first appear.[5] The concept of need defined as a medical problem requiring attention has become confused and entangled with demands and likes. Patient and doctor perceptions of the nature of a particular condition introduce a subjective and unstable element into the process of definition. Some patients present when their 'need' is not accepted by the doctor; others have demands which could be a need in some circumstances but, in conditions of financial restriction, cannot be said to constitute a need. Geographical location, access to hospital sites and fluctuation in hospital waiting-list patterns all impinge upon a definition of need. Therefore it is a prerequisite of an effective purchaser that it develops an operational definition of 'need' in order that it can then proceed to assess levels of need. Given that conceptual difficulty exists, it is likely that this will happen at a local level and idiosyncratic operational criteria will evolve. This is not in itself a bad thing since local circumstances may well be important in the placement of contracts for service. However, it is likely at least to result in an uneven pattern of response from DHAs in their capacity to represent the consumer.

The assessment of health-care needs is largely the domain and responsibility of the Director of Public Health. Clearly this process will be driven by epidemiological information and there is already a considerable body of such data (waiting lists, morbidity and mortality rates, etc.). However, the quality of this information is patchy and it is difficult, if not impossible, to develop a coherent purchasing strategy around this sort of information alone.

A final component of the needs-assessment process is for the DHA to determine its purchasing policy in terms of anticipated outcomes rather than simply in terms of quantifying inputs. The Health Service has, to a large extent, been caught in the trap of assessing its effectiveness in terms of the level of inputs made or the processes in which it engages. These can be important clues and the development of performance indicators makes use of this process of inference, that is, by assessing input we can make some estimate of likely output. But the future for purchasing lies in moving away from this approach to one of assessing health outcomes as a result of the health care it purchases. The reasons for this shift in position are underlying the whole purchasing structure. Outcome measures will enable the DHA to:

(1)   make better informed judgements on its priorities;
(2)   assess whether what it is doing is improving health or not;
(3)   consider whether a particular service should be retained, modified or abandoned;
(4)   establish whether the range of separate services purchased integrates properly into a coherent patient-oriented service.

One of the methods of making an assessment of health outcome is that of QALYs (quality-adjusted life years). It is a measure that considers both the years of life added and the quality of those years. The former aspect is based upon the prognosis of length of life with and without treatment and is clinically based. The latter aspect is much more subjective and perhaps therefore controversial. Numerous factors appear to come into play to destabilize the quality judgement. Most notably these are, first, the group chosen to make the decision about quality of life, that is, professionals differ from the general public; second, the capability of the professional staff involved in a particular intervention; and, finally, the specific condition of an individual patient. Perhaps for the reason of 'destabilizing factors' and also because of the resource implications in developing QALY information, the method remains a principle of what might be done rather than a prescription for practice.

The discussion has focused so far on the technical difficulties of making an assessment of need. There is the equally if not more controversial ethical issue of making explicit the treatments that will be purchased and those that will not. Even if in reality it is less clear cut than an either/or situation, it is likely that under fixed cash limits choices will have to be made about the amount of any service to be provided. In the day-to-day operation of this policy it will mean that for some individual patients certain kinds of treatment are not available. Clearly this is a difficult and uncomfortable decision. It is one that has probably induced the most vociferous reaction from the medical profession who have seen themselves being pushed into the front line in this decision-making process. They will, in fact, be agents of the health authority who will have taken a decision to fund a service to a particular level. It may, however, be the doctor who is forced to pass on this information to the patient.

One clear and probably irreversible change stemming from purchasing is the different relationship that has come to exist between hospitals (consultants in particular) and GPs. The pivotal position of GPs in the referral process meant that there was an obvious need for greater contact, collaboration and discussion as to the nature of services that should be purchased and also where these constraints should be placed. A simple but powerful example of the impact of this dialogue is the demand by GPs for greater access to services such as physiotherapy and chiropody – neither service being high in the priority rankings of hospital consultants.

Similarly there is a slow but increasing recognition that GPs are not only competent to assess the needs of their patients but in many instances are able to provide those services where traditionally they might have been referred to hospital. Specifically, treatment protocols for conditions such as asthma and diabetes have been developed to encourage GPs to take on an enhanced role in the provision of services. There is then more generally a shift to a primary health, preventive service where the interventionist model is increasingly being challenged.

One much vaunted achievement of the new purchasing arrangements is the ability of the purchaser to target specific categories of individuals on waiting lists. Early evidence would seem to suggest that the number of long-wait patients has been reduced. However, even here the overall list size may not have been reduced. Two important but adverse repercussions may result from this apparent improvement:

(1) The movement forward of long-wait patients may have happened at the expense of other patients who, although waiting for a shorter period, may be more severe cases.
(2) In order to avoid failing to meet their obligations under the Patient's Charter (no more than a 2-year wait) providers may refuse to accept patients on to their waiting list.

Contracting

Obviously the processes of purchasing and contracting are totally interwined. The mechanism by which purchasers influence and operate upon the market is by the placement of contracts. Initial government advice to ensure a smooth take-off to the Reforms meant that most contracts in 1991/2 were block contracts. These described the services to be provided but at a rather general level. This approach had the not inconsiderable benefit of ensuring that the purchaser would not suddenly be faced with an unforeseen financial demand from a provider who had 'been efficient' and exceeded the contract target. Thus, in terms of the questions raised at the beginning of this section, the contracting element of the market has so far done little to increase incentives for provider efficiency. It is unlikely that providers, especially NHSTs, will continue to accept block contracts. However, more precise cost-and-volume contracts will expose the purchaser to increased risk should demand exceed the planned levels. No guidance is as yet available as to how this potential conflict of interest will be resolved but it illustrates very clearly the continuing need, over the next few years at least, for a managed-market environment.[6]

Contracts were intended to provide more accessible and identifiable stand-ards and expected performance levels. However, the relative immaturity of purchaser organizations typically meant that they had inadequate resources (both staff and systems) for effective monitoring of the standards. This weakness was further compounded by a lack of good information about performance and delivery of the requisite service criteria. An opportunity for the future had been created.

A general limitation on the progress of the contracting process was the continuing ambiquity of the relationship between purchaser and DMUs.[7] It is hard to see how a purchasing authority could have pushed ahead with a set of contracts which might have jeopardized the stability of its own provider Unit, even if the pattern of service reflected in the contracts was felt to be desirable. The evidence for any radical change in the pattern of services purchased from that delivered under previous systems is virtually non-existent.[8] In part this is a reflection of what was intended. It also reflects the limitation of epidemiological data and the translation of this information into contracts. However, there may be some more lasting constraints which may operate even in a largely Trust-based provider sector. The critical factors here are:

(1) interdependence of clinical specialties;
(2) viability of a hospital Unit;
(3) geographical considerations;
(4) political acceptability.

If a purchaser should wish to operate in accord with the Type II internal-market model and 'shop around' for an advantageous situation, it is unlikely that all services in Hospital A would be consistently better or worse than the equivalent in Hospital B. More realistically, whether the criteria used are price, quality, access or whatever, it is probable that there will be an uneven picture with some specialties better than others. The competitive model would favour the dispersal of contracts to maximize the purchaser's advantage. However, a hospital unable to maintain its range of services may not be viable financially or medically. If we follow the logic of this purchaser-dominated example, the next stage for a non-viable general hospital is either specialization in a restricted range of services or closure. How will the former option fit into the total pattern of provision within a Region? What sense would there be in closure of a hospital serving a large rural area and what might be the reaction of local politicians to a proposed closure of the local hospital? Inner-city environments where over-provision may be said to exist may be able to sustain this market-oriented position but, on the whole, the use of contracts to secure significant competitive advantage may be fraught with great pitfalls. At least it would seem to call for some degree of regulation and management in the market-place.

Finally, in the context of contracting, we might ask how ECRs are faring as representatives of the market-forces Type II version of the internal market. Although only a small part of the total budget, ECRs do seem to cause a degree of tension. Phillips (1992) reports that ECRs are often being turned away because the authorities had already run out of money, adding that the DoH insists that these ECRs have been delayed so that patients wait an equivalent time to the period needed to obtain access to the hospital of the authority of residence. Clearly ECRs are attractive to providers as they receive real additional money for additional work. However, for DHAs they could prove very disruptive.[9] Planned programmes could be damaged by an excessive drain of resources to finance ECRs. Once again the operation of a free-market system does not seem entirely compatible with other aspects of the Service. Interestingly, authorities are taking quite different and opposing perspectives on this, with some moving to incorporation of ECRs into their scheduled contracts and others releasing more of the budget to the ECR provision. Once again we have the managed version versus the free-market version.

GP Fundholding

In some ways the GPFH scheme is a mini version of the whole market process in health care. The objectives of the scheme were stated as follows:

• to improve the quality of services on offer to patients;

- to stimulate hospitals to be more responsive to the needs of GPs;
- to enable GPs to develop their own services.

One of the fundamental objections to GPFH was the danger that a two-tier Health Service would be created, that is, that the benefits accruing to the patients of GPFHs would be provided only at the expense of patients of non-Fundholders. This fear remained even though provider Units were officially instructed to treat GPFHs in the same way as DHA purchasers. The greater freedom and negotiating flexibility of the Fundholder still suggests their patients will have greater choice as regards the place and time of treatment.

The second concern was essentially a financial one whereby fears were expressed that GPs would be affected in their clinical judgements by budgeting considerations. As Bull (1991) argues, this is to some extent a slur on the profession and there is no consistent evidence of a problem in this area. Neither is there a sense of a two-tier access system, although this may in part reflect the difficulties encountered in persuading patients to travel for treatment where it is available either quickly or more cheaply. One of the great assumptions of the health-care market's exponents is that patients will be willing to play their part and act like 'shop-around' consumers. On the whole, patients are expressing a strong preference for having their services locally based even if waiting times are longer.

On the whole GPFH seems to have exerted a positive force in the extension of primary care and in improving the responsiveness of hospitals and consultants. The Government is very keen to press ahead with the scheme and, after an evaluation study, Glennerster *et al.* (1992) are recommending extension. None the less, some general worries persist:

- the possible incentive for GPs to be more careful in their selection of patients;
- the possibility that GPs will reduce referrals inappropriately;
- a risk that resources will be allocated on the basis of demand and not need, thereby making it difficult to achieve material health goals and targets;
- a weakening of the strategic purchasing decisions of DHAs due to the reduction of their funds and fragmentation of purchasing decisions.

It is interesting to note that as GPFHs increase so there is discussion of how to coordinate disparate individuals. Consortia of GPFHs have been suggested as have ideas of GPFHs asking the DHA or FHSA to manage their budgets and purchase on their behalf.[10] Once again the free-rein market force is potentially directing itself back to a managed structure.

Consumer choice

The final aspect we might consider is the degree to which the internal market has facilitated a more responsive attitude to the consumer.

Consumerism as a private-sector model is somewhat wider than this aspect alone, incorporating:

- access;
- choice;
- information;
- redress;
- representation.

The purchaser has an obligation to represent the consumer in the determination of the nature of health-care services to be purchased and perhaps crucially as an index of the quality of the service available. However, despite a recognition of this involvement and of its desirability many purchasers have not really come to terms with how this is to be achieved. There are a number of formidable obstacles to this process. Fundamentally the patients do not in the normal sense exercise choice. The opportunity to examine the latest television set, tape-recorder or video in a range of suppliers is not paralleled in health care. Patients cannot assess the quality of the food they are likely to receive whilst in hospital, or the attitudes of the nursing staff or indeed the technical competence of the doctor in charge of their case. The patient can only exercise choice by proxy through the GP and even here the choice is based on very limited information.

Patients are not a homogeneous group. They are variously articulate, vocal, organized, sick or healthy and moreover they do not always know some of the options available or how to evalute them properly. The healthy majority might well influence purchasing policy to the disadvantage of the sick. Indeed experience from the USA with the 'Oregon approach' suggests the involvement of the public in priority setting may lead to some 'quirky' decisions (Dixon and Welch 1991). Patients may also opt for 'high-risk' options which could have longer-term costs much greater than the option advocated by professionals. A consequence of this would be that because of the increased subsequent costs another patient may not receive treatment. Can patient choice be allowed to operate in this unmoderated fashion?

The difficulties noted are not intended to decry the process of consumerism but to illustrate how yet again the transfer of commercial, retail practices to health (seen as a commodity) is not a simple process (Potter 1988). Undoubtedly health authorities must make strenuous efforts to engage the public in a dialogue about purchasing decisions. The effort must be directed to producing cost-effective, realistic and practical methods.

WHAT DEGREE OF MARKET MANAGEMENT?

Young (1991) raises the rather direct and awkward question of whether market-oriented systems will provide a better option for controlling health-care costs. He concludes, after a comparison of the initiatives in both the UK and New Zealand, that 'despite considerable cost to the taxpayer, the provision of health services by the State does seem to be more economical and equitable than that provided by an overwhelmingly private system'.

Interesting and thought provoking as this might be, it is not really the question we are addressing here. There is a commitment within the NHS Reforms to introduce a form of internal market. We have seen, however, that the form adopted is rather less radical in its degree of application than might first appear to be the case. The more immediate issue for the UK is how will the degrees of competition introduced impact upon health services and how will the interface between the various components of the model be managed?

Clearly these are not simple questions. Observers seem to be somewhat confused in their judgements, perhaps reflecting their own initial assumptions or their own subjective interpretation. Von Otter (1991) states rather boldly that it is a loss of faith in central planning that has been responsible in large part for the recent appeal of market principles in health care. He suggests that public organizations tend to assume a generally stable environment in which people make both personal and collective judgements about health care in a rational way. A very strong pressure towards this potential insularity is that until recently most public organizations have not had to test or validate their products against some form of external criteria. Of course the competitive process immediately attacks this fundamental omission and this in part is one of the great attractions of markets to their supporters. The Type I/Type II distinction made by Mullen is paralleled by von Otter who describes a demand-side form of competition where patients directly house their doctor or organization, as opposed to supply-side competition (as for the most part in the UK) where competition is between providers. Whatever the final balance, it is no coincidence that von Otter describes them both as 'planned markets'.

Similarly Ham (1992) describes the 'steady-state' approach of the Government to the Reforms as implementation in a 'managed' way. He suggests that the level of scrutiny and the desire to minimize emergent problems is less a market and more a 'command and control' bureaucracy of the type disappearing elsewhere in the world, of course just the type that von Otter describes as having failed.

The process of contracting has for many replaced the now outmoded concept of health-care planning. However, it is not entirely clear what the difference is between a managed market and a planned intervention. The clearest objective of the competitive process in the health-care context could well be argued to be greater efficiency in provider Units resulting in more health care being provided for the same level of resource. Even if evidence existed that this target was being pursued, there are a host of more negative possible effects. In circumstances of such uncertainty is it likely that any government would accept the social and political consequences of a hands-off, devil-take-the-hindmost approach? Numerous examples of tensions and potential problems have already been identified in the previous sections. Just as the internal market could deliver positive outcomes, equally possible are other more negative, perverse implications. For example:

(1)   Could the transaction costs (personnel, finance and information staff) be so high as to reduce the total amount of resource available for health care?[11]

(2)   If provider Units were to start operating as successful firms in a competitive environment might they well increase prices to maximize their market strength and as a consequence reduce the total amount of health care purchasers could require?

(3)   Might provider Units become the dominant market force thus reducing further the influence of consumers in shaping services?

If the internal market were to produce outcomes of the type outlined, a 'planned' intervention would be almost certain. There is then, for the foreseeable future, a very strong pressure for the market to be regulated and managed. This is not, of course, a negative conclusion. A managed market is not a failed market. It is more a process of avoiding the unacceptable and trying to build upon the potential positive influences of the internal market.

NOTES

1 Cf p.116.

2 See Chapter 14 for a detailed interview with a provider manager having to deal with a large-scale merger of purchasing Districts, and Chapter 12 for the view of a manager within a merging commissioning agency.

3 See p.263 for a similar view as outlined from a doctor's perspective.

4 The latter giving rise to ECRs, certainly a problematic feature in the DHAs already fraught efforts at effective planning in the Reformed NHS. See p.85 for a brief account of ECRs.

5 For an entirely sceptical view of needs and needs assessment by an academic doctor refer to pp.88–91.

6 But block contracts contain hazards as well as safeguards from the provider's standpoint. Refer p.218 for an illustration of the problems they can produce for providers.

7 Despite some statements to the contrary from both purchasers (pp.189–90) and providers (pp.212–13).

8 See p.108 for further evidence of this.

9 See pp.196–7 for an account of the effects of ECRs on one District in the first year of the Reforms.

10 Cf. pp.207–8 for a GP's view of the part GPs can play in partnership with the DHA in assessing health needs and forming commissioning plans.

11 For example, as described by a purchaser manager on p. 19. ECRs are costly to administer, that is, only 1% of the total spend for the District but taking up more than 5% of administrative costs.

REFERENCES

Arrow, K.J. (1963) Uncertainty and the welfare economics of medical care, *American Economic Review*, 914–73.

Bull, A. (1991) General practice budgets: opportunities and responsibilities, *Journal of Management in Medicine*, 167–70.

Dixon, J.D. and Welch, H.G. (1991) Priority setting: lessons from Oregon, *The Lancet*, April, 891–4.

Enthoven, A.C. (1985) National Health Service: some reforms that might be politically feasible, *The Economist*, 299 (7399), 19–22.

Glennerster, H. *et al.* (1992) *A Footnote for Fundholding*. Poole, Dorset: Bournemouth English Book Centre.

Ham, C. (1991) If it isn't hurting, it isn't working, *Marxism Today*, July, 14–17.

Ham, C. (1992) Managed competition in the NHS: progress and prospects. Paper presented to Manchester Statistical Society, March.

Mullen, P. (1990) Planning and internal markets, in P. Spurgeon (ed.) *The Changing Face of the National Health Service in the 1990s*. London: Longman.

Nichol, D. (1991) Opening address, in D.J. Hunter (ed.) *Paradoxes of Competition for Health*. Nuffield Institute for Health Services Studies, University of Leeds.

OECD (Organization for Economic Cooperation and Development) (1990) *Health Care Systems in Transition*. Social Policy Studies No. 7. OECD.

Phillips, M. (1992) A phoney war over health, *Guardian*, 7 February.

Potter, J. (1988) Consumerism and the public sector: how well does the coat fit? *Public Administration*, 149–64.

von Otter, C. (1991) The application of market principles to health care, in *Paradoxes in Competition for Health*. Nuffield Institute for Health Services Studies, University of Leeds.

Young, I. (1991) Internal markets: are they really the panacea for health-care provision? An Antipodean view, *Journal of Management in Medicine*, 16–22.

4
Creating Competition in the NHS: Is it Possible? Will it Work?

Alan Maynard

NHS POLICY FORMATION IN THE 1980s: THE TRIUMPH OF PRAGMATISM OVER IDEOLOGY

The dominant ideology in political discourse in the 1980s, epitomized by the rhetoric and some of the policies of Reagan and Thatcher, was libertarian with an emphasis on freedom of the individual and the decentralization of power to market mechanisms (as explored in Maynard and Williams 1984). This dominant ideology was contested in the health-care field twice during the Thatcher administration (1979–90). During her first term (1979–83), the 'think-tank', Central Policy Review group, of the Cabinet Office produced an (unpublished) report which advocated privatization and the rapid development of private health insurance. These views, and those of similar groups, were critically reviewed (see, for example, McLachlan and Maynard 1982) and the lessons from this process were used by Norman Fowler, the then Secretary of State for Health, in Cabinet to persuade Mrs Thatcher and her colleagues that the idea of privatization in health care was fundamentally flawed.

The consequence of this learning process was that Mrs Thatcher stated at the 1982 Conservative Party conference (and reiterated it in the 1983 general election manifesto of the Conservative Party) that 'The principle that adequate health care should be provided for all, regardless of ability to pay, must be a foundation of any arrangements for financing health care.' Such sentiments, clearly at variance with the apparent ideology of the Government, did not remove health care from the political agenda. A combination of parsimonious funding of the NHS, with continued pressure for 'efficiency savings' and the introduction of competitive tendering at the margins of the service, for example laundry, catering and cleaning, and increased demands for resources created recurrent 'crises' for the Government of adverse publicity about patient care. The DoH tried to persuade the Treasury to increase funding to meet demographic trends (the 'greying of the population'), technological change, the introduction of community care and the development of HIV/AIDS (Maynard and Bosanquet 1986). The Treasury admitted these claims to a limited extent and demanded improvements in the management of available resources. One response to this by Norman Fowler at the DoH was the Griffiths Inquiry and the reform of management in the NHS (DoH 1983; Griffiths 1992).

During the winter of 1987–8 there were renewed 'scandals' about the failure to treat particular patients and the consequent adverse media attention persuaded the Prime Minister, much to the surprise of her Cabinet colleagues, to announce in January 1988 on BBC TV's *Panorama* the creation of an NHS Review. The initial direction of this Review, carried out in secret by a small group chaired by Mrs Thatcher, involved the extension of private health insurance. However, this discussion, led by the Secretary of State, John Moore, was severely criticized by outside policy and research groups. By mid-1988 the NHS Review had made no progress and an impatient Prime Minister replaced Moore with Kenneth Clarke.

The new Secretary of State decided to retain a tax-financed NHS and to create a competitive market in the provision of health care. This is sometimes referred to as the 'internal market', something of a misnomer as public (NHS) and private suppliers of care were to be permitted to compete for NHS funding. The Government's outline proposals were published in January 1989 (DoH 1989a) and an ambitious programme was adopted to implement these preliminary ideas by April 1991.

These proposals to reform hospital care were complemented with changes in the organization and provision of primary care and community care. A new 'performance-related' contract was imposed on GPs in April 1990, although some of the services now required to be provided by GPs have been shown to have no basis in terms of proven cost-effectiveness (Scott and Maynard 1991). Also, and reluctantly because the Government regarded local government as inefficient and dominated by political opponents, it was agreed that community care, based on local authority social services as the purchaser, would be reformed from April 1993. Consequently, for the elderly, the mentally and physically handicapped, and the mentally ill living outside hospitals, the purchaser will identify client needs and buy appropriate services from competing public and private providers of social care (DoH 1989b).

The consequence of the ideological antipathy to the NHS within the right wing of the Conservative party in the 1980s was a recognition by Mrs Thatcher of its popularity with the electorate; the realization that the private finance option had failed to control costs and increase the efficiency of resource allocation in large markets such as the USA; and the adoption of a radical, barely articulated let alone designed, and unproven policy to create competition not only on the supply side of the NHS (for medical care) but also in the social care market.

THE 1989 REFORMS OF THE NHS

Introduction

The objective of the architects of the 1989 NHS Reforms was to create a competitive market in the provision of health care. A market is a network of buyers (purchasers) and sellers (providers) who exchange goods and services. The way in which markets function is determined by the rules of conduct which are created by public and private agencies. Public agencies use taxes, subsidies, laws, rules, and 'moral suasion' to manipulate the behaviour of public and private agencies. Private agencies use pricing, advertising and other policies such as cartels to manipulate the 'actors' they confront in their markets. Public agencies may operate to ensure a return in terms of political support by the maximization of votes. Private agencies may operate to ensure that they restrict competition, maintain market share and enhance profits; capitalists always and everywhere are the enemies of capitalism: 'People of the same trade seldom meet together, even for merriment and diversion, but the conversation ends in a conspiracy against the public, or some contrivance to raise prices' (Adam Smith 1976a, first publ. 1776: 145–6).

The way in which markets operate are, thus, determined by public and private regulations. All markets are managed by someone, sometimes by government and the private sector in cooperation to enhance their mutual interests of voting support and enhanced profits; as Stigler (1971) argued, government regulation can be used to buy votes and keep rival firms out of the market. The idea that 'free' markets can be created and sustained costlessly is naive; in health care, in particular, substantive regulation is unavoidable. The relevant issue is how, by whom, to what extent and at what cost markets are regulated. If regulations, implicit or explicit, are not created at the time of institutional change, the regulatory vacuum is filled by *ad hoc* initiatives, with rules that may create perverse behaviours and inefficient outcomes.

The nature of the Reforms

The Conservative Government separated the provider and purchaser functions in the NHS. The purchaser's roles are to identify the health needs of the local population, and meet those needs from the finite (public) budgets in a manner which is demonstrably cost-effective. The explicit allocation of these roles may make the purchasers more accountable, especially as they are employed on short-term contracts. The principal purchaser is the DHA. A secondary purchaser of hospital care is the GPFH. A small but increasing group of GPs, with a list size in excess of 9,000 in 1991 (7,000 in 1992), can elect for this status. It provides them with a budget to finance pharmaceuticals, diagnostic hospital services and some (non-emergency) elective surgery.[1]

The purchasers can use their resources to buy services from public and private providers. In the public sector there are hospitals which are DMUs and NHSTs. The latter have been created in cumulative annual 'waves' and are more autonomous but still State owned. They have, in principle at least, more access to capital and can implement their own labour contracts.

The purchasers and providers trade and fix contracts. These contracts are, in fact, agreements which cannot be enforced at law. They determine explicitly the volume, cost and quality characteristics of the services to be delivered and initially (1991–2) this process was very crude due to the absence of relevant data to specify contracts and to inform trading. Apart from services such as sub-Regional specialties, most service transactions in 1991–2 were block (volume/expenditure) contracts and only in 1992–3 are more detailed (but crude) pricing data beginning to merge slowly to inform price–volume negotiations between purchasers and providers. Whilst the development of the latter is slow, the process is focusing attention on the 'margins' and making providers anxious to, at minimum, maintain and hopefully increase patient 'traffic', and hence income.

Market characteristics

Until recently the UK NHS was run at the discretion of doctors and with little management. Few managers in post prior to the 1980s had much knowledge about how their hospital operated, for example they were unlikely to know how many patients were in their beds at any one time, and they had no data about the costs of services or whether those services enhanced the length of and quality of patients' lives. The NHS was and is not unique: managers and clinicians in all health-care systems are ill informed and resources are used in ignorance of their health consequences.

For a market to use scarce resources efficiently the competing purchasers and providers need to know the nature of the rules for exchange and be better informed; in particular, they need to know about prices, the rules for exchange, quality, the capacity of the system to provide care, whether the choices of consumers are met, and how equity is affected.

Prices
In markets prices serve a central function in allocating resources. When demand increases, without a change in supply, prices tend to rise, rationing purchasers' demands and inducing providers to consider increasing supply. When demand falls, prices tend to fall, and providers are encouraged to reduce supply and switch resources to those services which are in greater demand. Prices are a signalling device which inform the decisions of purchasers and providers and initiate changes in the use of scarce resources.

The Reforms create trading relationships which are not only ill informed because of the paucity of price data[2] but may also be distorted by the power of local monopolies. In London, Sheffield, Newcastle and other large cities there are NHS hospitals which may, in fact, compete. However, in many other places there is a local monopoly for most services. And monopolies can raise prices to levels in excess of costs and, by doing so, may distort market signals and use resources inefficiently.

The Government was slow to recognize this problem after the publication of its White Paper (DoH 1989a) and, when it did, Ministers set a rule which limited the rate of return on assets to 6%. Thus a hospital can set its prices but, because of Government regulation to countervail monopolies, the signal to purchasers and providers may be distorted because those prices cannot generate a return in excess of 6%. So prices, as a signalling device to market traders, are not free to reflect scarcity and surplus in the reformed NHS. As in the USA (Robinson 1991; Enthoven 1991), government-created barriers to price competition have meant that the impact of competition on resource allocation has been difficult to detect.

Service capacity
This price control may induce perverse market behaviours. In the US health-care market and in the pharmaceutical market worldwide, there is little price competition. Usually competition in these markets is based on crude indicators of quality. US hospitals compete by buying the latest technologies and deploying them liberally in the absence of proof about their cost-effectiveness. The pharmaceutical industry spends much on the colour, name and marketing of its products. Competition by 'quality' can be inflationary (Robinson and Luft 1988).

Such competition may increase the capacity of the system to levels in excess of patient need. Thus competing NHS hospitals may make individual decisions about elective surgery capacity, for example in orthopaedics and ophthalmic surgery, to reduce waiting lists and, in so doing, may duplicate provision and produce excess capacity.[3] Such hospitals may recognize that there are economies of scale to be achieved from large investments in diagnostics facilities and invest in pathology and scanning facilities, and surgical capacity in the absence of a market for these services.

Duplication and over-capacity is wasteful. It can be curtailed by vigorous purchaser policies which will regulate the size, location and nature of investments which affect its market. Purchasers are unlikely to permit providers to invest freely. Such freedom, if loss making, would affect adversely the financial structure of hospitals and one of the purchaser's aims is to ensure financial viability and continuity in supply by regulation of providers. However, the technical knowledge base to inform purchaser decisions of this nature is poor and they appear somewhat reluctant to remedy these differences.

A crucial tenet of competition is that there will be 'winners and losers'. Some providers will thrive in the market if they have comparative advantage in producing patient care. Some providers, due to inefficiency or just bad luck, will be driven out of business. Governments welcome the former benefits ('health gains') but can suffer electorally from the latter. In the USA the introduction of DRGs (diagnostic-related groups), a system of prospective hospital reimbursement, reduced length of stay and threatened the viability of rural, poor and teaching hospitals. The Federal Government could not cope with the political backlash and now makes $5 billion extra-DRG payments to keep them in business and politicians in office!

In the short time in which the UK Reforms have been in operation the Government has shown a similar unwillingness to let the 'weak' go out of business. It exempted the Special Hospital, for example the Royal Marsden in London, from competition altogether, fearing the effects a market might have on them. It has made special payments, for example, to the Brompton, to keep some favoured London hospitals in this group in business. Rather than let the market drive London hospitals out of business the Conservative Government set up a commission of inquiry to report after the 1992 general election. The resultant report by Sir Bernard Tomlinson will require significant bed closures in London and closure of major hospitals.

The rules for exchange

Whilst the Reforms have separated purchaser and provider, market transactions inevitably bring them back together.[4] What is the nature of the trading relationship: adversarial or collaborative?

The simplistic economic model emphasizes adversarial competition. Thus Adam Smith argued:

> It is not from the benevolence of the butcher, the brewer and the baker that we expect our dinner, but from their regard to their own self interest. We address ourselves, not to their humanity but to their self-love, and never talk to them of our necessities but to their advantages.
>
> (Adam Smith, 1976a, first publ. 1776)

More recently, and more controversially, it is alleged that Roy Kroc – the creator of the McDonald's empire – when asked what he would do if he saw a rival drowning, is alleged to have replied 'put a hose in his mouth'! This is competition 'red in tooth and claw' which is sometimes endorsed by liberal advocates of market mechanisms.

However, many market relationships are not of this nature. Sainsburys and other food retailers have detailed, long-term contracts with their providers. Other retailers (Marks and Spencer, for example) have similar relationships with their suppliers which are detailed and collaborative. In these markets each partner, purchaser and provider wishes to thrive and be assured of continuity of supply and revenue, for high-quality goods and services. These requirements for contracting between purchasers and providers are evident in the US health-care system and raise issues about the efficiency of the newly created purchaser–provider divide in the NHS. Adam Smith recognized this interdependence of buyers and sellers:

> Those general rules of conduct when they have been fixed in our mind of habitual reflection, are of great use in correcting the misrepresentations of self-love concerning what is fit and proper to be done in our particular situation . . .
> The regard of those general rules of conduct, what is properly called a sense of duty, is a principle of greatest consequence in human life, and the only principle by which the bulk of mankind are capable of directing their actions.
>
> (Adam Smith, 1976b, first publ. 1790: 160–2)

Cooperation and custom may be more cost-effective means of managing markets than anarchistic, atomistic adversarial competition where the weak are driven out of business. This is evident in the arrangements of market transactions which emphasize mutual interdependence and quality control, for example in Japan (Morishima 1982). Competition in many successful markets is restricted for efficiency reasons. As Sen (1987) has argued, self-interest is not the great redeemer and collaborative transactions, particularly in doctor–patient relationships, may be more efficient. Indeed, competition may undermine professional mores and enhance cost inflation and inefficiency (Fuchs 1987; Relman 1992).

Quality in health care

Exchanges between purchasers and providers in health-care markets are poorly informed not only about resource consequences (prices and costs) but also quality. No health-care system has information about the effects, if any, of health-care interventions on the patient's length and quality of life.

The search for such measures has been long and similar to the quest for the Holy Grail! Frances Clifton, physician to the Prince of Wales, wrote in the eighteenth century in his book *The State of Physick*:

> In order, therefore to procure this valuable collection, I humbly propose, first of all, that three or four persons should be employed in the hospitals (and that without any ways interfering with the gentlemen now concerned), to set down the cases of the patients there from day to day, candidly and judiciously, without any regard to private opinions or public systems, and at the year's end publish these facts just as they are, leaving every one to make the best use he can for himself.
>
> (Frances Clifton, 1732)

The editor of the *Lancet* rediscovered the importance of outcome measurement in Victorian times: 'All public institutions must be compelled to keep case-books and registers, on a uniform plan. Annual abstracts of the results must be published. The annual medical report of cases must embrace hospitals, lying-in hospitals, dispensaries, lunatic asylums and prisons' *Lancet* (1840–1).

The 1844 Lunacy Act required the managers of psychiatric hospitals to measure outcomes. Data on whether such patients were dead, relieved or unrelieved were kept throughout the nineteenth century. Florence Nightingale adopted this classification in her book *Some Notes on Hospitals* and concluded:

> I am fain to sum up with an urgent appeal for adopting this or some uniform system of publishing the statistical records of hospitals. There is a growing conviction that in all hospitals, even in those which are best conducted, there is a great and unnecessary waste of life . . . In attempting to arrive at the truth, I have applied everywhere for information, but in scarcely an instance have I been able to obtain hospital records fit for any purpose of comparison. If they could be obtained, they would enable us to decide many other questions besides the ones alluded to. They would show subscribers how their money was being spent, what amount of good was really being done with it, or whether the money was doing mischief rather than good.
>
> (Florence Nightingale, 1863)

The US Federal Government rediscovered the need for outcome measures in 1987, publishing mortality rates for all hospitals which had Medicare patients. This work was criticized, as was that of Paul Kind (1988) which used NHS data. Kind showed that in-patient death rates in England varied considerably: Grimsby, South West Durham and North Tees Health Authorities, for instance, appeared to perform badly.

Such data beg more questions than they answer: there is a need to adjust them, for example for age, sex, severity and economic class. Furthermore, even after such adjustment, there is difficulty in explaining the variations in mortality because of the small number of cases for individual doctors. However, the merit of these data is that they focus the attention of clinicians and managers on outcomes.

Managers need to be informed not only about survival of in-patients but also, with record linkage, about survival over time in the community. The quality of survival is also important to patients and purchasers and can be informed by collection of data with valid and robust measures. There are two types of quality-of-life (QoL) measure: disease specific and generic. There are hundreds of disease-specific QoL measures which have been validated and replicated to varying extents; a discussion of these can be seen in Spilker (1990) and a special edition of Spilker *et al.* (1990). Generic QoL measures, such as Short Form 36 (SF 36) (Ware and Steward 1992), are used across disease and treatment categories and may facilitate allocation decisions if translated into measures which combine both duration and quality of survival guesstimates, such as quality-adjusted life years (QALYs), for example see Williams (1985).

The collection of outcome data is crude and can be improved by agreeing best practice for the collection of a nationally agreed core data set.[5] This should not be about process issues alone (patient satisfaction, recurrence rates, postoperative infection) but should also be focused on health benefits. If this route is adopted, it will facilitate the production of 'best practice' advice to purchasers and clinicians. Such data will improve the regulation of the market to ensure that cost-effective care is provided. Its absence now means that the efficiency of market-induced changes in resource allocation is unknowable.

Consumer Choice
In the Reformed NHS, consumers have little choice as the patients' guardian, the purchaser, decides treatments on behalf of his or her clients.[6] The architects of the 1989 Reforms paid lip-service to patients' choices and real change will occur only if purchasers measure customer preferences and use this information vigorously and imaginatively to determine choices. This outcome is similar to that produced in the 'competitive' US health-care market where 'managed care' programmes cover increasing portions of the population but use insurers and Health Maintenance Organizations (HMOs) as the guardians of the patient.

Equity
Resources to fund health care are allocated on a per capita basis with a weighting for need, proxied by the number of elderly in the local population and standardized mortality ratios (SMRs). Thus purchasers with more elderly and high death rates get more resources.[7] SMRs are used as a proxy for absent measures of morbidity and mean that, if purchasers kill off more of their population, they get more resources! It would be more efficient if resource allocation reflected the capacity of local purchasers to buy treatments which would improve health cost-effectively.

Whatever the formula used to allocate health-care resources, their equal distribution does not ensure that health inequalities are reduced. In the

NHS, resources are allocated between competing patients, in principle at least, in relation to their capacity to benefit, that is, enhancement in health. The capacity to benefit of competing groups of patients may vary, for example the poor may benefit less, per unit of expenditure, than the rich because, for instance, of their genetic endowment, their work, leisure and household behaviours, and their education, housing, income and wealth. Consequently, if resources are allocated to those who benefit most, the poor may get less care and health inequalities may be increased.

Equity issues such as these cannot be ignored in a publicly funded health-care system. The competitive market, if it is successful in allocating resources, on the basis of capacity to benefit, will be constrained by public regulation in order to meet socially determined equity targets.

CONCLUSIONS

The 1989 Reforms were apparently designed to introduce a competitive market in the production of health care. In fact the Government has regulated the Reforms closely with central control, facilitated by the NHSME, being greater than before. In 1991–2 managers were instructed to maintain a 'steady state', and the guidance in 1992–3 is for 'managed change'. Planning or management, the regulation of resource allocation, is inevitable in health-care markets. Whichever party is in power, regulation will dominate the way in which networks of buyers and sellers trade. The issue of whether the 'internal market' preferred by the Conservative Party or the 'planning' process preferred by the Labour Party is superior, is an empirical issue which should be determined by evaluation rather than rhetoric. In practice they may vary little and be confronted by the same obstacles to change, and both parties will be reluctant to adopt their preferred option and 'confuse' policy formation with evidence!

The NHS Reforms in 1989 have changed the attitudes and behaviour of managers and clinicians for the better and begun the process of a rapid escalation in management costs. Investments in personnel and information technology are considerable, running into hundreds of millions of pounds. Clinical practice is being challenged and considerable resource is being spent on medical audit, an unproven and poorly conceived process. Thus the Reforms are producing advantages and disadvantages and the balance of these effects is unknown.

Are the Reforms efficient? If they were, enhanced efficiency in treatment practices would produce health gains which would offset the resource costs of creating the new management structure. No proper evaluation of the Reforms has been carried out and it is impossible to determine whether competition in health care is efficient. The US evidence about managed care (Miller and Luft 1991) is absent or incomplete: competitive mechanisms are advocated but with, as yet, little empirical support. Indeed, Hadley and Langwell (1991) suggest that, if efficiency gains are produced in the USA by managed care, they may be offset by the higher administrative costs of such market mechanisms. This outcome may be replicated in the UK where the absence of evidence about the efficiency of the Reforms is coupled with a refusal of the Government to evaluate their progress.

The absence of evidence about the efficiency of competition in health care is accompanied by an increased recognition that regulation of competition is pervasive and increasing. After an initial 'freeing up' of attitudes and behaviour the reform pressures in the NHS appear to be declining. Whether it is called managed care (as in the USA) or competition (as in the UK), the use of market mechanisms in health-care systems involves large increases in management costs with as yet unproven benefits in terms of resource allocation. Maybe the introduction of competition in health care will not work; certainly it should carry a Government health warning! Perhaps competition is unnecessary and improved management of resources, without the separation of purchaser and provider functions, may better achieve those elusive goals of Government policy: efficiency, equity and cost containment. However, that, like the claims of the advocates of the many variates of competition, can only be sustained by evaluation and evidence. Whatever the words used to describe reform – competitive, regulated or managerial – better outcome measurement to facilitate *glasnost* and *perestroika*, and continuous questioning of existing structures and processes are essential.

NOTES

1 The Reforms are enhancing the status of GPs, not only in the role of direct purchasers (GPFHs), but also as consortia of GPs willing to influence and advise on commissioning decisions. This is acknowledged by a commissioner on pp.193–4.
2 Cf. pp.197–8 and pp.217–20.
3 For another case where over-capacity has been a result of the market, see pp.210–1.
4 For two accounts of the degree of separation between purchaser and provider as perceived by a commissioning manager and a provider manager respectively see pp.189–90 and pp.212–3.
5 Cf. p.194 where a commissioning manager also points out the need for national evaluations on treatment outcomes.
6 Doctors from yet another viewpoint argue that the concept of consumer choice is untenable as the commodity does not have the knowable qualities of other products, i.e. the patient may not know what may be in their best interests in matters of health care. See p.236 for more on this argument.
7 For more on the effects of this type of funding allocation refer to pp.213–4, where, despite much deprivation in one District, the merged commissioning agency has tried to standardize the resource losses across its three Districts. This is a good example of a District where morbidity data would be more useful than SMRs, as its needs are reflected less in its age profile than in other statistical indicators.

REFERENCES

Clifton, R. (1732) *The State of Physick, Ancient and Modern Briefly Considered*. London.
DoH (Department of Health) (1983) *NHS Management Inquiry*. London: HMSO.
DoH (Department of Health) (1989a) *Working for Patients*. London: HMSO.
DoH (Department of Health) (1989b) *Caring for People*. London: HMSO.

Enthoven, A. (1991) Market forces and health care costs, *Journal of the American Medical Association*, 2751–2.

Fuchs, V. (1987) The counter revolution in health care financing, *New England Journal of Medicine*, 1154–6.

Griffiths, R. (1992) Seven years of progress: general management in the NHS, *Health Economics*, 61–70.

Hadley, J.P. and Langwell, K. (1991) Managed care in the US: promises, evidence to date and future directions, *Health Policy*, 91–118.

Kind, P. (1988) *Hospital Deaths – the Missing Link: Measuring Outcome in Hospital Activity Data*. Discussion Paper No. 44. Centre for Health Economics, University of York.

Lancet (1840–1) Editorial, 650–1.

Langwell, K. (1990) Structure and performance of Health Maintenance Organizations: a review, *Health Care Financing Review*, 71–80.

McLachlan, G. and Maynard, A. (eds.) (1982) *The Public Private Mix for Health*. London: Nuffield Provincial Hospitals Trust.

Maynard, A. and Bosanquet, N. (1986) *Public Expenditure on the NHS: Recent Trends and Future Problems*. London: Institute of Health Services Management.

Maynard, A. and Williams, A. (1984) Privatization and the National Health Service, in J. Le Grand and R. Robinson (eds.) *Privatization and the Welfare State*. London: Allen & Unwin, 95–110.

Miller, R.H. and Luft, H.S. (1991) Perspective, diversity and transition in health insurance plans, *Health Affairs*, 37–44.

Morishima, M. (1982) *Why has Japan Succeeded?* London: Longman.

Nightingale, F. (1863) *Some Notes on Hospitals*. London: Longmans Green.

Relman, A. (1992) What market values are doing to medicine, *Atlantic Monthly*, 7 March, 98–106.

Robinson, J.C. (1991) HMO market penetration and hospital cost inflation in California, *Journal of the American Medical Association*, 2719–23.

Robinson, J.C. and Luft, H. (1988) Competition, regulation and hospital costs, 1982 to 1986, *Journal of the American Medical Association*, 2676–81.

Scott, T. and Maynard, A. (1991) *Will the new GP Contract Lead to Cost-Effective Medical Practice?* Discussion Paper No. 82. Centre for Health Economics, University of York.

Sen, A.K. (1987) *On Ethics and Competition*. Oxford: Basil Blackwell.

Smith, A. (1976a) *An Inquiry into the Nature and Causes of the Wealth of Nations*. (First published 1776.) Oxford: Clarendon Press.

Smith, A. (1976b) *A Theory of Moral Sentiments*. (First published 1790.) Oxford: Clarendon Press.

Spilker, B. (ed.) (1990) *Quality of Life Assessments in Clinical Trials*. New York: Raven Press.

Spilker, B. *et al.* (1990) Quality of life bibliography and indexes, *Medical Care* Supplement.

Stigler, G. (1971) The theory of economic regulation, *Bell Journal of Economics and Management Sciences*, 3–21.

Ware, J.E. and Steward, A.L. (eds.) (1992) *Measuring Functioning and Well Being: The Medical Outcomes Study Approach*. Durham, NC: Duke University Press.

Williams, A. (1985) Economics of coronary artery bypass grafting, *British Medical Journal*, 326–9.

5

Understanding Internal Markets in the NHS*

Ewan Ferlie, Liz Cairncross and Andrew Pettigrew

MARKET-LIKE MECHANISMS AND THE NHS

The NHS is currently introducing far-reaching measures designed to introduce a quasi or 'internal market' element into resource allocation processes
previously dominated by planning and by line-managerial hierarchies (DoH
1989). These are changes which are now apparent throughout much of the UK
public sector, but have a particular visibility in the NHS which is often seen as
its 'jewel in the crown'. While the NHS will continue to be publicly funded,
component parts will be expected to behave more competitively within a
market-like framework (it is argued) to reduce costs, provide incentives for
performance and improve quality. The time scale for these changes has been
very ambitious with pleas for pilot schemes being rejected.

Given that a possible danger is of an excessive action orientation, there is a
need for thinking as well as doing. In particular, there has been little strategic
discussion so far about the type of market that is likely to emerge in the new
order. The nature of such markets may vary from locality to locality and from
specialty to specialty. We suspect, for instance, that internal market pressures
are likely to be more severe in metropolitan areas (and especially London) than
in rural areas. We also take the view that the market-like model fits relatively
discrete specialties such as elective surgery more neatly than less bounded
specialties such as psychiatry or oncology.

But we may also need to generate more conceptual thinking about the
nature of markets. The relationships between the four key groups of producers, consumers, purchasers and regulators can be modelled in a number
of different ways. In the case of the NHS, market-like transactions are likely

* This is an amended and redrafted version of a paper first given at a conference on strategic
change processes within organizations held at the University of Venice in May 1991. Thanks
are due to the discussant, Gerard de Pouvourville of the Ecole Polytechnique, Paris, and to
Jenny Griffiths, Oxfordshire FHSA, for comment on a later draft.

It has emerged from a research and development project that has been funded by the National
Health Service Training Directorate working in conjunction with the National Association of
Health Authorities and Trusts.

to take place in complex organizational settings very different from simple notions of economic exchange between individual consumers and producers. Indeed markets may be consciously created by regulators so as to induce competition, by grouping hospitals together in certain ways. Markets may be best seen as closely linked to a series of economic and social institutions rather than as a freestanding aggregate of individual transactions. It may be useful to consider possible parallels in the creation of a single European market, where many government institutions are also heavily involved (Shipman and Mayes 1990).

The construction of market typologies is a theme in many research settings. The conventional distinction between monopoly, oligopoly and perfect competition is one example of such a typology within economics. Levacic (1990: 22) compares the neo-classical view of the market with that of the Austrian school who reject the idea of market structure as irrelevant and see market coordination as much more of a dynamic process in which entrepreneurship plays a key role. Within the NHS, Mullen (1990) has distinguished between a 'Type 1' internal market (purchaser-led) and a 'Type 2' internal market (patient-led).

The next step is to build our own typology of possible models of an internal market, identify key assumptions and also outline some associated 'signs and symptoms'. How, in other words, would we know that the world was beginning to look like this model, were it indeed to do so? We assume for the purposes of this chapter (and for no other reason) that health-care 'products' can indeed be usefully analysed as provided along market-like lines, although this remains a fiercely controversial area (e.g. Laughlin 1991).

FOUR ALTERNATIVE MARKET TYPES

In this section we outline literature which sheds rather different lights on the possible development of any internal market in health care.

An unregulated neo-classical market

Following in the steps of Adam Smith, the proponents of the neo-classical market contend that it has advantages over the bureaucratic system in terms of its greater internal and allocative efficiency and increased consumer choice. The market of the neo-classical economists is set in a world of perfect competition where a multitude of sellers compete for the business of an equally large number of buyers. The market is one where the product is easily identifiable and of uniform quality, intermediaries play a minor role and there is no question of ignorance among buyers and sellers about the market price.

These arguments were often thought to lack descriptive validity in health care: it was thought that no health-care market could possibly look like that. However, in the USA of the 1980s the Federal Government (Robinson 1990) initiated more vigorous pro-competition policies in order to contain health-care costs. The main planks of this initiative were the introduction of cost-sharing arrangements to make consumers more aware of the costs of health care, anti-trust legislation which aimed to remove supply-side constraints, and the development of managed-care systems such as Health Maintenance Organizations (HMOs) which offered alternative forms for the delivery and finance of health care.

Critique of the neo-classical model

Of course, the neo-classical model has itself been subject to a number of important criticisms. As long ago as Robinson (1933) there have been attempts to develop more complex typologies of market structure to complicate the simple dichotomy between free market and monopoly such as monopolistic competition and oligopoly. In the NHS the number of buyers and sellers may be small (Williamson 1975, 1985) and this may result in market failure.

Second, within functioning markets there is the requirement for contestability (Baumol 1982; Baumol *et al.* 1982), that is, a credible threat that alternative producers are lurking in the wings, and that they could come on stage as soon as a monopoly or oligopoly producer raises their price above the market price. However, there may be considerable entry and exit costs in health care as hospital construction and other aspects of health-care provision may involve massive new capital investment or sunk costs, and large-scale hospital bankruptcy seems a remote prospect.

Third, there is the principal–agent problem. Is the consumer really sovereign? In the internal market, consumer 'proxies' (such as GPs) exert a critical gatekeeping role, and the individual patient has little direct role in the purchase of care. The principal–agent problem is that the objectives of principals and agents may diverge and that information levels may also be different. This draws attention to the potentially problematic relationship between patient and GP, and between GP and DHA/FHSA.

Fourth, and using here a transaction–costs perspective, there may be considerable contracting costs involved in any shift from hierarchies to markets (Williamson 1985), especially for those contracts which cannot be handled on a block basis. There is an expectation in the British system that the contracting system will progressively move from a block contract basis to cost-and-volume contracts and indeed cost-per-case contracts. Such a shift in the predominant mode of contracting would heavily increase the work load.

As well as the increasing volume of contracting work, there is also the question of developing the analytical base behind the contracting process. What do we mean by 'quality' in health care and how do we recognize a 'quality' service? Quality as well as price-based competition emerged as of some importance in the US experience of the 1980s (Robinson 1990) and the role of quality competition may be even more important in the 1990s (Schumacher 1989).

Assumptions of the neo-classical model

Thus, within the neo-classical model, a number of distinguishing assumptions are made:

- There would be a large number of buyers and sellers.
- There would be a credible threat of market entry by new producers.
- There would be little automatic recontracting, and many 'one-off' contracts.
- Purchasers would respond rapidly to evidence of changing demand; consumer proxies would operate with roughly equivalent agendas to consumers themselves.
- There would be evidence of strong competitive forces operating, with clear winners and losers.
- Cost and information systems would be robust enough to support formally based decision-making processes; there would be well-developed measures of quality, clinical as well as non-clinical.
- Consumers would themselves have access to good information, would be in the position to make well-informed choices between providers and would also be relatively mobile between them.

It seems unlikely that even the restructured NHS will fit all or even many of these assumptions.

An unregulated relational market

The relational-markets literature has developed out of the concerns of marketeers, and is perhaps best associated with the Scandinavian work of the 1980s (Ford 1990). It was felt that the conventional view of an active marketeer, passive consumers and an atomistic market restricted understanding of what actually happened in markets. The neo-calssical model assumes that markets are populated by individuals or simple firms, yet economic life is often dominated by a small number of large and complex firms which behave in a different way.

A number of important implications follow from this new perspective. Unlike individual consumers, corporate buyers would often interact with sellers. The relationship between companies might be complex, close and long term, including a mixed history of adaptation, commitments, trust and conflict. Such buyer–seller relationships are, however, but one example of a much wider group of relationships in which a company would operate: seller–seller relationships must also be considered as well as buyer–seller relationships which have as their primary focus product or technology development rather than the conventional sale.

So the interaction process does not solely revolve around the product/service exchange, or even information or financial exchange, but also includes social exchange, undertaken so as to reduce uncertainty and to build trust or clannishness (Ouchi 1980) which is a distinctive organizational form where there are common values and source loyalty. There is a tendency to 'keep things in the family'. Buyers, once locked into a set of relationships, may be relatively inert in seeking new sources of supply.[1]

Power, trust and influence emerge as important concepts in such network analysis as well as efficiency. It thus contains an important behavioural component. However, such network analysis has been criticized (Mansfield

1987) for being limited and rather static. There is often insufficient attention to how networks are created and are maintained over time. In addition, the social component to relational markets is worth investigating in much richer empirical detail. How are coteries of buyers and sellers formed? What are the social institutions which shelter such groups? What are the socialization mechanisms?

The pattern of negotiations between actors in a relational market may well be shaped by a 'rule system' (Shipman and Mayes 1990) which places boundaries around acceptable forms of behaviour. Some of these rules will be enforced externally, by the courts or by government (the arbitration function played by RHAs is one conflict-resolving 'rule'). Some may be set by a small group of power holders. Others are internally generated and enforced through convention. The emergence of any such 'rules system' may of course pervasively shape the operation of any internal market.

Some assumptions of the relational-market perspective include:

- There are a relatively small number of well-established buyers and sellers locked into long-run contracts or repeat buying.
- Buying decisions are made on the basis of soft data (trust) as well as hard information. It is difficult to secure formal information to support decision-making.
- Inter-organizational cooperation may be apparent between producers or between purchasers.[2]
- Purchasers have a developmental as well as a controlling role *vis-à-vis* their providers; it is difficult to maintain an 'arm's length' relationship.
- There are social groupings or institutions which bring providers and purchasers together informally. These groupings provide a covert 'safety net' for losing providers as it becomes psychologically impossible to drive them into bankruptcy.
- Historical or inherited referral patterns are of continuing importance.
- 'Reputation' is a key intangible asset on which purchasers trade, offsetting cost disadvantages.
- 'Rules systems' emerge, either imposed or negotiated to structure contracting. There is a link between rule setting and the possession of organizational power.

A regulated market

Both the accounts developed above describe different ways in which an essentially unregulated market may operate. This may prove an unrealistic assumption, and so we may also need to access and develop theories of market regulation, both by public regulatory bodies and self-regulation by professionals.

Governmental regulation
In the US context, regulatory theory has been developed as the scope of government regulation expanded from early concern with anti-trust policy and the regulation of a few industries with natural monopoly characteristics

to affect more and more sectors of the economy. Early assumptions that regulators acted in the 'public interest' and to correct market failure were challenged by other theories (Stigler and Friedland 1962) which suggested that regulation may act as a device to transfer income and power to well-organized groups that often capture the regulatory process. Theoretical work now seems to be moving on again from a simple capture model to a recognition that the regulatory arena involves multiple and competing interests (Romer and Rosenthal 1987).

The nature and effects of regulation emerged as a major British theme of the 1980s, partly in response to the pro-competition policies pursued by the Government which sought to roll back public ownership and to construct new markets which were then subjected to regulatory regimes. The new GP contract of 1990 can be seen as a classic attempt by the Government to regulate a profession, carried to extremes. At a policy level, there is also now substantial experience on which to draw in the regulation of newly privatized industries by such bodies as Ofgas and Oftel. Some of the key problems in regulatory theory have been discussed by Vickers and Yarrow (1988) which concluded that there had been important efficiency weaknesses from the point of view of competition policy apparent in the newly privatized utilities. Crude forms of price regulation had often been adopted, and information flows were poor, giving wide discretion to the regulated firms.

Although there may be a policy switch from direct line management to regulation as a means of control, the nature of the regulatory regime may itself also evolve over time. As Bowen and Jones (1986) point out, deregulation was a characteristic of US industrial policy in the 1980s and this could change the basis for competitive behaviour in an industry (as in the airline industry). Financial services also underwent deregulation in the Britain of the 1980s, with some unanticipated demand side-effects.

We need to know more about how decision-making processes are influenced by various regulatory regimes. Cook *et al.* (1983) have attempted to develop a theory of organizational behaviour by US hospitals when confronted by regulatory regimes. The response of hospitals under light regulation was thought to be confined to peripheral areas, and only under heavier and more prolonged regulation would changes to core services and structure take place.

Analogous work is now badly needed in the British context. A common view here is that any market would need to be heavily regulated to prevent possible market failure. For example, the scenario-building exercise undertaken by the Office of Public Management (1990) for East Anglia RHA indicated the breakdown of service systems which might be apparent as a result of introducing quasi market reforms without effective 'market management'.

Heavy regulation creates, however, its own source of compliance costs. In the Netherlands, for example (van de Ven and Wynard 1989), traditional detailed government regulation is now seen as unworkable and there is now a move from government regulation to market and self-regulation. Instead of direct government control on volume and prices, the government will now create the necessary conditions to let the market achieve societal goals. The emphasis of government regulation will therefore be on anti-cartel, quality control and information-disclosure measures.

Professional self-regulation

Medicine has often been seen as the ideal typical profession, at the heart at which lies a socially accredited claim to power and autonomy on the basis of the possession of a special expertise and social function. Control is here exerted through self-regulatory bodies such as the General Medical Council which has successfully managed to fend off demands for radical reform while implementing more piecemeal change (Stacey 1989). Such a high degree of self-regulation might be expected to shape, and possibly weaken, the operation of internal market forces.

During the late 1970s and 1980s, however, there has been a search by third-party payers for measures to control the behaviour of physicians as costs of health-care systems have escalated, especially in the US context. These measures include peer review, but go far beyond such self-regulatory mechanisms.

We need to consider the role of market-based incentives in changing the pattern of professional behaviour.[3] For neo-liberals and classic Marxists alike, ideology reflects economic interest, assuming a crude theory of motivation. However, for neo-Marxist writers such as Lawson (1977), a crucial question revolves around the relationship between professionals such as clinicians and the market. Are they 'free marketeers' or are they part of an anti-market 'counter movement' using protective legislation, restrictive associations and other instruments of intervention? For Durkheim (1964), professionals provided a model which would include the ethics and rules needed in a complex division of labour and thus save modern society from anomie. Professionals were seen as having a sense of social identity and shared values (even mission), organizing themselves within a 'college' and emphasizing non-contractual social relations.

Perhaps the challenge to medicine's professional status was taken furthest in the USA of the 1970s and 1980s (Elston 1991). Marxist writers even claim to detect the 'proletarianization' of doctors as their control over the work flow is eroded (Oppenheimer 1973). Non-Marxists more modestly detect 'deprofessionalization' (Starr 1982) based on changes in the doctor/patient relationship. Increased rationalization of medical practice and knowledge, the development of 'alternative' medicine, a social trend to assertive consumerism and a greater willingness to litigate have all led to a decline of the authority of US medicine. Elston (1991) asks whether this pattern is also likely in the UK but concludes that this is as yet unlikely.

If this assessment is correct, and the social prestige and power of British medicine is largely undisturbed, then doctors are likely to retain considerable powers of self-regulation with which to shape – and presumably to soften – the force of the internal market. Indeed, GPFH essentially puts a group of professionals in charge of small corners of the market. The obstacles to the development of a general-management role in primary care perhaps illustrate how much control has been established elsewhere.

Some questions and propositions deriving from these two regulatory ideal types can be readily identified:

- How are rules of competition established? What is the role of higher tiers in setting and maintaining rules and incentive structures and what is the basis of competition that is established (quality, price, reputation)?
- How are markets constructed? (There may need to be at least two groupings of roughly equivalent mass in any area for competitive forces to operate.) What is the degree of competitive pressure which is tolerated or indeed encouraged? (This may vary by locality, and there are expectations that the degree of competition will be stronger in metropolitan areas such as London than in rural areas.)
- How tightly regulated is the labour market? Traditionally pay and conditions have been agreed through national pay bargaining machinery, but there are now moves to bring in local pay bargaining. The NHSTs may be particularly important here.[4] At the same time the DoH has also publicly expressed concern at the possible spiralling of managerial salaries in the new Trusts and the need for a 'steady state' at the beginning of the transitional period.
- How tightly regulated is access to capital? NHSTs were promised greater freedom to borrow, but many have been disappointed with the initial borrowing limits announced by the Department.[5]
- Are there explicit or implicit rules for intervention for the higher tiers (Ham 1990)? For example, how are disputes at lower tiers arbitrated?
- Who regulates? Is there an independent regulator? Does the Department regulate? Is the task handed back to the Regions or are new mechanisms found especially as the number of NHSTs and GPFHs increases?
- What is the role of professional self-regulation in shaping the operation of the internal market? In particular, are there rules or norms which act to restrict the degree of competition?

The 'pseudo market': reorganization as relabelling

Here we are contemplating an extreme ideal typical case of politically dominated 'heavy regulation': in effect we may be seeing the introduction of the internal market as a symbolic reform which makes little substantive change to the inherited pattern of relationships. Often previous reorganizations within the public sector achieved only modest change (March and Olsen 1983), and perhaps should indeed be seen as symbolic rather than substantive reform efforts. An implication for the NHS might be that politicians or their surrogates (the DoH, Regions) would continue to intervene in politically sensitive matters, despite superficial changes to the formal system (Culyer 1990).

Brunsson (1989) indeed argues that, while organizational reform is often presented as a radical change, reform is better seen as a repetitive activity which is easy to start but difficult to finish. Reforms may be oversold, or lead to a perception of fresh problems for which still newer reforms are needed. Reforms come in cycles, in part because strong fashions in the stock of managerial knowledge guarantee that the practices of organizations will periodically appear old-fashioned. Reformers are aided by the fact that most organizations forget more than they learn.

Much of this wider debate about the limits of reorganization can also be seen, perhaps in a particularly dramatic form, in the health care sector where, for instance, the repeated failure of attempts at reform in New York was explored by Alford (1975).

It must be said, however, that the 1980s have witnessed a rather different pattern of events where the pace of change has sometimes been greater than sceptics expected. March and Olsen (1989) now argue that institutions may be intentionally transformed through processes of radical shock, where it is hinted that the Thatcher experiment may represent an exemplar.

Specifically within health care, Pettigrew *et al.*'s 1992 study of the relationship between the introduction of general management and the pace of strategic service change also found that at least in some localities and in some issues there was evidence of substantial acceleration of the pace of change by the late 1980s. Service issues that had drifted for many years – such as the reprovision of psychiatric services – were at last being tackled.

Some more specific propositions which emerge from this stream of literature can be identified as follows and can be tested empirically:

- The attention of politicians is unlikely to remain on the reform process itself but will move on to still newer issues.
- Existing personnel are successful in 'relabelling' themselves so as to conform outwardly to the new demands, while retaining old beliefs and behaviours. There is a high continuity of key personnel.
- Health care is not 'depoliticized' as an issue but rather local and central politicians are still taking key decisions about what gets on the agenda; when crises blow up in the new order (e.g. unplanned ward closures), there is still political intervention; difficult problems are put on ice by the politicians (e.g. the planning of health care across London).
- Old norms of conduct are not eroded and are resistant to change, e.g. meeting in public; old roles and relationships gradually re-emerge, for example, regions reinvent themselves as regulators.[6]

RESEARCH AGENDA AND CONCLUDING DISCUSSION

A research agenda

The authors are part of a team at the Centre for Corporate Strategy and Change, University of Warwick, which is currently undertaking a major empirical study of how the new health authorities are making strategy in the internal market (Pettigrew *et al.* 1991). The study combines national postal questionnaires conducted at three points of time (thus generating a longitudinal data set) covering all health authorities and their members, together with intensive case studies of decision-making in 12 sites.

These localities together comprise two interrelated geographical clusters, drawn from Regions, Districts, DMUs, Trusts and FHSAs. There are wonderful opportunities in this study to observe the behaviour of the new authorities in action, including sitting in on a large number of authority meetings. It is also unusual to find a large-scale study which so combines quantitative and qualitative approaches to the study of decision-making.

An important component of this Project will be to further the understanding of how these authorities are operating in the new world of 'managed competition'. We will be able, for instance, to trace the development of the new purchasing function in our localities, or the birth and evolution of Trust hospitals. In order to do this effectively, however, we need to have some concept of market type at a more strategic level. This chapter has indeed signalled some of the new streams of literature needed in health-care management research and has also begun to operationalize these perspectives, in effect by asking, What would the world look like, if it looked like that?

Implications for theories of strategic change in the public sector

Often explanations of strategic change in public-sector settings (or its absence) have relied essentially on theories of bureaucratic behaviour, such as budgetary incrementalism or the elegant model advanced by Downs (1967). This was perpetuated into the 1980s, even though then the focus was increasingly on how bureaucracies did sometimes manage to change (see Körman and Glennerster's (1990) account of an ambitious hospital closure programme which, despite their own initial doubts, was implemented). Market-style pressures were not really considered within these analyses as a source of change, given that these institutions were after all largely insulated from such considerations at the time the data were gathered.

So the introduction of an internal-market model may have far-reaching implications for the way in which strategic-change processes come to be understood in the public sector. They may, in a word, become rather more like private-sector change processes. As such, it will be increasingly important for researchers undertaking work in health-care settings to be able to tap into generic organization theory.

The first point is that, while some of the growing literature on health-care management research has been open to the more generic strategic-change literature (e.g. Ferlie and Bennett 1992), there have always remained important differences with much private-sector work. Resources in the public sector were historically allocated through hierarchies rather than markets. Given the lack of economic or market-based pressures for competition (although hospitals have always competed in other ways for political clout or for reputation), hospitals could not really be seen as 'firms'.

Now, however, the Trust hospital, in particular, operates much more as a firm than hitherto, responsible for generating business and trading in competition with other providers (although the nature and intensity of this competition will vary). This is a new and blurred organizational form which crosses the conventional divide between the private and public sectors. So literature on the behaviour of the firm will have much more resonance in health-care settings than has previously been the case. In particular, there is likely to be greater interest in questions of competitive performance, and why it varies from one site to another. How NHSTs come to understand the nature of competition, and how this basis of competition may change over time, is another important theme (Pettigrew and Whipp 1991).

We suspect also that the pace of strategic service change is likely to accelerate in the Trusts and other health-care organizations. In some localities there is now talk of very significant reconfiguration over the next 3 to 5 years. Although ambitious, the change agenda may also be less dependent on outside constituencies than hitherto in the NHS (Pettigrew *et al.* 1992): inter-organizational complexity may have been reduced somewhat. In addition, a strong ideology of independence is already apparent in some Trusts. NHSTs have more potential to manage their own strategic-change processes, but failure may also carry severe financial penalties. Based on their private-sector study, the question posed by Pettigrew and Whipp (1991) – 'Does the way a firm manages strategic change make a demonstrable difference to its competitive performance?' – now also becomes central to the future of the NHSTs. Clearly we need to reconsider just how it is that we conceptualize the process of strategic change in the public sector as such market-based models continue to take hold.

NOTES

1 Refer to p.63 for a description of a similar market model.
2 For an account of apparently just such cooperative behaviour between providers see pp.131–2.
3 For a provider Unit manager's view on the impact of the internal market on his clinician's behaviour see p.224.
4 For further discussion of the industrial relations implications of the internal market refer to Chapter 11.
5 See pp.123–4 for an account of one Trust hospital that was disappointed in this way.
6 For two opinions, one by a commissioning manager and the other by a provider manager, on a new role for the Regions, see p.192 and p.211.

REFERENCES

Alford, R. (1975) *Health Care Politics*. London and Chicago: University of Chicago Press.
Baumol, W.J. (1982) Contestable markets: an uprising of the theory of industry structure, *American Economic Review*, 1–15.
Baumol, W.J. *et al.* (1982) *Contestable Markets and the Theory of Industry Structure*. New York: Harcourt, Brace, Jovanovich.
Bowen, D.E. and Jones, G. (1986) Transaction cost analysis of service organiza-tion–customer exchange, *Academy of Management Review*, 428–41.
Brunsson, N. (1989) Administrative reforms as routines, *Scandinavian Journal of Management*, 219–28.
Cook, K. *et al.* (1983) A theory of organizational response to regulation: the case of hospitals, *Academy of Management Review*, 193–205.

Culyer, A.J.(1990) *The Internal Market: An Acceptable Means to a Desirable End*. Discussion Paper No. 67. Centre for Health Economics, University of York.

DoH (Department of Health) (1989) *Working for Patients*. London: HMSO.

Downs, A. (1967) *Inside Bureaucracies*. Boston: Little, Brown.

Durkheim, E. (1964) *The Division of Labor in Society*. New York: Free Press.

Elston, M.A. (1991) The politics of professional power: medicine in a changing Health Service, in J. Gabe *et al.* (eds.) *The Sociology of the Health Service*. London: Routledge, 58–88.

Ferlie, E.B. and Bennett, C. (1992) Patterns of strategic change in health care: District Health Authorities respond to AIDS, *British Journal of Management*, March, 21–38.

Ford, D. (ed.) (1990) *Understanding Business Markets*. London: Academic Press.

Ham, C. (1990) *Holding on While Letting Go*. Project Paper No. 86. London: King's Fund.

Körman, N. and Glennerster, H. (1990) *Hospital Closure*. Milton Keynes: Open University Press.

Laughlin, R. (1991) Can the information systems of the NHS internal market work? *Public Money and Management*, Autumn, 37–41.

Lawson, M.S. (1977) *The Rise of Professionalism: A Sociological Analysis*. London: University of California Press.

Levacic, R. (1990) Markets: an introduction, in G. Thompson *et al.* (eds.) *Markets, Hierarchies and Networks*. London: Sage.

Mansfield, R. (1987) Commentary on Chapter 7, in A. Pettigrew (ed.) *Management of Strategic Change*. Oxford: Basil Blackwell.

March, J.G. and Olsen, J.P. (1983) Organizing political life: what administrative reorganization tells us about government, *American Political Science Review*, 281–96.

March, J.G. and Olsen, J.P. (1989) *Rediscovering Institutions: The Organizational Basis of Politics*. New York: Free Press.

Mullen, P. (1990) The NHS White Paper and internal markets, in G. Thompson (ed.) *Markets, Hierarchies and Networks*. London: Sage.

Office of Public Management (1990) *The Rubber Windmill*. London: OPM.

Oppenheimer, M. (1973) The proletarianization of the professional, *Sociological Review Monograph*, 213–37.

Ouchi, W.G. (1980) Markets, bureaucracies and clans, *Administrative Science Quarterly*, March, 129–41.

Pettigrew, A.M. and Whipp, R. (1991) *Managing Change for Competitive Success*. Oxford: Basil Blackwell.

Pettigrew, A.M. *et al.* (1991) The leadership role of the new Health Authorities: an agenda for research and development, *Public Money and Management*, April, 39–43.

Pettigrew, A.M. *et al.* (1992) *Shaping Organizational Change*. London: Sage.

Robinson, J. (1933) *The Economics of Imperfect Competition*. London: Macmillan.

Robinson, R. (1990) *Competition and Health Care*. Research Report No. 6. London: King's Fund Institute.

Romer, T. and Rosenthal, H. (1987) Modern political economy and the study of regulation, in *Public Regulation: New Perspectives on Institutions and Policies*. Cambridge, Mass: MIT Press, 73–116.

Schumacher, D. (1989) Organizing for quality competition: the coming paradigm shift, *Frontiers of Health Services Management*, 4–30.

Shipman, A. and Mayes, D. (1990) *Changing the Rules*. Discussion Paper 199. London: National Intitute of Economic and Social Research.

Stacey, M. (1989) The General Medical Council and professional accountability, *Public Policy and Administration*, 12–27.

Starr, P. (1982) *The Social Transformation of American Medicine*. New York: Basic Books.

Stigler, G. and Friedland, C. (1962) What can regulators regulate: the case of electricity, *Journal of Law and Economics*, 1–16.

van de Ven, A. and Wynard, P.M.M. (1989) *A Future for Competitive Health Care in the Netherlands*. Occasional Paper 9. Centre for Health Economics, University of York.

Vickers, J. and Yarrow, G. (1988) *Privatization: An Economic Analysis*. Cambridge, Mass: MIT Press.

Williamson, O.E. (1975) *Markets and Hierarchies: Analysis and Antitrust Implications*. New York: Macmillan.

Williamson, O.E. (1985) *The Economic Institutions of Capitalism*. New York: Free Press.

6

Commissioning: An Appraisal of a New Role

Louis Opit

Commissioning in the NHS means the quantitative and qualitative specification of the health-care services required to meet the assumed health-care needs of a given population over a defined time (usually 1 year). In attempting to convey how this process of commissioning is being implemented in the UK, we run into two other problems. The first of these is that the reorganization has atomized the structure of the NHS so that the flow of public knowledge about the details of implementation has slowed to a trickle. The reasons for this are, in part, the present political control of information but it is also a direct consequence of the atomization itself. The second problem is that, although the ideological intentions of the Reforms were clear or at least discoverable, the technical and intellectual means required to achieve the changes had hardly been considered at all. As a consequence, there appears to be great diversity in the mechanisms of implementation and nationally the ground rules seem to be changing almost monthly. Thus, public knowledge about the implementation of the Reforms tends to be mainly gossip or available only in the most general forms.

Despite these difficulties, this chapter attempts to give a coherent account of the process of commissioning as it has arisen in the most recent reorganization of the NHS. In order that this account be self-contained, it will be located, albeit briefly, in relation to some of the other structural, functional and ideological changes introduced in the White Paper *Working for Patients* (DoH 1989.) The chapter will also suggest improvements and alterations to the commissioning process where these appear to be called for.

THE NEED FOR COMMISSIONING OF HEALTH-CARE SERVICES

The new NHS envisaged in the White Paper (DoH 1989) and many subsequent documents from the NHSME is centred around an 'internal' market conjured out of the existing organization by separating two previously fused responsibilities. The key reform of the NHS is the separation of the task of obtaining health care from that of actually delivering this care. Commissioners of care, or purchasers of care, were thus to be managerially and financially independent of those who provided the activities of health care.[1] The health care required for a given population is now commissioned prospectively and then the services required are formulated as contracts with chosen providers. As set out in Figure 1 in the Introduction two types of existing health-care agencies – DHAs and GPFHs – were given the main task of commissioning health services while three types of organization – DMUs, NHSTs and private-sector providers – were designated as potential suppliers of services. This supposedly brought into existence both 'buyers' (commissioners) and 'sellers' (providers), the contractual relationship between them arising out of the process of health-care commissioning. The ultimate size of this market is controlled mainly by the financial allocation made to the NHS and distributed to DHAs by the Regions.

THE COMMISSIONERS

Under the new arrangements the major commissioner was developed by restructuring the DHA management to create an agency with responsibility solely for specifying and obtaining the health-care services for their resident populations. In some areas these agencies now operate on behalf of several contiguous districts.

The other commissioning agencies developed by the Reforms were certain general practices themselves; initially these were restricted to large practices (more than 11,000 registered patients) who could demonstrate the necessary management capacity. These GPFHs can directly commission elective health care from their own choice of health-care providers and each practice has been given a budget for the purchase of care. The preconditions for such Fundholding practices are steadily being relaxed and it is the clear intention of the present Government to make the GPFHs a major element of the commissioning mechanism.[2]

This seemingly elegant organizational structure, however, overlooked a simple reality – that the public does not consult the DHA commissioner about illness. Instead individual people refer themselves, or consult a GP who acts as a referral agency about illness. In this way, whatever priorities or theories the commissioners have about health-care needs can be subverted by what patients or their GPs actually want, and commissioners who wish to develop contracts restricted to certain providers must then either coerce their local non-Fundholding GPs to use previously selected providers or make due allowance for other referrals. These purchasing arrangements have already created a succession of problems which require discussion.

EQUITY AND OTHER PROBLEMS IN THE EVOLVING COMMISSIONING SYSTEM

Whose choice?

The political rhetoric of the last 12 years has been dominated by the notion of choice. It is appropriate to ask whether the reorganized NHS has increased public choice in health care because there is certainly no direct increase in individual users' choice since they can still only influence the market through their existing relationship with other health-care workers such as the GP and the DHA commissioner. Indeed, because the patients' referral agents, the GPs, have had their choice constrained, there is potential decrease in choice. General practitioners within Fundholding practices make their own choice of hospitals and consultants for referral but it is unclear to what degree they are or will be influenced by their patients' wishes in this respect. Gains were foreseen for Fundholding practice patients because such practices certainly expected to be able to propel their patients into jumping NHS queues by specifying priority treatment in their commissioning contracts. On the other hand, the majority of people are presently registered with practitioners who are not GPFHs and, in these circumstances, their choice of referral is constrained by the commission contracts arranged by the DHA commissioning agency. In some cases this may now result in exclusion even from NHS hospital or specialist care for certain types of illness (Godlee 1991).

In sum then both GPs and their patients may be constrained in their choice of referral site and, overall, there is a risk of loss of choice with the emergence of arbitrary inequity. As these effects of the commissioning mechanism have emerged into the public debate, the resultant political tensions have obliged the DoH to reformulate the rules (Ross 1991). In the end the key choice for the individual could become Fundholding practice or not. This may well be an implicit intention of the Reforms.

Conflict in clinical priorities

As the previous arguments suggest, whatever clinical priorities a DHA commissioning agency adopts can easily be subverted by Fundholding practices, particularly if the system for GPFHs is so structured by the DoH that meeting their own patients' demands becomes an economically rational strategy. In that circumstance every practice can evolve its own particular priorities. Most DHA commissioning agencies have, for example, restricted the number of NHS-funded terminations of pregnancy (OPCS 1989) but where this has happened, GPFH pratices in the same district can now decide to finance all or none of these terminations in their own client population.

The allocation of funds is being changed from RAWP to a capitation basis for each DHA's own resident population.[3] Thus, the DHA must cope simultaneously with this change and the likehood that some of its money be removed to finance any GPFHs within its catchment. Each practice budget is determined by the appropriate RHA and, in theory, this is based on records of the practices' pattern of utilization. Since the data for these calculations are mainly of poor quality, there is a strong element of direct negotiation in this allocation; thus individual practice allocations vary for both demographic and other reasons. Funding is provided only to cover the practice contracts for elective acute-service care, although sums are allocated for drug use and other purposes. On the other hand, the DHA commissioning agency has to finance (through its contracts) all emergency and long-term care for the whole resident population as well as elective care for patients registered with non-Fundholding practices. The fairness then of this GPFHs' allocation is critical to the DHA commissioner's task.

A simple test of this allocation is to gross-up the GP allocation, assuming that every practice is Fundholding and see what remains of the District's allocation. This approach suggests that overall the Fundholding practice allocations have been overgenerous and that, by inference, the cash remaining for the DHA is likely to be insufficient to cover their service commitments. This likelihood is compounded by the capacity of GPs, with or without the collusion of hospital staff, to redefine the boundaries between elective and emergency cases. This has always been the case but its significance is now much greater. Evidence that the Fundholding allowances were excessive is now beginning to emerge as some Regions report considerable underspends in Fundholding practice allocations (Anon 1991a).

Extra-contractual referral (ECR)

It is a critical assumption of District commissioning and contracting that non-Fundholding GPs will refer their patients to provider Units already chosen by the DHA. It soon became necessary, even before implementation, to decide how to proceed in the event that some GP referrals go to other providers.

These are now called ECRs. It was always recognized that there might be difficulty in forcing the complete compliance of non-Fundholding GPs – the majority – to refer elective cases to predetermined hospitals or other services. The reasons for such behaviour can be many, ranging from acceding to patient wishes, judgements about the suitability or responsiveness of different consultants, convenience or just cussedness. Every DHA commissioning agency was advised to reserve contingency funds for this eventuality and to put in place a bureaucratic process to adjudicate on the circumstances of ECRs in case the receiving hospital management declined to accept responsibility for the referral or its consequences. It is already clear that problems are emerging and that they will extend as more GPs are encouraged into becoming Fundholding. There are no publicly available systematic reports of the clinical or financial problems created by ECRs,[4] yet the tip of the iceberg is clearly visible as Districts find themselves unable to pay for all ECRs incurred on behalf of their populations (Anon 1991b, 1991c).

Our next task is to examine the provider structure created within the reorganized NHS and examine how the separation affects the process of commissioning health care.

PROVIDERS OF CARE IN THE NEW NHS

Three types of health-care provider organizations were defined within the White Paper (DoH 1989). First was the NHST, a hospital or other service agency which had no direct relationship with any DHA. Trusts are responsible only to their boards of management and, through them, to the DoH. Second, even where no Trust exists, the DMUs have been made managerially separate from the DHA. It is very hard to gauge to what degree real separation has occurred for it is clear that in many DHAs the boundary between their functions of commissioning and service provision is very permeable as senior DHA executives struggle to keep their personal options open. Finally, the White Paper envisaged the use of private hospitals or organizations as potential providers of NHS services although, in many respects, this relationship between NHS and the private health-care organizations had begun to develop before the White Paper was published.

THE CONTRACT

The relationship between commissioner and provider Units is crystallized in the form of a contract which is not, however, legally binding. The contract specifies such items as the guaranteed availability of facilities or services and the volume and price of services to be provided. The White Paper and its subsequent documents envisaged three types of contracts: block contracts, cost-and-volume contracts or cost-per-case contracts. To date, almost all contracts have been specified by clinical service type and are crude block contracts. A contract to general surgical providers will specify the facilities which should be available and the work load as total in-patient admissions, day cases and out-patient contracts. For this block of work, an agreed sum of money is paid.

Although the inclusion of quality indicators in contracts was also encouraged, using such parameters as waiting time or mean length of stay, it appears that relatively few contracts have specified these standards. GPFH service contracts have been more demanding as practitioners attempted to create contracts which guaranteed selective access for their own patients. The political tensions created by this when it became public caused a rapid retreat by the NHSME. Some of the professed 'market' benefits envisaged by the White Paper have already been rejected as implementation has proceeded (Jones 1991).

The commissioner is critically dependent on the provider in relation to information about utilization. Almost all Health Service data are created at the point of service use so that only the provider Units can capture information about the levels of demand or service quality. It is not difficult to see that, as provider Units become separated from the commissioning system, their focus of interest in data collection will change. Their concern is likely to be price setting and it is possible that there will be a reduced interest in recording epidemiological data relevant to commissioning. Furthermore, exchange of data may be inhibited by provider arguments about the need for secrecy with price competition. In theory this problem could be addressed by the commissioner insisting on appropriate data being returned in an accurate and timely fashion as part of the contract. It remains to be seen whether this will occur or whether there will be pressure to validate such data.[5]

Now that we have briefly examined the commissioning process and set it within the context of the Reforms more generally, we can pass to the technical problem which prospective work-load determination creates. Ideally the commissioning process was expected not only to specify the future service work loads but also to allow for local debate and decision about priorities and quality of care. Without doubt, this was a daunting intellectual and technical problem even with good-quality epidemiological and utilization data; in their absence, the problems multiply exponentially.

In the following section we will examine the technical and methodological problems of commissioning, first and mainly with respect to the task of assessing the likely volume of clinical services which need to be purchased. Because the DHA remains the major commissioner of secondary health-care services, our discussion will be limited to this agency. Indeed, it is not at all clear how the Fundholding practices can reliably commission in advance or how the DHA allows for the purchases made by GPFHs. The only feasible approach at present is for the DHA to reduce its resident population by the number of persons registered with Fundholding practices within the District. Even this strategy is not entirely free of problems and our earlier discussion highlights some of the difficulties and assumptions which the multiple commissioning system entails.

The determination of the expected service volume of care is the first critical step on which the whole market depends. Given the squeeze on resources available to the DHA, even this estimate is very likely to require difficult negotiation to determine priorities. The public is now expected to have a voice in this (NHSME 1992).

Finally, the rhetoric of the White Paper and the documents that have followed it stresses the capacity of the internal market to enhance the quality of and public satisfaction with health care. This is achieved theoretically by trade-offs between volume, cost and quality and is supposedly incorporated in the choice of provider and the conditions set in the contract between commissioner and provider. Since the whole approach rests upon the determination of volume of service which needs to be purchased, we will commence our account of the implementation with this. It seems appropriate now to turn to the *fons et origo* of all wisdom in this matter, namely, the guidance issuing from the NHSME and the DoH.

GUIDANCE FROM THE DEPARTMENT OF HEALTH CONCERNING COMMISSIONING

The commissioner's overriding problem is the task of finding some instantly implementable basis for the choice of the appropriate type and volume of health-care services which need to be purchased on behalf of the resident population. We will ignore, at this stage, the difficulties referred to earlier of the effect of competition between providers and simply concentrate on how the District commissioner determines what services to purchase from the provider.

A number of documents have now been issued by the Management

Executive to RHAs and DHAs, to assist them in this task (NHSME 1991a, 1991b, 1991c). These documents generally espouse a naive theory of what is called health-care needs assessment. In general, they concatenate the issues of service volume, quality and effectiveness but provide no operational models of the process of commissioning. The approach is best illustrated by quoting from these recent publications.

Health needs assessment

In May 1991 the NHSME issued a document entitled *Assessing Health Care Needs* which purported to set out the approach to the task of commissioning (NHSME 1991b). At the outset the document acknowledged the confusion surrounding the notion of needs and then proceeded to offer its own version of the key definitions. These are worth quoting verbatim, even if the syntax leaves much to be desired:

Need:　　What people could benefit from;
Demand: What they ask for (or in a market are prepared to pay for), or what their
　　　　　health professional prompts them to ask for; and
Supply:　What is provided.

(NHSME 1991b)

The next section 'refines' the concept of need further as:

- The *population's* ability to benefit is the aggregate of individuals' ability to benefit but, for any health problem, depends on the incidence of (different degrees of severity) of the condition and the prevalence of its effects and complications.
- The *ability* to benefit does not mean that every outcome is guaranteed to be favourable. But it does mean that there is only a need where this is a potential benefit, i.e, where the intervention and/or the care setting is effective.
- The *benefit* measured should include:
  (i)　　clinical status compared with that without the intervention;
  (ii)　　reassurance, both the individual and professional, that avenues of potential benefit have been explored, i.e. confirming the diagnosis;
  (iii)　　supportive care and the relief of pressure on other carers.
- Health *care* includes prevention and promotion, diagnosis, treatment, continuing care, rehabilitation and terminal care – all taken within the context of their setting.

(NHSME 1991b)

This is one of the most impenetrable accounts of the problem of 'needs' ever to be formulated. The next document, *Purchasing Intelligence*, issued in this series (NHSME 1991c), carries forward this conceptual framework. Here types of 'intelligence' are suggested as the basis for needs assessment and commissioning. These are described as:

- epidemiological assessments; no further clarification offered;
- comparative assessment of health status, utilization rates, prices and performance;
- corporate views which, roughly speaking, seems to be what various key participants think.

(NHSME 1991c)

There are now several documents in this Management Executive series, all of the same degree of confusion, all promoting the same approach but none giving usable operational advice. In support of these concepts, a number of disease or clinical-state reviews have also been issued or commissioned from 'experts'. These technical reports are supposed to give guidance to commissioners. These documents are important both because they may reveal hidden purposes of the NHS Reforms and because they show the political, social, technical and intellectual distance between the Reformers and those who have to implement commissioning and provide the new service. Even more academically focused accounts seem unable to steer free of abstractions or offer some method or approach presently usable (Stevens and Gabbay 1991).

A critique of the Management Executive guidance

One is left with the feeling that a key purpose of commissioning is to constrain the existing demand for health-care services; this intention was also apparent in much of the evolving quality-of-care debate which began in the USA 40 years ago (Opit 1991a). Essentially we are seeing a return to the issue of 'unnecessary care'. The belief that 'need' is an unambiguous and operationally usable concept is clearly a product of economists' thinking. Really it is much more about cost–benefit or cost-effectiveness, merely a flaccid extension of the earlier notion of QALYs, quality-adjusted life years (Williams 1985).

In reality the concept of need being advanced in the NHSME documents is barely understandable and is not usable for the following reasons. First, it requires a vast body of reliable information which can be interpreted unambiguously by the commissioner. Second, the concept of need as potential benefit merely transfers the problems of need to that of benefit. Whose notion of benefit – even if we can measure it – is paramount? Is it that of the patient, public opinion, professional, manager or economist? In any case, as *Assessing Health Care Needs* (NHSME 1991b) acknowledges, benefit is an actuarial notion. Two simple examples from the real world will suffice to indicate the confusion inherent in this approach when applied to health-care commissioning.

First, a recent study of a population prevalence of venous disease gave rates of 23% for men and 49% for women (ages from 20 to 75 years) (Franks *et al.* 1992). However, if the general practitioner morbidity study for 1981/2 is consulted, the incidence rate of consultation for varicose veins for the same age range could be estimated as approximately 0.6% and 1.2% respectively (Royal College of General Practitioners 1986). Many of these persons are not referred to hospital services where treatment rates are closer to 0.2%.

The second example is the study of the needs for residential care in children with mental handicap (Pahl and Quine 1986). Three different categories of professionals offered similar general principles of need applicable in client selection but these did not square with the actual decisions made by the individual professionals in choosing which children went into residential care.

We are obliged to ask in both these illustrative cases how the definition of need postulated by the Management Executive papers would have helped and whose concept of potential benefit was most relevant.

In conclusion then, although the effectiveness of treatment is clearly an issue of importance in determining the health-care commissioning process, incorporating this complex idea into the notion of 'needs' is confusing rather than helpful. The concept of 'needs' is and always has been a negotiated one, socially constructed between patients or clients and their professional advisers. This may be unsatisfactory for those who wish to impose some central control on 'needs' but this reality will have to be accepted. Commissioners may define 'needs' but they do not make the decisions which cause these needs to emerge as operationally visible demand. In reality, we will never know in the abstract what the 'need' is for most of the services that are the bread and butter of health-care provision.

One potential destination of the health-needs assessment approach recommended by the NHSME can be seen in the Oregon experiment (Dixon and Welch 1991; Smith 1991). In this scenario, a defined hierarchy of health-care interventions is created by so-called public debate and economic analysis. This then becomes the basis for meeting, or not meeting, the demand for individuals' health care. Even in Oregon it should be noted this scheme would only be applied to the 30% of population too frail or poor to have adequate health insurance. The Oregon programme has created considerable interest in some UK circles although, to date, it is not yet being publicly recommended. Quite apart from the profound technical and philosophical problems of creating an acceptable hierarchy, its explicit general application to NHS commissioning would be likely to generate public, political and professional mayhem. Although rationing has always been a fact of life in the NHS, it has been mainly implicit and ambiguous in its form, the ultimate power of choice being located in professional hands. In many ways, this has suited the political and bureaucratic systems. Giving this power to the faceless commissioner or the public-health minion does not look like a viable option.

At the end of the day, the commissioner is left with the pressing urgency of the volume of demand for health care arising directly or indirectly from the public's perception of the value of health-care services whether or not these are 'scientifically' or 'economically' valid. Attempting to deal with the problems of volume, quality or effectiveness simultaneously has merely created confusion at the coal-face and complacency at the centre.

From the information which is currently available, it is quite clear that for the first two annual rounds of commissioning by DHAs, only the crudest methods of estimating service demands have been used to create contracts.[6] In the main, DHAs have simply used their most recent year's (1989/90) local demand data to formulate contracts with, or usually without, any allowance for growth in demand. A good deal of energy has been spent on looking at patient flows into and out of the District from other Districts or Regions.

This has required some DHA commissioners to formulate a very large number of contracts, many concerned with quite small volumes of clinical work and at the same time they have attempted to convince or coerce non-Fundholding GPs to use provider institutions with whom contracts have been made.

In the next section, we will explore a more realistic and potentially more rewarding approach to determining service volumes. The major part of our discussion will, however, be focused on the commissioning of acute-hospital care but there will be some discussion of commissioning for other client groups.

COMMISSIONING CARE FOR THE ACUTE SERVICES

If the concept of health needs is, as I assert, not usable at the present time for commissioning the volume of Health Service provision, is there some feasible alternative? For the last 30 years the NHS has been collecting statistics of Health Service utilization and, in many respects, these data have become deposited in a sort of data cemetery. The gross under-use of these routinely collected data has also ensured that the data quality is poor since timeliness, completeness and accuracy of data can only occur when they are subjected to repeated use and scrutiny. In spite of this deficiency, every DHA has available a large body of statistical information about the expressed demand on its Health Service providers, particularly on the demand for in-patient acute general services. The variation in the utilization of hospital services is, however, well documented both in the UK and elsewhere (McPherson *et al.* 1981; Andersen and Mooney, 1990). If such demand data are to be used as a basis for commissioning then it is necessary to identify some critical sources of this variation.

Variability in demand

One critical source of variability is located in a wide range of data errors, incomplete records, misuse of data definitions or poor coding (usually associated with incomplete narrative data or loose rules about data precedence). Five other significant factors which cause variability relevant to the use of demand data for commissioning are:

- socio-demographic differences in the catchment population;
- differences in resource availability – either beds, staff or operating theatres – at the provider level;
- differences in local clinical practice and custom;
- variations in disease distribution;
- presence of unmet expressed demand as queues.

The key to unravelling such a tangle of possibilities is to attempt to construct an analytical basis for expected normative demand using demography and service availability as independent variables and then to identify the exceptions. It is a fundamental tenet of this approach that any single DHA cannot determine whether its pattern of work is usual or exceptional. Only by such comparisons with other Districts is it possible to have insight into this for, as I have indicated earlier, there is virtually no theoretical basis for ascertaining Health Service needs.

Local factors

Local service organization and history give some understanding of the effect of local rules on the service pattern of demand. These are best illustrated with three examples, all of which show the flexible nature of medical specialties.

(1) Where there is no designated urology service, the general surgery case load will contain a substantial component of urology. This can be estimated and allowed for in the analysis of both general surgical and urology services but it also raises the commissioning policy issue of who should be entrusted with certain categories of clinical work.

(2) The existence of nominated geriatric medical services, thoracic medicine or even cardiology can act as substitute services for acute general medical services so that the real general medical demand may require aggregates of the work loads of all of these services. As in the previous example, this could also promote discussion of the type of medical or geriatric service preferred and contracted for by the commissioner.

(3) Some particular categories of clinical problems may be dealt with by different services in different districts. The admission of head injuries is a good example because this can be carried out in general surgical or orthopaedic beds, according to specific local rules, so that comparison of service demands requires knowledge of, and allowance for, such local behaviour.

Where this level of local information is available, it is possible to use regression analysis to identify normative levels of demand for clinical specialties as defined in this locality or, alternatively, to use bed occupancy rates for such specialties to predict demand, after making allowance for such things as outliers, patients located in the ward of another specialty. This type of analysis gives crude but useful baseline estimates for the commissioning process but it can also help to raise commissioning policy issues for discussion. Where utilization levels are high or low in relation to the normative estimates based on the population and *prima facie* where significant data errors have been excluded, this would constitute *prima facie* evidence that some characteristic of local practice needs investigation. Here one can envisage discussion between appropriate clinicians, commissioners and GP groups. The upshot of this discussion should be a commissioning policy which accepts or rejects the local explanation and expresses this in its purchasing contracts.

This approach can also be extended to examine the expected resource requirements for individual services if normative assumptions about expected levels of productivity are made in relation to out-patient activities, bed turnover rates, staffing levels and level of operating theatre use. This analysis can be carried out in a variety of ways and at different levels of sophistication. For instance, most simply one could base this just on the elective/emergency mix, or age-specific admission or treatment rates for single or aggregated specialties. A more detailed technical account of this approach and its application within a single Region is available (SE Thames RHA, 1991a, 1991b, 1991c).

The focus on elective surgical admissions contained in the White Paper and subsequent documents has encouraged consideration of a more detailed breakdown of the clinical work load, with particular attention being paid to common surgical problems figuring heavily on the waiting lists. This obliges the commissioning agent to analyse the admission data in much more detail and to find some way of simplifying the pattern of illness which appears to generate admission and treatment. This has become known as case-mix analysis.

CASE-MIX ANALYSIS FOR ACUTE SERVICE COMMISSIONING

Each patient admission can generate up to four diagnoses and four coded surgical treatments in the standard NHS record so that unravelling of the case mix is a complex problem. One approach to simplification has been to import analytical computerized technology from the USA. The best known of such classification technologies is the DRG (diagnosis-related group) but others do exist (Sanderson et al. 1986).

The DoH has favoured the use of DRGs and has pursued further development of this classification system for use in the NHS. It is not clear what point has been reached in this process, but there is some evidence that enthusiasm for DRGs is waning and there are certainly problems with its use (Sanderson et al. 1989). It was developed to create hospital reimbursement categories and, as such, attempts to define 'iso-resource' groups of admissions, that is, those categories of illness at the same level of resource utilization. It is not, however, especially coherent as a commissioning classification and there is little evidence that commissioners are using this case-mix analysis for purchasing services. One alternative is to develop specialty-specific, local case-mix classifications for this does force the purchaser to decide how specific the purchasing strategy needs to be. It represents quite a difficult and labour-intensive task but can be accomplished at the regional level (Opit 1991b).

One important benefit from such local case-mix initiatives is that they help to tie the commissioning process to medical audit. If there is to be a serious management input into the question of service quality and effectiveness, the classifications used in medical audit and commissioning must match. Clinical areas that require investigation in this context can often be identified by normative analysis of demand. For example, if a District has an unusually high or low treatment rate for certain problems in its resident population which are not explained either by demographic or data differences then the commissioner may have identified an area where audit can help in deciding the appropriate purchasing strategy. In most cases we do not know what the correct level of 'need' should be and, as I have already stressed, in many cases this concept is not itself very meaningful. Such discussion of 'abnormal' expressed demand will be complex and difficult and should involve provider specialists and GPs. Nevertheless, this will be one important way forward in the debate about effectiveness and quality.

Finally, it is necessary to say something about the overall growth in demand for health care. Ever since the beginning of the NHS, there has been a steady growth in both met and unmet demand for care. This has occurred because of changes in demography, technology and patient expectation. Few Districts then will be in a steady state so that commissioning based solely on historical data will be misleading. Most have existing queues of unmet demand in the form of waiting times for out-patients or waiting lists for in-patients. Some allowance must be made for this. Indeed, it is not clear at present with the new system who is responsible for the 'old' waiting lists. Much money and bureaucratic energy have been expended on reducing the numbers waiting more than 1 year for admission in order to 'level the playing field' before the implementation of the reorganization. These queues, however, remain a big problem that is not likely to go away without either excluding certain clinical problems from NHS care or increasing the financial allocation to the NHS. The seeds of the next NHS crisis are already visible herein as demand for health care continues to outstrip the financial provision made to deliver it.

COMMISSIONING CARE FOR LONG-TERM CLIENT GROUPS

The preceding account deals almost exclusively with the problems of purchasing acute health-care services, since this was the focus of *Working for Patients* (DoH 1989). The reorganization of the NHS as an internal market, however, has involved significant changes in the organization of both primary care (DHSS 1988) and long-term social care.

The proposals set out in the White Paper *Caring for People* (DoH 1990a) will make local authority social services responsible for most long-term health and social care for the elderly, the young disabled, the mentally ill and handicapped. The proposals transfer the financial and administrative responsibility for social security-financed residential care to local authorities. Social service departments are also being asked to develop and specify their formal links to the NHS locally. In this way, then, the internal market is being extended and the notion of a prospective purchasing strategy continues to be paramount.

The implementation of *Caring for People* (DoH 1990a) has been delayed until 1993 but the conceptualization of purchasing which appears in departmental documents remains vague and unhelpful. Official documents issuing from the DoH about community care are long on rhetoric and short of implementable advice (DoH 1990b). Once again, in some as yet unspecified way, local authorities are expected to assess 'needs' and allocate contracts to achieve the rhetorical aims of increased efficiency, improved quality and 'consumer' satisfaction, all within severe cash limits.

A normative demand model, suggested earlier for acute-service commissioning, is unlikely to be usable for long-term care for the following reasons:

- The boundaries between formal health and social care are impossible to define.
- A very great number of persons and formal caring agencies are often involved in the support required or given to individuals.
- Data about such activities are frequently absent, inappropriate or of poor quality.
- Even where such demand data are available, they are usually held separately and incompatible in type or format, making aggregration hazardous.
- The creation of an equitable and efficient purchasing strategy requires knowledge of who is not receiving services since there is ample evidence that certain problems such as incontinence, blindness or deafness are markedly under-represented in most demand data.

Although there are strenuous efforts in place to improve the availability and use of information about social-care demand, this is unlikely, by itself, to enable the development of a coherent, prospective commissioning strategy to meet current political expectations. The problems of target efficiency (Knapp 1984) will remain because it is necessary to know not only about those who receive services but also about those who do not.

POSSIBLE ALTERNATIVE APPROACH TO COMMISSIONING

One approach being adopted or encouraged is the *ad hoc* local survey of 'needs'. This is a time-consuming, expensive and methodologically inadequate way of defining the purchasing requirements for health or social care. A much more usable framework for commissioning has been available for many years.

Over the last 40 years there have been at least three large national surveys of disability which could constitute the basis of local DHA or social service commissioning. The most recent of these is the OPCS Disability Survey in 1985 (OPCS 1989). This survey contains a wealth of data including socio-demographic data, specific disability, availability of informal carers, income, expenditure and the present use of both health and social-care services.

These data can be used as the basis of a synthetic model for forecasting both the extent and levels of disability and to give a picture of the way in which health and social care are targeted. The OPCS survey provides a random sample of people in whom both socio-demographic and clinical features are known. Since the clinical problems are strongly correlated with age and other socio-demographic characteristics, it is possible to derive statistical models to forecast the clinical features in another population for whom only the local socio-demographic characteristics are available.

This approach has been developed for use as a 'needs' based local planning model for purchasing (Opit 1991c). It produces a far more robust model than the usually inadequate local survey and clearly is far cheaper. Also it can be used to explore the nature of actual or theoretical service targeting as it evolves in community-care plans (Opit and Opit 1991).

In due course, if reliable, consistent demand data are generated by the reorganized community-care services, it will be possible to compare the theoretical estimates from the synthetic model with the information arising from records of this expressed demand. This should lead then to a review of the adequacy of service targeting and to exploration of the important service quality and acceptability issues. As I have argued in the section on acute-service commissioning, the estimation of the volume of services which have been met or which can be thought of as representing normative demand is a critical prerequisite to debates about policy or quality. In due course it may become possible to examine both actual and expected benefits in the form of outcome measures but this should not be confused as the starting point of the commissioning process.

CONCLUSIONS

It is still too early to make any certain judgements about the viability of prospective health or social service commissioning. In some respects we could think of commissioning as merely a form of sensible forward planning in which the discussion of competing priorities begins to intrude. The way in which commissioning has been evolved from the ideological framework of the NHS Reforms, however, imposes particular difficulties. The 'competition' expected from several 'buyers' and 'sellers' for a single population has created political problems, reduced individual choice and made inequity more rather than less likely.

All these political and managerial problems have been compounded by the quality of the technical advice being offered to commissioners and by the Management Executive's insistence on health-needs assessment, a commissioning model which is both questionable in concept and overly complex in practice.

In the absence of timely, reliable and unambiguous demand data, the outcome of the rhetorical approach has been mainly the evolution of a very crude system of block purchasing and contracting which effectively replicates and, due to the necessity for contracts, freezes historical demand. The political context of the Reforms also appears to be shifting. The old imbalance between supply and demand in both social services and the NHS remains unchanged even if the reorganization and the process of commissioning has temporarily disguised it. It is the re-emergence of this old problem and the way in which the internal market copes with it that will determine the long-term viability of the present NHS reorganization.

NOTES

1 Chapter 9 contains a lengthy discussion of this relationship.
2 Some predict a dominant commissioning role for GPFHs. See, for example, p. 116 and especially Figure 7.8.
3 Cf. p. 65.
4 Refer pp. 196–7 for a commissioner's account of problems around ECRs.
5 Refer pp. 215–7.
6 See pp. 192–5 and pp. 214–7 for more details on this area.

REFERENCES

Andersen, T.F. and Mooney, G. (eds.) (1990) *The Challenges of Medical Practice Variations*. Basingstoke: Macmillan.

Anon (1991a) Regions report GP Fundholding underspends, *Health Services Journal*, 24 October, 7.

Anon (1991b) New ECR waiting list as money runs out, *Health Services Journal*, 24 October, 3.

Anon (1991c) Overspend HAs seek ECR top up, *Health Services Journal*, 29 August, 6.

DoH (Department of Health) (1989) *Working for Patients*. London: HMSO.

DoH (Department of Health) (1990a) *Caring for People*. London: HMSO.

DoH (Department of Health) (1990b) *Community Care in the Next Decade and Beyond*. London: HMSO.

DHSS (Department of Health and Social Security) (1988) *Promoting Better Health*. London: HMSO.

Dixon, J. and Welch, H.G. (1991) Priority setting: lessons from Oregon, *Lancet*, 891–4.

Franks, P.J. *et al.* (1992) Prevalence of venous disease: a community study in West London, *European Journal of Surgery*, 143–7.

Godlee, F. (1991) Minor procedures off the list, *British Medical Journal*, 311.

Jones, J. (1991) GPs agree to truce in dispute over NHS, *The Independent*, 20 June.

Knapp, M. (1984) *The Economics of Social Care*. Basingstoke: Macmillan.

McPherson, K. *et al.* (1981) Regional variations in the use of common surgical procedures within and between England and Wales, *Social Science and Medicine*, 15A, 273–88.

NHSME (National Health Service Management Executive) (1991a) *Moving Forward: Needs, Services and Contracts*. London: Department of Health.

NHSME (National Health Service Management Executive) (1991b) *Assessing Health Care Needs*. London: Department of Health.

NHSME (National Health Service Management Executive) (1991c) *Purchasing Intelligence*. London: Department of Health.

NHSME (National Health Service Management Executive) (1992) *Local Voices: The Views of Local People in Purchasing for Health*. London: Department of Health.

OPCS (Office of Population Censuses and Surveys) (1989) *Legal Abortions 1988: Residents of Regional and District Health Areas*. Monitor services AB89/4. London: OPCS.

OPCS (Office of Population Censuses and Surveys, Social Survey Division) (1989)

Survey of Disabled Adults in Private Households, 1985 [computer file]. Colchester: ESRC Data Archive.

Opit, L.J. (1991a) The measurement of Health Service outcomes, in W.W. Holland *et al*. (eds.) *Oxford Textbook of Public Health*. Oxford: Oxford University Press, 160.

Opit, L.J. (1991b) *Commissioning of General Surgery for the West and East Kent Consortia*. Centre for Health Studies, University of Kent.

Opit, L.J. (1991c) *Elderly Care Planning Model, Wessex Regional Health Authority*. Centre for Health Studies, University of Kent.

Opit, L.J. and Opit, L.W. (1991) *Needs-Based Community Care Purchasing for the Elderly. Handbook to accompany Wessex interactive computer model*. Centre for Health Studies, University of Kent.

Pahl, J. and Quine, L. (1986) The 'need' for long-term care among mentally handicapped children living at home. Unpublished paper. Health Services Research Unit, University of Kent.

Ross, A.P.J. (1991) Consultants, contracts and Fundholders, *British Medical Journal*, 1479–80.

Royal College of General Practitioners (1986) *Morbidity Statistics from General Practice*. Series MB5, No. 1. London: HMSO.

Sanderson, H.F. *et al*. (1986) Using diagnostic groups in the NHS, *Community Medicine*, 37–46.

Sanderson, H.F. *et al*. (1989) Evaluation of diagnosis-related groups in the National Health Service, *Community Medicine*, 269–78.

Smith, R. (1991) Rationing: the search for sunlight, *British Medical Journal*, 1561–2.

SE Thames RHA (South East Thames Regional Health Authority) (1991a) *Conceptual Framework for Analysing Acute Services*. London: SETRHA.

SE Thames RHA (South East Thames Regional Health Authority) (1991b) *Modelling the Demand for Acute Services, Urology*. London: SETRHA.

SE Thames RHA (South East Thames Regional Health Authority) (1991c) *Modelling the Demand for Acute Services, Gynaecology*. London: SETRHA.

Stevens, A. and Gabbay, J. (1991) Needs assessment needs assessment, *Health Trends*, 20–3.

Williams, A. (1985) Economics of coronary artery bypass grafting, *British Medical Journal*, 326–9.

7

Competition and the NHS: Monitoring the Market

John Appleby, Paula Smith, Wendy Ranade, Val Little and Ray Robinson

INTRODUCTION

A new market in health care

After more than 40 years the NHS planning system which had guided and informed health-care developments, and the organizational and managerial structure of the Health Service, underwent a transformation on 1 April 1991: a new economic framework was installed; decision-making and power were devolved; new types of hospitals were created; the financial-allocation and capital-accounting systems were overhauled. At the centre of the Reforms, however, was the creation of a quasi market for health care. Whilst the basis of this key change was theoretically straightforward, in practice it was highly complex, involving not only a radical reshaping of the economic environment but also a fundamental change in managerial, and indeed clinical, cultures.

The main thesis of the White Paper *Working for Patients* (DoH 1989) was that the perceived ills of the NHS were not related to the size of its budget; more money was not the answer.[1] Rather, the NHS needed a new set of incentives – incentives provided by a market – to encourage more efficient delivery of health-care services. And it was Alain Enthoven's ideas for a limited form of managed market for the NHS (Enthoven 1985) which provided the basic framework for the NHS Reforms. Enthoven argued that the problems of inefficiency in the NHS could best be addressed by importing some of the rigours and incentives of competitive markets. He considered that one of the necessary (but, it should be noted, not sufficient) conditions for a market – the separation of purchasers and providers or the creation of buyers and sellers – would mean that purchasers 'could buy services from producers who offered good value. They could use the possibility of buying outside as bargaining leverage to get better performance from their own providers' (Enthoven 1985). Here, Enthoven reveals the ultimate consumer power in any market: the threat to buy from someone else. He also implicitly reveals that markets do not operate automatically. Greater efficiency and increased choice – the oft-quoted twin virtues of markets – are not guaranteed; they are

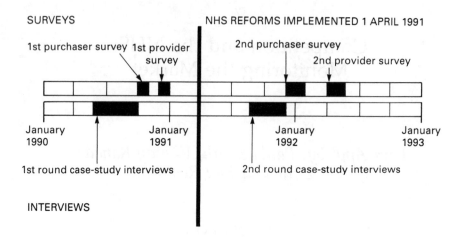

Figure 7.1 The timing of the pre- and post-Reforms implementation surveys and interviews in our study

a possible outcome of an interaction between buyers and sellers. In the case of the NHS, the interaction between purchasers and providers is complex, and the outcome by no means certain.

The material presented in this chapter addresses this uncertainty. It draws on an empirical study we have undertaken of the introduction of a limited form of market competition into the NHS – the Monitoring Managed Competition Project of NAHAT in conjunction with West Midlands RHA and Newcastle Polytechnic. The Project has been funded by the King's Fund Institute for a period of 3 years.

Data have been drawn from a number of sources, but primarily from national and Regional surveys, and in-depth, face-to-face interviews with managers and clinicians in four case studies of DHAs. Figure 7.1 shows the timing of the pre- and post-Reforms implementation surveys and interviews undertaken by the study. Postal surveys of purchasers covered all DHAs in England and Wales (excluding one piloted Region) with response rates of 72% for the first and 67% for the second survey. The surveys of providers (i.e acute DMUs and NHSTs) were conducted in one Region only. The response rate for the first survey of providers was similar to the national survey of purchasers.

Competition and the NHS: monitoring the market

In this chapter, divided into four sections, we report on selected results gathered during the first 2 years of our study and, in particular, concentrate on various aspects of competition in the NHS. The first section of the chapter looks at the separation of providers and purchasers and describes the attitudes of DGMs and UGMs to the Reforms and, in particular, the idea of a market in health care; UGMs' assessments of competition; factors affecting the placing of contracts; the implementation of the purchaser/provider split itself. The second section describes the 'structure' of the new health-care market as purchasers and providers come together to complete transactions through the bridging document of the contract.

With competition – even the limited form of 'managed competition' – at the heart of the Reforms, it is clear that quantifying the difficult and definitionally slippery concept of competition would provide a valuable indicator to correlate, for instance, with measures of efficiency such as unit costs. Section three describes one approach to quantifying competition using an industrial 'concentration index'.

Finally, we look at some possibilities for the future of managed competition in the NHS. The future will be uncertain not only because of potential health-policy changes by central government but also because of uncertainties inherent in the Reforms themselves. To what extent will the managed market be allowed to evolve; to what extent might it be further constrained?

THE SEPARATION

The separation of providers and purchasers has been a necessary but, as we noted above, not a sufficient, step in creating a market in the NHS. Divorcing providers from a guaranteed source of income and giving purchasers a freer hand in determining health-care priorities are nevertheless important factors in Enthoven's 'leverage' argument. Implementation of this split has not necessarily been easy, however, and attitudes to, and interpretations of, the Reforms by managers will play a crucial role in determining how this split, once established, actually works in practice.

Here, we look first at managerial attitudes, preparations for implementing the Reforms and potential changes in service provision of Units/providers in one Region, the West Midlands. As indicated in Figure 7.1, the data have been drawn from a survey carried out in November 1990 and face-to-face interviews with managers, clinicians and Unit management team members carried out during the summer of 1990. Second, we look at purchasers, drawing on national and Regional data collected before and after the implementation of the National Health Service and Community Care Act 1990 (DoH 1990) on 1 April 1991.

Providers

All 32 acute provider Units in the West Midlands Region were surveyed and 24 UGMs replied, a response rate of 75%. The attitudes of UGMs towards the National Health Service and Community Care Act 1990 were broadly the same as those expressed in a similar survey of DGMs in the Region, although there was even greater approval of the purchaser/provider split (92% compared to 84%) and the 'market concept' in health care (60% compared to 55%).

About one-fifth of the UGMs had taken steps to quantify the level of competition their Units were likely to face, ranging from 'informal assessments' to SWOT analyses (strengths, weakness, opportunities and threats).[2] The specialties believed to face most competition were general surgery (48% of responding Units) closely followed by orthopaedics and ENT (35% of responding Units.) A Unit in an adjoining District or a proposed NHST hospital were the most frequently perceived sources of competition. The least perceived threat was posed by the private sector.

UGMs were asked about Unit intentions to change levels of provision (that is 'introduce', 'expand' or 'reduce') in four selected specialties: general surgery, gynaecology, trauma and orthopaedics, and ophthalmology.[3] This question generated fewer replies than any other, and perhaps reflected a reluctance to reveal business intentions. Of those who did answer, none planned to introduce a specialty not already provided but 10 planned to expand their provision of trauma and orthopaedics (a third of all West Midlands providers) and 7 planned to increase provision of ophthalmology. These intentions were based on the fact that 71% of providers felt they had spare capacity. If carried out, such plans represented considerable expansionary pressure, since there was no counterbalancing intention to reduce provision in these specialities by other Units. How far this could be accommodated within total Regional purchasing power was an open question.

In assessing the effects of competition on their Unit, confidence was high. Three-quarters agreed that they were 'confident that this Unit can take on the competition'. None disagreed; a fifth were neutral; and two-thirds believed that their Unit was in good shape to do so. Although one-third acknowledged that 'there is a greater likelihood of financial insolvency for this Unit as a result of the NHS Act', two-thirds did not see this as a real threat and agreed that 'in reality this Unit will not be allowed to close'.

The four case-study Districts and their main acute providers allowed us to get behind these generalized statements and study the local factors which affected perceptions. The four had been chosen to reflect a wide variety of 'competitive' situations and circumstances. The factors taken into account included geographical size, range of facilities, quality of capital stock, cross-boundary flows and the proximity of competition.

At the time of the first interviews in June 1990 the Authorities were grappling with the devolution of services to Units, and the separation of purchasing from providing. Achieving the correct balance between 'holding on while letting go' (Ham 1990) was never painless, even in Districts with highly devolved management styles, and conflicts sometimes emerged around the issue of self-governing status. Many respondents were surprised how quickly the different interests of Units and Districts had manifested themselves: 'I think Unit plc now'; 'There are already flashes of independence from the Units.'

Attitudes to market opportunities and threats depended both on the local context and management culture. Only one District, District A, was highly optimistic about its ability to increase its share of the market based on its entrepreneurial record, spare capacity and efficient departments. This District already had considerable experience in contracting with other Districts and the Region for earmarked money from the national waiting-list initiative. The UGM spoke gleefully of 'hammering the competition' in some of the Regional specialties.

The acute Units in the two rural Districts had a virtual monopoly of business from their host District, but their perceptions of future threats and opportunities differed greatly. One felt totally unthreatened: 'We have no Regional specialities and no speciality which logically we shouldn't have in terms of patient flows and the population served. No reason for anyone to threaten us or vice versa.'

The Unit did, however, have a brand new community hospital on the fringes of the District for which it had to find half the revenue consequences by attracting patients from across District boundaries. In the main, however, their aspirations were confined to making relatively modest service improvements. One-third of their residents were treated in other Districts and no one seriously questioned the feasibility of changing existing patient flows substantially.

In the other rural District, District C, the DGH was the only hospital over a huge geographical area. It provided acute services for a neighbouring District without a DGH and this already represented one-quarter of its business. The opportunities for providing innovative packages of care to rural communities were considerable, and individual respondents in both the acute and community Units were alert to these opportunities. However, attitudes to the Reforms in the acute Unit were divided, and at District level pessimistic.

By contrast, District D, an inner-city authority, did face considerable competition which they perceived to be threatening the viability of some of their providers. The main acute Unit had a large number of Regional and supraRegional specialities serving over 120 Districts, high average costs and a small 'resident' population accounting for only 17% of its business in 1989/90. The Unit faced a difficult situation. The Unit team were realistic about this but reasonably confident of their ability to compete on grounds of reputation and quality.

Purchasers

The nature of the NHS Reforms – evolutionary rather than revolutionary; planned but without a blueprint – meant that attitudes, especially the attitudes of those most involved with implementation of the changes – managers – take on a particular importance in influencing the shape and direction of the Reforms. Given this, we examined District managers' attitudes towards the central theme of the Reforms, the market.

The first national survey of purchasers (i.e. DHAs), carried out in October 1990 revealed support for the concept of a market in health care. Just over half of DGMs surveyed agreed that 'the market concept would work successfully in health care'; two-thirds disagreed with the statement that the market concept of the Act was not in the best interests of patients. Almost half did not agree that the market would cause a 'shunting around' rather than a genuine reduction in waiting lists. There was considerable support for the purchaser/provider split, with 87% agreeing that it was a good idea. There was also support for the Reforms' emphasis on health needs and maximizing health gain.

Despite the considerable support for the separation of roles, in the first year the vast majority of Districts remained managerially accountable for the vast majority of providers (where the latter did not opt for Trust status). Material from our case-study Districts illustrates how they coped with this situation.

In the first case-study District, District A, all services provided by its own Units were deemed to be 'core' by the DGM and were to be supplied within the District 'come hell or high water'. This approach was influenced by a belief that the District existed to support the Units who would be free to compete and increase their market share as long as this did not jeopardize work for their 'home' District.

District B intended to use their newly acquired purchasing responsibility to 'tweak the Units' tail' to get action on long-standing problems such as waiting times. Their impression was that Units were expecting a cosier relationship than was, in fact, envisaged by the District.

In the other rural authority, District C, relations between Units, and between Units and District, were reported to be more adversarial. However, in this District the DGM felt that 'competition in a meaningful way [was] not going to be a factor' and the White Paper was therefore seen as 'irrelevant'.

The major preoccupation for District D was the viability of their own providers who were perceived to be facing more competition than other authorities due to the large proportion of specialist work undertaken for other Districts. Whilst there was support for the split in responsibilities between those who provided health care and those who decided what and how much health care should be provided (although, interestingly, there was less support for the idea of a market as such), exercising change through these new roles was clearly seen as fairly limited, at least in the short term.

Our survey identified 10 factors influencing decisions on where to place contracts in the first year of the Reforms. Factors given a high ranking (first, second or third) included: existing patient flows (93%); GPs expressed preferences (74%); ease of travel for residents (40%) and previous experience of the provider (39%). Only 22% felt that competitive prices were a significant factor affecting the decision on where to place contracts. This may have been due to the problems obtaining comparative cost data that were being experienced by 80% of Districts. On the issue of quality the fact that a provider may have a 'well-developed quality assurance' programme was only seen as a significant factor in terms of contract placement by 12% of purchasers.

Overall, evidence on the first year of the Reforms confirms that the new competitive environment was, in essence, competitive in name only and that a combination of a tight implementation timetable, inappropriate accounting systems, inadequate information systems and the emphasis on 'steady state' conspired to maintain the status quo.

But in the second year of the Reforms, to what extent are purchasers moving towards what Ham calls 'real' purchasing: needs assessment, involving the public, evaluating services and the beginning of purchasing power being used to change how services are provided (Ham 1991)? Initial results from our second purchaser survey (carried out during December 1991 and January 1992) revealed that a majority (73%) were planning to change their health-care priorities for 1992/3 as a result of their health-needs assessment.[4] Just over a quarter were not.

Many were also planning to alter their 1992/3 contracts: 62% were planning to cease a contract that existed for 1991/2; 71% to contract with a provider where no contract existed for 1991/2; 50% to reduce volumes more than 10% with an existing provider; and 78% to contract for a greater volume of care per pound spent. Whilst this suggests a tremendous modification to contracts, not knowing the monetary values these changes represent makes it difficult to assess their significance. Evidence from the case-study Districts suggests that, as in the first year, change will occur, but largely at the margin.

There were also shifts in emphasis on factors influencing decisions on where to place contracts. Factors given a high ranking in the second survey were: GPs expressed preferences (85%); existing patient flows (80%); previous experience of the provider (46%); and ease of travel for residents (40%). The percentage giving competitive prices a high ranking (24%) had risen slightly, although the same proportion were experiencing problems in obtaining comparative cost data as in Year One. Fewer (7%) gave a well-developed quality assurance a high ranking, and only 34% ranked it in their top five factors. In our second survey, 81% of DGMs gave protecting their own provider Units a low priority, a significant contrast to the picture presented by the case-study material in Year One.

How significant are these changes and how far were these actions influenced by competition? In our second survey just over half of DGMs attributed the perceived benefits of the purchaser/provider split to the market, disagreeing with the statement, 'We don't need a market to get the benefits of the purchaser/provider split.' Almost a third agreed with this statement. On the status of Units, NHSTs or DMUs, opinion was more equally divided: 46% agreed with the statement, 'We don't need Trusts to get the benefits of the purchaser/provider split', and 44% disagreed. However, 28% were experiencing difficulties coping with the new District/Unit relationship compared to 23% in the first survey.

A majority (81%) felt that contracting had led to improvements in service quality for residents. For example, they cited the heightened awareness of quality as an issue; improved attitudes of provider staff towards patients; and the reduction of waiting times and waiting lists. The extent to which it was the Reforms and not the extra resources directed to reducing waiting times over the last 3 years which led to this latter benefit is, however, debatable.

Purchasing, the role of the market and competition in health care are clearly complex issues and, as the earlier evidence from our study shows, purchasers are not reacting to the new economic environment in a simplistic way. Moreover, not only are price signals very weak, they are generally ignored in favour of what purchasers perceive to be more reliable and important indicators, for example GPs preferred referral patterns.

THE MEETING

Providers and purchasers get together

The separation of providers and purchasers of health care is, in reality, the separation of providers from a guaranteed allocation of resources, together with a transformation of the allocation process. But in pulling apart – teasing out new roles – purchasers and providers need to establish new ways of coming together, of cooperating within their new economic environment.

One important aspect of our study was the practical effects of this meeting of purchasers and providers in terms of the structure of the market and particularly how this structure is likely to change over the next few years.

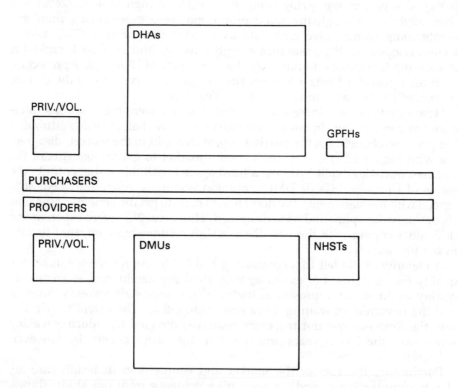

Figure 7.2 The relative size of the actors in the health-care market, Year One, 1991/2

The market actors

Figure 7.2 provides a representational view of the (English and Welsh) acute health-care market in terms of expenditures/budgets (purchasers) and incomes/receipts (providers).

Figure 7.2 shows the relative size in financial terms of the 'actors' in the market in the first year of the Reforms, 1991/2. On the purchasing side there are two main groups: the private and public sectors. Within the public sector there are two sets of purchasers: DHAs and GPFHs. On the providing side there is a similar split between private/voluntary and public sectors, together with a further split within the public sector between DMUs and NHSTs.

Contracts: the link between purchasers and providers

There are two other pictures of the market which provide an interesting perspective on its structure and which also provide quantifiable indicators of change as the market develops. Tables 7.1 and 7.2 are taken from our second survey of DHAs and show the types of contracts let and with whom in the first year of the Reforms.

Covering nearly 60% of all DHA purchasers in England and Wales, Table 7.1 shows that block contracts plus variants on block contracts accounted for 83% by number, and 94% by value, of all contracts let. More detailed cost-and-volume and cost-per-case contracts accounted for only 5% of the value of all contracts and largely reflects the relative paucity of adequate

Table 7.1 Contracts for acute services, 1991/2, by contract type ($n=101$)

Contract type	Number	Value (£ million)	Per cent of number	Per cent of value	Average value (£ million)
Block	1,131	4,346.5	40.7	60.4	3.84
Block with ceilings and floors	1,179	2,434.5	42.4	33.8	2.06
Cost and volume	169	314.1	6.1	4.4	1.86
Cost per case	108	17.6	3.9	0.2	0.16
RHA agency on behalf of DHA	191	85.9	6.9	1.2	0.45

Source: National survey of English and Welsh DHAs, conducted in December 1991.

Table 7.2 Contracts for acute services, 1991/2, by provider type ($n=101$)

Provider type	Number	Value (£ million)	Per cent of number	Per cent of value	Average value (£ million)
NHS provider within District	488	5,610.1	17.8	78.6	11.50
NHS provider outside District	2,161	1,503.4	78.6	21.1	0.70
Private sector	13	1.5	0.5	0.0	0.12
Voluntary sector	67	9.4	2.4	0.1	0.14
Other	19	1.2	0.7	0.2	0.63

Source: National survey of English and Welsh DHAs, conducted in December 1991.

cost information necessary to formulate such contracts. There is evidence (NAHAT 1991) that both purchasers and providers plan to move towards cost-and-volume and cost-per-case contracts over the next few years.

Table 7.2 clearly shows that contracts were overwhelmingly let within the NHS (99.7% by value, 96.4% by number). Over three-quarters of the total value of contracts were with NHS providers within the District. These were often large block contracts, as the average contract value indicates. Contracts with NHS providers outside Districts' borders were more numerous but of a much lower average value.

MEASURING COMPETITION

With competition as the core theme of the Reforms and with hard evidence as to the benefits of competition – increased efficiency, improved quality, etc. – at best equivocal (Robinson 1989) as well as the lack of a comparable 'control', the key empirical question in terms of monitoring the reforms is to what extent competition *per se* is responsible for any changes in, for example, efficiency. And addressing this question requires a quantified measure of competition.

We began to examine this issue by a study of the degree of competition in general surgery facing each of 39 hospitals in one Region offering this service in 1988/9. Of any specialty, general surgery was reckoned by UGMs to face the greatest competition. Base data of all finished consultant episodes, FCEs, for in-patients and day cases in the specialty were used for a study comprising three main stages:

- identification of each hospital market and the hospital's market share within it;
- identification of its 'competitors' within each of these geographical markets;
- production of an overall index of competition for each hospital.

Defining hospital markets

Morrisey *et al.* (1988) discuss the concept of economic and anti-trust markets and their empirical measurement in the hospital context. Neither an economic definition of market (based on costs of transporting the product) nor anti-trust market definitions (which focus on product price changes) has direct applicability in the UK health-care context where the patient, not the product, travels and where there are no price data. However, we can use patient flows as a form of 'shipments' data to gauge geographical hospital markets. The degree of resolution of the market definition will be finer or coarser dependent on the level of spatial referencing of the patient flow data. In the West Midlands study, the DHA was used as the unit of analysis. While this is a relatively high level of aggregation (compared with a ward or census enumeration district) it is, none the less, the 'purchasing' unit under the new arrangements for the NHS.

Following Melnick and Zwanziger (1988) a District was included in a hospital's market area if it contributed at least 3% of the hospital's total episodes. For most hospitals this defined an area containing around 80% of the hospital's episodes.

Competitors

Again following Melnick and Zwanziger (1988) a cut-off point of 3% was taken, that is, if a second hospital drew out at least 3% of any District total episodes from at least one of the Districts in the first hospital's market area, it was considered to be a competitor.

Degree of competition

Having established the hospitals competing within each district, it is possible to summarize this in an index – the Herfindahl–Hirschman Index (HHI) – which reflects both the number of competitors and the degree of concentration within each District. These can then be combined to assess the degree of competition facing each hospital.

The HHI (Miller 1982) is obtained by summing the squares of the market shares of all competitor hospitals within a District. The HHI is widely used by the US Department of Justice in assessing market competitiveness in anti-trust cases and ranges from 0 (a large number of competitors all with small market shares) to 1 (a single monopoly supplier). For anti-trust purposes the index value is customarily multiplied by 10,000.

Each hospital's market area is made up of a number of Districts, each of which may have different concentrations of competing hospitals. The final stage is, therefore, to calculate the weighted sum of the HHIs for each District within each hospital's market area. The weights are the proportions of the hospital's patients drawn from that District. So, we arrive at an index showing the degree of competition facing each hospital.

How much competition?

Table 7.3 shows the hospitals in the West Midlands ranked in order of the degree of competition faced, based on 1988/9 data. One test of the competitiveness of the market is the US Department of Justice guidelines which state that markets with an index value in excess of 1,800 are considered highly concentrated, that is, they tend to be monopolistic. If this standard were applied to the West Midlands hospitals in Table 7.3 it would suggest that a quarter operate in markets where monopoly or oligopoly power may exist and, further, these hospitals account for nearly two-fifths of the total number of patient episodes. Nevertheless, the results suggest a potential for competition in general surgery in a sizeable segment of the Region (75% of hospitals covering 60% of episodes).

However, this may be an overstatement of the true potential for two reasons. First, the District as the unit of analysis for market areas may be an inappropriately high level of spatial aggregation. Basing hospitals' market areas on zones such as electoral wards will increase the degree of concentration though the 'right' level of spatial aggregation remains a matter of judgement rather than objective analysis. As the spatial resolution becomes finer, the market area reduces and tends towards monopoly.

Second, the use of data on general surgery episodes assumes that these are homogeneous but 'general surgery' covers operative procedures as diverse

Table 7.3 Hospital competition indices for general surgery, West Midlands, 1988/9

Hospital (host District)	No. Districts* in market area	No. of competitors facing hospital in market area	Degree of competition
†St Cross (Rugby)	3	1	6,790
†George Eliot (N. Warks)	2	1	6,570
†County (Hereford)	2	1	6,450
†RSH (Shropshire)	2	1	5,980
†WRI Ronkswood (Worcester)	1	1	5,120
†Walsgrave (Coventry)	2	1	4,510
†KGH (Kidderminster)	3	4	4,000
†Warwick (S. Warks)	1	3	2,680
†Alexandra (Broms./Red.)	2	4	2,450
†Sandwell DGH (Sandwell)	2	6	2,100
†Stafford DGH (Mid Staffs)	1	5	1,770
†Selly Oak (S. B'Ham)	3	5	1,590
†NSRI (N. Staffs)	2	9	1,510
The Royal (Wolverhampton)	4	8	1,190
City General (N. Staffs)	3	9	1,130
†Russells Hall (Dudley)	3	12	1,090
†New Cross (Wolverhampton)	4	8	1,020
†East B'ham Gen. (E. B'Ham)	3	5	920
†Good Hope (N. B'ham)	4	9	880
†Manor Hospital (Walsall)	2	5	840
†Dudley Road (W. B'ham)	4	8	820
General (Walsall)	3	10	720
Burton General (S.E. Staffs)	2	4	680
General (C. B'ham)	6	6	570
Wordsley (Dudley)	3	12	560
Warneford (S. Warks)	1	2	540
Queen Elizabeth (C. B'Ham)	8	9	520
WRI Castle St (Worcester)	2	2	480
Staff. Gen. (Mid Staffs)	1	5	450
†Solihull (Solihull)	3	5	420
Tenbury (Kidderminster)	3	3	350
†Burton DHC (S.E. Staffs)	3	9	330
Longton (N. Staffs)	2	8	310
Guest (Dudley)	2	6	280
Stratford (S. Warks)	3	5	270
Tamworth Gen. (S.E. Staffs)	3	9	230
Corbett (Dudley)	4	14	160
Biddulph Gr. (N. Staffs)	3	9	120
Lichfield Vic. (S.E. Staffs)	4	9	90

* Flows from other English regions treated as an additional district.
† District general hospitals.

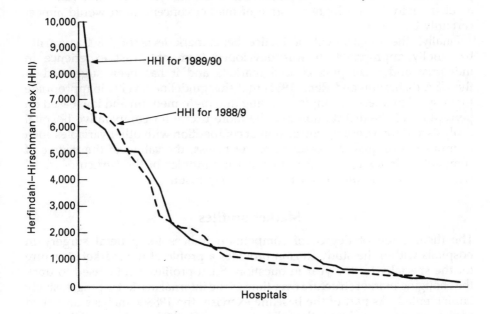

Figure 7.3 Market profiles: general surgery, 1988/9 and 1989/90

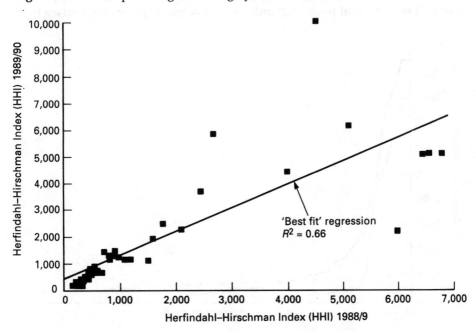

Figure 7.4 Comparison of Herfindahl–Hirschman Indices (HHIs) for general surgery in 1988/9 with 1989/90

as hernia repair and kidney replacement. If the analysis were undertaken at a subspecialty level a higher degree of market concentration would almost certainly be found.

Finally, the Department of Justice benchmark level of 1,800 may not be wholly appropriate. It was developed from anti-trust experience in industrial and retail price-cleared markets and it has been suggested in the USA (Schramm and Renn 1984) that this guideline level is inappropriate for hospital markets. A simple grouping into high, medium and low based on percentiles of the distribution may be more useful for comparative hospital analysis and for assessing correlation of competition with other variables such as unit costs or quality measures. Nevertheless, the values of the degree of competition index can be used to construct profiles of the 'structure trade' within the West Midlands for temporal comparison.

Market profiles

The distribution of degree of competition indices for general surgery in hospitals within the study Region provides a profile of the market structure for the specialty for the year in question. Such profiles can be used to track the changing market structure over time as the internal market is progressively implemented. As part of the baseline exercise, the 1988/9 analysis described earlier was compared with the following year, 1989/90. As Figure 7.3 shows, some change in the profile can be detected. Whilst one of the changes (the move of one hospital from high index to a position of monopoly) arises from

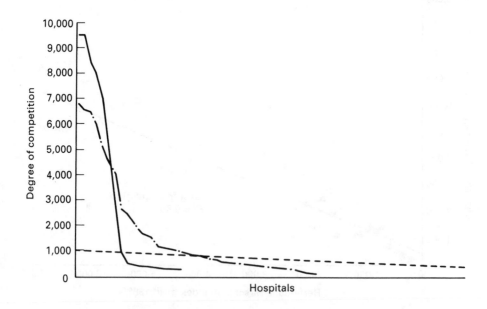

Figure 7.5 Which way will the curve shift? —— WM general surgery data; —— low competition; – · – · high competition

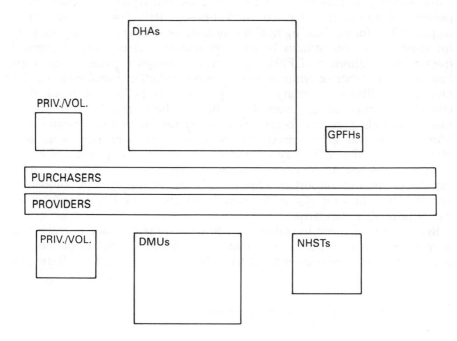

Figure 7.6 The relative size of the actors in the health-care market, Year Two, 1992/3

the statistical base used, the remainder reflect changes in hospital provision in the Region, primarily the opening of a major DGH in one District.

Whilst there is some year-on-year change (Figure 7.4) prior to the introduction of the internal market, the question was how the curve will move over time. Will it become flatter, with more competitors entering the market? Or will it steepen as hospital Units merge and competition diminishes (Figure 7.5)? The continued empirical measurement of the structure of the internal NHS market will be an essential prerequisite for effective market regulation and examination of the extent to which hospital performance in efficiency and quality bears any relation to the degree of competition faced.

A FUTURE FOR COMPETITION?

A new, managed market in health care

At the beginning of this chapter we described the NHS Reforms introduced through the National Health Service and Community Care Act 1990 (DoH 1990) as a fundamental reshaping of the economic environment within which the Health Service operates. Certainly the proposals contained in the White Paper *Working for Patients* (DoH 1989) and the subsequent Act held out the prospect of a radically reformed, market-based NHS. The separation of the responsibility for purchasing health care from providing it offered the scope for supply-side competition between providers seeking service contracts from health authorities, GPFHs and private insurance plans. There were, however, a number of critics who questioned whether health-care markets met the conditions necessary for supply-side competition to result in an efficient allocation of resources. In particular, the local catchment areas of many hospitals gave rise to concerns that spatial monopolies would arise. Moreover, it was emphasized that health-care systems pursue multiple objectives and that efficiency is only one of them. The pursuit of equity, in terms of access to services, and the maintenance of acceptable quality standards are two important objectives. Even if supply-side competition succeeds in achieving efficiency, there is no guarantee that it will achieve equity or quality standards.

Recognition of these limitations led to Government policy moving away from more extreme forms of competition in order to emphasize the need for regulation or management of the market. In the first year of the Reforms, this

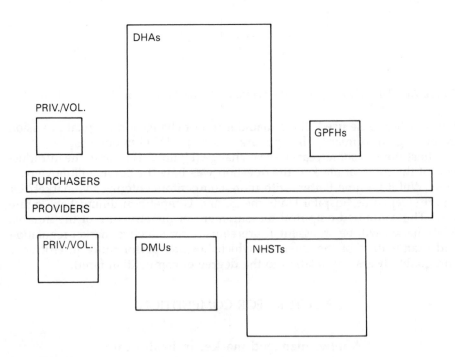

Figure 7.7 The relative size of the actors in the health-care market, Year Three, 1993/4

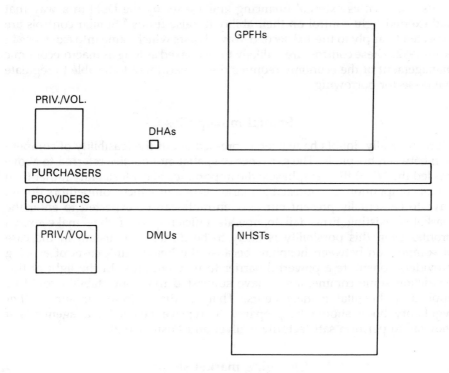

Figure 7.8 The possible relative size of the actors in the health-care market, Year Five, 1995/6

was reflected in the NHSME directives which emphasized the need for 'steady state', that is, new systems should be implemented but no dramatic changes should take place in patterns of service delivery compared with those of the previous year. At the same time, however, specific forms of regulation which could be expected to have a more lasting life were put in place.

Market regulation: the example of NHSTs

One vivid example of stronger regulation has been provided by the treat-ment of NHSTs. When the NHS Reforms were introduced, Trust status was presented as a means of offering greater freedom and autonomy for individual hospitals to manage their own affairs. They were presented as an important part of the competitive supply-side. The freedom to borrow from both public and private sectors in order to finance capital expenditure was seen as an important element of their newly acquired autonomy. In the event, however, this freedom has not materialized. As part of the public sector, Trusts' borrowing forms part of the public-sector borrowing requirement. As such, the Treasury has taken a close interest in their activities. Each of the 57 Units which became first-wave Trusts in April 1991 had their borrowing limits – known as external financing limits – set by the DoH in a way that had exerted tight control on their ability to raise funds.[5] Similar controls are expected to apply to the 103 second-wave Trusts which came into existence in April 1992. These controls are unlikely to be relaxed as long as macro-economic management of the economy requires the Government to be able to regulate public-sector borrowing.

Spatial monopolies

More generally doubts have been expressed about the feasibility of competition between hospitals. The existence of spatial monopolies referred to above has led the NHSME to emphasize the importance of contestability rather than actual competition. A contestable market is one in which competitors do not have to be actually present but new entrants can be expected to enter the market if existing firms fail to operate efficiently or if they make excess profits. Even this possibility is likely to be difficult to sustain in the case of competition between hospitals because the heavy sunk costs of existing providers constitute a powerful barrier to new entrants. In the light of this restriction some commentators have suggested that contestability could be applied to hospital managements. That is, the NHSME or some other regulatory body should be prepared to replace hospital managements if they fail to perform satisfactorily (Culyer and Posnett 1991).

Changing market shape

Whilst making predictions about the future development of the internal market is hazardous, there are clear indications of the trends in the 'shape' of the market. Following through the changes in terms of the relative financial size of the actors from the first to the third year of the Reforms (Figures 7.6 and 7.7), reveals a growth in GPFHs at the expense of DHAs on the purchasing side of the market. By 1993/4, there will be around 5,500 to 6,000 individual GPs involved in Fundholding, controlling a total budget of between £1.2 billion and £1.5 billion (1991/2 prices). These budgets are direct deductions from DHAs' purchasing budgets.[6]

On the provision side of the market the change is more dramatic. By 1993/4, NHST hospitals are likely to account for two-thirds of all public-sector provision. Figure 7.8, tentatively labelled Year Five, shows the outcome of the trends over the previous years; DHAs reduced to little or perhaps nothing in terms of purchasing power; GPFHs controlling virtually the entire public-sector health-care expenditure; and all DMUs transferring to Trust status.

Balancing policy conflicts

Predictions are difficult but, as we have shown, major change has taken place already although conflicting pressures have led to quite strong modification and refinement of plans during implementation. This seems to be the most likely course for the future. Regulated competition will continue to evolve with policy-makers seeking to balance the sometimes conflicting objectives of efficiency, equity, quality and choice in particular contexts.

NOTES

1 Cf. pp. 91–2.
2 See pp. 214–5.
3 Refer p. 215.
4 For a critical view of the value of health-needs assessment refer to pp. 88–91.
5 See pp. 123–4 for an account of a first-wave Trust under such tight controls.
6 This is still not without its critics. For one in the medical world see p. 54.

REFERENCES

Culyer, A.J. and Posnett, J. (1991) Hospital behaviour and competition, in A.J. Culyer *et al.* (eds.) *Competition in Health Care*. London: Macmillan, 12–47.

DoH (Department of Health) (1989) *Working for Patients*. London: HMSO.

DoH (Department of Health) (1990) *The National Health Service and Community Care Act*. London: HMSO.

Enthoven, A. (1985) *Reflection on the Management of the National Health Service*. London: Nuffield Provincial Hospitals Trust.

Ham, C. (1990) *Holding on While Letting Go: A report on the Relationship between Directly Managed Units and DHAs*. London: King's Fund College.

Ham, C. (1991) Purchasing: past, present and future. Paper given at NAHAT/King's Fund conference, 17 October.

Melnick, G.A. and Zwanziger, J. (1988) Hospital behavior competition and cost-containment policies: The Californian experience, 1980 to 1985, *Journal of the American Medical Association*, 2669–75.

Miller, R.A. (1982) The Herfindahl–Hirschman Index as a market structure variable: An exposition for anti-trust practitioners, *The Anti-Trust Bulletin*, Autumn, 593–618.

Morrisey, M.A. *et al.* (1988) Defining geographical markets for hospital care, *Law and Contemporary Problems*, 165–94.

NAHAT (National Association of Health Authorities and Trusts) (1991) *Autumn Survey of the Financial Position of District Health Authorities and Provider Units*. Birmingham: NAHAT.

Robinson, R. (1989) *Competition and Health Care: A Comparative Analysis of UK Plans and US Experience*. London: King's Fund Institute.

Schramm, C.J. and Renn, S.C. (1984) Hospital mergers, market concentration and the Herfindahl-Hirschman Index, *Emory Law Journal*, 869–88.

8

Four Providers' Strategic Responses and the Internal Market

Juan Baeza, David Salt and Ian Tilley

The purpose of this chapter is to sketch out the strategic response of four NHS hospital providers to the environment in which they operate. In the process of doing this, care will be taken to see how that broad response is influenced by the internal market. In other words, are the two things linked; if so, what parts of the strategy are affected by 'managed competition'; is the relationship direct or indirect; how strong is it; and how basically does it work?

In the official documents relating to the Government's health Reforms such as the White Paper *Working for Patients* and the new NHS Act (DoH 1989, 1990), the internal market has a prominent place. It appears as a critical force for change, perhaps even the central engine, driving the other aspects of the Reform package. On the other hand, we are told in Chapter 7, for example, that two-thirds of UGMs in their sample did not see any serious threat from the internal market.[1] Likewise a recent survey of provider managers' views of the market, in its second year of operation and as 'steady state' faded from the picture, was reported in the *Health Service Journal* under the heading, 'Managers' verdict: internal market does not yet exist' (Agnew 1992). Where does the truth lie? Can it be in a real sense caught in such generalizations? In their different ways both this and the previous chapter consider these complex questions.

OUR APPROACH

This chapter is an interim report summarizing one facet of the University of Greenwich Business School's study of the impact of the current health initiatives on hospital[2] provider Units. The overall study is concerned with all aspects of the initiatives and the implementation process and is not focused on the internal market as is the present chapter. Thus, the wider University of Greenwich study includes a look at how NHSTs, medical audit, RM, Project 2000 and the Patient's Charter work in practice.

Although based in four hospitals, the study's principal component is a comparison between an inner London teaching hospital Trust with another such hospital which is not yet an NHST. To deepen the comparative analysis a smaller amount of data gathering is being undertaken at two hospitals distinctly different from the two main sites. The two subsidiary locations are a London suburban Unit and an out-of-London teaching hospital Trust. In terms of methodology the wider University of Greenwich research project has both qualitative and quantitative dimensions. The main form of qualitative data gathering is semi-structured interviews with managers, doctors, nurses and other Health Service staff, chiefly at these four Units, but also at District, Regional and other levels of the NHS in order to locate our Unit-based studies.

Given our aims in this chapter, we will only draw here upon our semi-structured interviews and largely those of managers at Unit level. What we offer, therefore, is four mini case studies based on our four research sites. Unless otherwise indicated the direct quotations in the chapter come from field interviews. Our intention is to protect the anonymity of our individual respondents and their institutions and so pseudonyms have been used when referring to the latter. The positions held by our managerial respondents and some of the detailed facts and figures of each case likewise will not be fully given where this would be likely to increase the chances of identification.[3]

If our aim is to use the semi-structured interviews and other material to depict briefly the main features of our four Units' strategic responses to their particular environments, what we mean by strategy needs to be clarified.

The nature of a strategic response

Strategy is a potentially useful, though it has to be said problematic, idea used increasingly by social researchers[4] in their many fields of inquiry. It is problematic because some of the theoretical and methodological matters it raises have yet to be fully resolved. As Crow (1989: 2) says, 'No consensus exists concerning such fundamental issues as what is to qualify as a strategy, the nature of the relationship between strategies and agency, or the relationship between strategies and rationality.' Whilst acknowledging this, the present chapter can only address such matters empirically. In other words, the proof of its usefulness in this chapter can only be whether it aids in the organization of our material and produces some useful conclusions.

Our starting point derives from Mintzberg:

> defining strategy as a plan in advance of taking action is not sufficient; we . . . need a definition that encompasses the resulting behaviour, the strategies actually pursued through those actions. To put this another way we need to understand the strategies organizations really have achieved, not just the ones they intend to pursue.
>
> (Mintzberg 1988: 14)

Thus, it is most important for readers to realize that by strategy and strategic response we are not referring to the consciously worked out

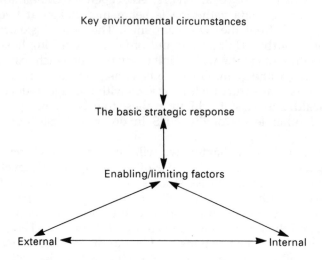

Figure 8.1   The elements of the Unit's strategic response

policies expounded by the dominant coalition in the hospitals, although such policies are part of the data used analytically to construct, or infer, the strategic response.

What we see as the Unit's basic strategic response is the first step in its reaction to its environment or the key perceived features of that environment. The response may then be complicated by various other external and internal factors that enable and limit the operation of the basic strategic response as shown in Figure 8.1. Clearly, as situations and perceptions of them change, so does the response. We can only offer here what we were able to infer based on the evidence available to us at the time of writing.

For analytical purposes an NHS hospital's strategic reaction can be viewed in two parts. First, the key perceived features of the hospital's environment call forth what we have defined as the basic strategic response. To a significant degree this will be mediated by past strategic responses and anticipated future ones.

The second part involves consideration of the external environment again, but also dwelling on the internal workings of the organization. However, both are considered only in terms of how factors involving each might enable or constrain the straightforward deployment of the basic strategic response.

The best way to proceed is to start by identifying the most decisive, in outcome terms, of these enabling and limiting factors, introduce it and note how the basic strategic response solidifies, alters or is transformed by its introduction, then move on, in like manner, with the other enabling/limiting factors.

The resultant picture offers a focus for subsequent investigations and, as these occur and a more refined understanding of the organizational and other processes emerges, this more detailed knowledge can be bounced back on to the initial sketches of the Units' strategic responses and used to improve those sketches.

In this chapter, however, all that can be offered is the basic sketches themselves and, given the concerns of this book, the place that the internal market or 'managed competition' occupies in them. In fact, as the first two hospitals are our main research sites and the next two just subsidiary ones, only the first two mini case studies will even offer a summary encompassing all the elements in Figure 8.1 above. The third mini case study will not cover the enabling/limiting factors and the final case study of the only out-of-London Unit studied here is restricted even further, to the key environmental circumstances and basic strategic response but only partially and in the ways that these differ from the three London Units.

However, the first two case studies will give some coverage of external and internal enabling/limiting factors. The internal side refers to the different professional and other interest groups inside the hospital, their particular agendas and resources. Such resources are financial and symbolic, including the differing status and knowledge bases of managers, doctors, nurses and paramedics. Restricting our discussion of such limiting and enabling factors to the first two mini case studies does not imply that they are unimportant: quite the contrary. As Willcocks and Harrow (1992: xxvi) point out, studying NHS management is very much about looking at such internal factors and the 'alternative agendas' and 'multiple systems' they spawn, if only because '"management" occurs in all [the different professional] domains whether or not it is recognised as such'.

In our Business School study as a whole we are keen to consider what 'general management' from Griffiths (1983) onwards actually means and, conversely, what the supposed departure from the earlier, public model of 'consensus management' might mean in the circumstances of particular NHS Units. Thus, inter- and intra-professional relations will be important and studied effectively in a given hospital. For example, if financial cuts are part of the basic strategic response, how such cuts are implemented and what share, say, is borne by the different medical specialty budgets, and why, are all important research questions for us. Whilst this is true for the research project in its entirety, for reasons of space it will only be possible to say anything about such matters in the first two mini case studies, and for the same reason this will be brief.[5]

The purpose of this subsection was to define terms and offer a general explanation of what we mean by strategy and how we will deploy the idea here. Further explanation of strategy, the central organizing notion for Chapter 8, is best left to emerge from the actual mini case studies themselves. Before turning to them, two other matters require attention:

(1) There is a clear London focus to our studies. Why and how does this affect the conclusions we can validly draw?

(2) Linked to (1) above, what is the relationship of this chapter to others in the collection, specifically the one that precedes it?

Our London focus

The research team is London based and, clearly, studying London hospitals is the easiest approach for us to undertake. However, this pragmatic consideration was not the decisive one in our largely selecting hospitals in the capital. Rather it sprang chiefly from our decision to make the hospital our basic unit of analysis.

Daunted by the number of NHS hospitals in Britain but desiring to make a detailed comparative study of only several of them, we soon realized that the team's location in London was actually fortuitous. Right from the start it was clear to most commentators that the NHS Reforms were going to have their largest impact in the capital. This London primacy was something the DoH itself was well aware of and is, for instance, suggested in an internal Departmental memorandum quoted by Professor Ham (1992: 250) which also predicts some of the misfortunes that are actually recounted in our London case studies: 'Health Authorities outside London might decide to treat patients locally instead of referring them to London's teaching hospitals . . . The effect would be to destabilise hospital provision in London, leading to piecemeal closures and cutbacks.'

Our argument is that, for good or ill, London is, for purposes of the health Reforms, something of a 'social laboratory' where the changes are the more transparent due to their relative intensity. Furthermore, the NHS, despite its importance, remains under-researched in terms of hospital organization. Therefore London is a useful location for studying such questions at this stage in terms of that whole research enterprise. Our concern therefore was one of gaining access to different types of London hospital that would facilitate effective comparative analysis. Our choices were indicated earlier.[6]

Given the diversity likely to exist in Units outside the capital, we were, however, aware that focusing on London hospitals could also distort as well as help illuminate. Our response to that was twofold: (1) the limited one of bringing in one out-of-London teaching hospital Trust; and (2) viewing as vital to our study that it be supplemented by, and itself supplement, the work of other researchers working in different locations and with different methods. The prime candidate in this reader is Chapter 7, although the collection as a whole also rounds out our conclusions.

Our relationship to the preceding chapter

Chapter 7 presents part of the results, those pertaining to the internal market and competition, of an important large-scale study of the NHS Reforms. It also reports on some more detailed case studies of the effect of the Reforms in different types of District. Given that they are in the same collection of readings on 'managed competition', Chapter 7 is, in effect, a companion chapter to the current one and hopefully the converse holds too. It seems to us that each chapter adds to the other's coverage. Chapter 7 makes it clear in which way our findings are specific to London. We hope our chapter adds details to Chapter 7 which, given its focus and methodology, could not be brought out within one chapter. Further, despite clear methodological differences, both chapters see the interpretations the leading groups of protagonists place on the Reforms and the internal market as of significance in terms of how the purchase/provider split actually works. Further, some of the findings of the two chapters are quite similar. The conclusion to the present chapter will therefore include, among other things, a brief enumeration of those findings broadly common to both.

Before we move to our four mini case studies we will pose the central research questions the chapter considers. Doing this both concludes the present section and provides a focus for the remainder of the chapter.

Our central research questions

We reported earlier[7] how depictions of the internal market have, in the space of a few years, ranged from it being portrayed as the engine of change driving the whole Reform package, through to those that are sceptical of its importance at this stage.

From this we derive the basic question the chapter examines: Can the place of the internal market be in any sense portrayed by either of these generalizations? What role does it have in the strategic responses of our four Units? What can we glean about its modes of functioning?

THE MINI CASE STUDIES

Managing a long-term income restriction

Our first mini case study concerns the Inner London Trust (ILT), a large London teaching hospital. It was one of the first-wave Trusts of 1991–2 and, as well as being the only provider in its whole District, has a remit covering both acute and community services. A large proportion of ILT's resident population is from the ethnic minorities and the incidence of social deprivation is particularly high. For the past few years the ILT has suffered from a lack of capital funds. This was not immediately alleviated by gaining Trust status as many within the Unit had hoped. A top manager of the Trust stated in an interview with us that

> The then Secretary of State made much of greater access to capital in persuading people to join the first wave of Trusts; but it turned out, of course, to be somewhat of a chimera because the amount of capital for the whole NHS is no more than it was before.

In its first year as a Trust ILT received from the DoH an external financing limit (EFL) which caused great disappointment. For 1992–3 ILT is permitted to borrow nearly four times its first EFL. This will enable it to carry out its proposed site rationalization policy. This policy involves the centralizing of the accident and emergency (A&E) and acute services on one site, and concentrating all the community and mental health services on another. This will eventually result in the closure of one A&E department and some psychiatric services currently operated by the Trust. ILT hopes to have completed these plans within a few years despite strong opposition from certain sections of the local population, including many of its local GPs, none of whom is a GPFH. This absence of GPFHs is an important feature of ILT's environment and something not shared by the Units in the other three case studies. The absence of Fundholders certainly reduces the uncertainties faced by the ILT but its GPs appear to exercise significant influence through the local DHA.

It should be pointed out that the local residents and, more importantly, GPs – due to their greater power – have provided considerable resistance, first, to the creation of the Trust, and latterly to these planned site closures. Closures of NHS facilities tend to be quite fraught, drawn-out, even acrimonious affairs. However, it is not yet typical to see a significant proportion of local GPs, placards in hand describing their position as local doctors, in a demonstration outside a hospital. This, none the less, is precisely what ILT's managers have faced and, as one somewhat wryly observed, 'We don't have a good relationship with GPs and that is something we will have to work on.'

Some of the GPs have also queried whether the Trust may be meeting overspends in acute services by diverting funds from its community budget. This the Trust management has denied. It is worth noting in passing that the DoH has now ruled that new Trust aspirants will in future be 'strongly discouraged' from lodging applications which join acute and community services within the one Trust (Dobson 1992b).

As mentioned earlier,[8] our first step in defining a Unit's strategic response is to find out the key perceived circumstances of its environment. In ILT's case many of these are concerned with funding matters. The NHS funding formula has changed from RAWP to weighted capitation, the latter resting on the size of the population which is weighted by age and the standard mortality ratios of the area. It is probable that ILT's host District is a net gainer from this important change to the basis for allocating funds. We say probably as the funding received is based on the census figures which, in deprived ethnic areas, tend to understate the actual population. If the census enumeration is substantially correct that will indeed mean ILT's District gains, albeit slightly. If, on the other hand, the count produces a definite understatement of the actual population, this will effectively make the District, and thence ILT, a loser, again only slightly. Thus, in contrast to the next mini case study, the alteration to the method of funding is not an important environmental circumstance for ILT, strategically speaking.

However, if the total level of funding has only altered marginally, the same cannot be said of its division between the acute and community sides of the Trust. The local commissioner has moved several millions of pounds of contracts from the acute sector – the focus of this chapter – into the community budget.

Clearly in our terms the District's switch of contracts from one area to another is a significant environmental circumstance, yet it had little to do with the internal market directly. It was more to do with the purchasing selections of the local DHA which reflected an enhanced status for community health care in Government policy generally.[9] The role for the internal market in this situation was one of being the mechanism, if you like the transmission belt, via contracts, for effecting changes deriving from another part of current health policy.

The internal market did, however, exert a direct financial impact on ILT which manifested itself in the shape of other surrounding DHAs pulling back some of their work to their own hospitals. These lost contracts added up to a few million pounds or around half what ILT's acute services 'lost' to community provision. What the suburban DHAs pulled back was routine 'lumps and bumps' work that their 'own' hospitals could do at a cheaper price than inner London teaching hospitals. As the DGM of ILT's District said to the local press, 'A number of London hospitals are facing cash problems as health authorities outside London find they can treat people closer to home.' These DHAs also felt that they could exert more non-price controls, for example in terms of quality, on their local hospitals than they could place on the ILT.

However, in a short-term financial sense at least, ILT effectively recovered this lost revenue caused when part of their previous work load moved back to neighbouring DGHs. This came in the form of Regional Transitional Monies designed to provide short-run mitigation to providers incurring substantial cutbacks of this kind. The relief came from a £46 million stabilization reserve set up by the four Thames RHAs in order 'to help them [providers] with the effects of population-based funding and [, as ILT experienced,] a shift in referral patterns to hospitals' favouring suburban and rural providers (Dobson 1992a: 5).

We billed our ILT mini case study as about managing a long-term income restriction. To date we have focused on the short term, the revenue reduction next financial year. First, to summarize, the short-run position: as the loss to hospitals in other Districts was covered by Region, the aggregate short-term cut – viewed from the perspective of those running acute services – is the several millions lost when the home DHA moved funds from the hospital to the community services of the Trust as a whole.

But the restriction is not merely a short-term problem and it is not clear how long the Regional Transitional Monies will be available to mollify part of the income loss. Dealing with the overall income restriction involves making changes to the organizational and cost structure of the hospital that will take time and a long-term strategy to alter. To begin to understand its basic strategic response, it is useful to think about the main options available to ILT for dealing with the changes in the acute work load resulting from changes to contracts by *both* the home and surrounding DHAs – as both must be addressed as soon as possible. These options are:

(1) To raise revenue by seeking new contracts from the home District and/or from nearby inner London Districts or other suburban ones. Over time they might, for instance, add new specialities or work from the existing ones but endeavour to compete in price or skill terms, the latter perhaps being possible in outer suburban Districts.[10]

(2) To cut provision and its related expenditure. This is a slow and painful process, given the high level of fixed costs[11] and the likely resistance from the specialties affected. Cost cutting also poses the policy 'choice' as to whether the burden could be borne equally by specialties or otherwise. The question of how costs are borne, how Regional Transitional Monies are deployed and so on are of real significance in understanding micro-organizational behaviour and the relationships between and within the different professions represented in the hospital.

ILT's basic strategic response for acute services could, in principle, be based on (1) or (2) above or some combination thereof. The managers adjudged all variants of option (1) as unfeasible.[12] Rather they are pursuing option (2) in the form of reducing the current provision in areas where contracts have been lost and cutting costs there and more generally. As made clear, this is likely to be a slow, difficult process requiring a long-term solution. Given the time-spans involved in reducing or eliminating provision and the possibility of some further erosion of contracts, ILT's acute managers anticipate they face a gap between income and expenditure which will widen and by 1993–4 might possibly amount to as much as twice the level of 1992–3 contracts lost by the acute sector.

The first instalment of managerial action to reduce costs was their announcement of a vacancy freeze throughout the Trust. The Trust board declared several hundred posts were to be cut, fewer than half entailing redundancies, only a small percentage of which will be compulsory.

The cost cutting has involved all specialties but surgery has been worst affected as it was this service that lost the most contracts. All occupations have suffered losses with the notable exception of doctors. One manager thought this was because 'nobody wants to touch the doctors' and she added that 'morale will be at rock bottom if somebody doesn't bite the bullet about the medical staff'.[13]

Thinking about the enabling and limiting external factors in Figure 8.1, an influence on ILT managers during these events, certainly something requiring their careful attention, has been to avoid or minimize adverse national media publicity arising from the retrenchments. NHSTs have frequently been in the media spotlight rendering such a task not particularly easy. Although the ILT received some bad press locally around such policies as their site rationalization,[14] and more recently upon announcing their cuts in provision and expenditure, the latter only evoked momentary national media attention. In part at least this must be due to fairly rapid and vigorous action by management to begin to face their problems promptly.[15] They avoided the lengthy delays which heighten speculation and pain internally, and increase the likelihood of being accompanied by sustained media interest. ILT's approach kept all this to a minimum.

Moving to 'internal factors', our interviews carried out after the cuts reflect, not unexpectedly, a considerable degree of resentment by staff of the Trust management's handling of the problems. How quickly this will dissipate is unclear at this stage. One complaint we heard was about the way many staff first learnt of their hospital's difficulties. One ILT consultant commented 'the first I heard of it [the financial problems] was on the news on Saturday morning at home. . . . So there was extremely inadequate dissemination of information within the institution beforehand.'

The Trust's reduction in provision had to be made within quite tight limits. Whilst the guiding principles were to trim expenditure to income and as soon as was possible, these principles had to be put into action with care so as not to impair ILT's capacity to fulfil the contracts actually won. Contraction in provision could not be allowed to jeopardize the ILT's strong local market which provides over half its work.

First, there is a threshold below which services cannot be cut if they are to remain viable. Second, there is the further problem of matching the Unit retrenchment plans with those of purchasers. Although the hospital management might see the need to eliminate a particular service on economic grounds, the purchaser may resist this.[16] The interdependency between services means that they cannot be assessed in isolation.

Because in common with most NHS Units, even in Year Two of the internal market, ILT lacks the detailed knowledge of the behaviour of its costs, the hospital has found it difficult to make accurate financial predictions upon which to plan for the cuts.[17] This became apparent when the plans first drawn up were found, on closer examination, to be unreliable. They were scrapped, adding to existing anxieties at what was already an uncertain, difficult time for all. It seems important to reiterate that it appears most Units within the NHS would still find it difficult to manage such cost restrictions with what are, for most, rudimentary management accounting systems.

Another internal limiting factor on the basic strategic response may come from the medical school. Actually their influence is likely to pull in different directions: on the one hand, the existence of such a school required the Trust to keep a wide range of medical work, including that of a routine kind for training student doctors. Besides this, for reasons of prestige and to enable it to attract top doctors, the medical school is also likely to exert pressures to retain and expand high-tech specialities which may sometimes not be justified on economic grounds alone.

One potentially enabling option which this particular Unit has not taken is making savings by holding down wages and salaries to staff.[18] As an NHST, it has the power to negotiate such matters locally. The ILT management has a lengthy history of valuing loyalty, commitment and longevity of employment from their staff. This means they are likely to follow rather than lead in terms of making changes on this industrial relations front. A senior executive confirmed this view when he said that 'the process of moving into determining your hospital's own pay and conditions involves a significant change and is something we are beginning to actually exercise only very slowly and very sensitively'.

One final point: the Tomlinson Report (1992) will have significant impact on this hospital, although it is not one of the Units under threat. This could well complicate and alter ILT's strategic response.

Trouble on the home front?

The second of our mini case studies is the South London Teaching Hospital (SLTH) which is currently a 'shadow Trust'. Thinking about SLTH's perceived environment, the first factor of note is that it has one commissioning body that provides two-thirds of its business. That is in no way unusual, however, unlike ILT's purchaser, SLTH's commissioner is a merged body covering several DHAs and a number of other providers apart from SLTH. In theory at least, SLTH might, to some degree, be in competition with the other providers within the enlarged purchasing area. To date this has not occurred. Fears that it might are a part of the SLTH management perception of its environment.

Of much more immediate importance and in contrast to ILT, SLTH is a significant loser in the change in funding from RAWP to weighted capitation. Along with the other local providers SLTH has received the first of a series of budget cuts to begin to effect this. For 1991–2 at least, SLTH has been able to secure relief from this budgetary pressure from the same Regional Transitional Monies ILT drew upon. However, these monies are intended merely as a bridging device to enable its beneficiaries to find long-term ways of dealing with their problems. Thus, the change in the funding formula remains very much a key environmental factor.

Recently the Secretary of State informed SLTH it would definitely become an NHST from April 1993. Prior to that, securing Trust status had been a major managerial goal and one that affected their policy choices. Before receiving their notification, the desire to secure a favourable outcome on the Trust question pushed SLTH's financial position even more to the forefront than it would otherwise have been on the management agenda. Managers were of the opinion that to ensure success on Trust status, they had to show they had effective financial management control systems operating and could produce a balanced budget by the end of the 1992–3 fiscal year. But apart from the difficulties caused by the change to weighted capitation, there had been substantial fluctuations in SLTH's monthly performance reports. Like ILT and many other NHS Units, the Reforms have been implemented at a speed that made it impossible to strengthen and develop the hospital's financial information system fast enough. All these factors together heralded a period of real tension and the constant search for budget savings over the months before Trust status was confirmed.

Until the Tomlinson Report (1992) actually emerged, this tension was added to by rumours and speculation during 1991–2 about how this Inquiry might affect SLTH. To a degree these fears were founded on the damage the hospital's reputation had suffered periodically from negative coverage in both the local and national press. Once again management's fears were not realized; Tomlinson said nothing about SLTH.

Other circumstances that have played a part in determining the Unit's strategic response include the fact that the SLTH faces an acute accommodation problem as well as being a provider based on two sites. The present two-site operation increases costs because of duplications on hotel services and the difficulty of moving patients between sites. Like ILT, SLTH has a site rationalization plan but it has been delayed by the fall in land prices in the property slump. In the short term SLTH may therefore retain and use both its sites.

This leads us to SLTH's basic strategic response. The first part involves the long-term moves of cutting both provision and costs in response to the loss of funds by its main purchaser, and thence SLTH, because of the introduction of weighted capitation. The second and subsidiary part of its response is, unlike ILT, to endeavour to expand outside its home area.

There are at least two external limiting factors which have a direct impact on this expansion policy. The first is the increasingly 'protectionist' tendency of DHAs towards their local providers and, second, the small but growing number of GPFHs. At present only a few per cent of SLTH's contracts are with GPFHs but managment sees the issue as of significance in view of the Government policy decision to lower the entrance criteria and increase their numbers. Surveys of local GPs have been carried out so that the SLTH is in a position to know what GPs as a whole, and GPFHs in particular, require.[19] This was a proactive move in the face of the possibility of some heightening of competition within the merged purchasing area.

Whilst holding down costs, SLTH must also maintain the standards associated with a London teaching hospital if it is going to ensure it retains supra-Regional and national specialties. In common with the ILT, the SLTH's strategy is influenced by its medical school in that it must keep a wide range of specialties if it is going to continue as a teaching hospital. This is a stated aim of senior management who, fearful of local competition, assert 'a district general hospital is not a long-term strategy' for SLTH.

The chapter will now move on to London District Hospital (LDH) which is neither a teaching hospital nor, at the time of writing, a Trust. Our presentation will be restricted to LDH's key environmental circumstances and its basic strategic response; the enabling/limiting factors will not be offered.

Pressed on all sides

As it is in London, LDH has been affected to a certain degree by the Tomlinson Inquiry. Yet, as a smaller non-teaching hospital, it did not expect to be directly affected by the Report's findings, nor was it when they recently emerged. However, while the Inquiry was underway, it introduced uncertainty into London hospital services generally including LDH. One recent notable change is that the Unit applied for and was granted Trust status and will be in the third wave of new NHSTs.

Other salient facts include, first, it is a two-site provider Unit with similar problems to SLTH in terms of duplication of service and higher costs. Second, LDH is positioned between the inner London teaching hospitals and the out-of-London district hospitals. This is important as it could potentially lose contracts to providers outside London offering lower-priced services, as well as their local DHAs employing a 'protective strategy' towards those same providers in their 'home' areas. It is also facing some competition from the large teaching hospitals in inner London who, like SLTH, are seeking to expand into other areas. Such hospitals have an acknowledged expertise in certain specialisms which GPFHs and DHAs may want to take advantage of. These teaching hospitals may also be protected to an extent by their local commissioning bodies. A senior manager at the LDH stated that 'We lost a contract to [a London teaching hospital] despite the fact that on cost LDH was more competitive. The local commissioning body [for that teaching hospital] saw its local needs as paramount and they wanted to support their local hospital.'

Furthermore, the LDH expects that it might lose part of its contract with a neighbouring authority which wants to protect its local provider. The lost contracts could amount to as much as a fifth of the work load of the smaller of its two sites. LDH's basic strategic response is to develop this smaller Unit as an elective resource site reducing it in time to only a fraction of the beds it currently has and leaving the other hospital as the main site containing, among other things, all the A&E resources in the District. When the changes have been effected at the smaller second site and it emerges as a much reduced elective Unit, it will have become, in management's view, an effective operator in the quite difficult internal market it faces. It will be able to meet its admission times and dates as there will be no emergencies competing for beds. In fact, as a senior manager remarked to us: it 'can be run like a sausage factory'. Not only is LDH beginning to lose part of its contracts to neighbouring health authorities but, like SLTH, it is forfeiting a significant amount of contracts over the next 5 years because of the changes in the funding from RAWP to weighted capitation. As a manager remarked to us, 'The old gainers [under RAWP] will gain again. Brighton, for example, will develop a local specialty in cardiology so that there will be fewer referrals to the District specialites and London hospitals.'

LDH also has Regional specialties at its smaller site, which are likely to be relocated in nearby inner London teaching hospitals.

As a result of all the above pressures from inner and outer London hospitals on LDH, it acknowledged in its Trust application an expected falling-off in work. The management of LDH see 80% of their total work load as being entirely safe but possibly as much as 20% being at risk.

In fact, there are favourable developments that may well mean the actual contract losses are less severe than this. LDH's main purchaser, in common with DHAs up and down the country, is merging with a neighbouring DHA and FHSA. This could mean a pruning back of the smaller site's loss of contracts. The enlarged commissioning agency should be in a position to 'protect' its provider Units in the same way that the combined body did for the SLTH above. Conversely LDH will need to be even more in tune with this more powerful purchaser.

As we are comparing our London Units one with the other, it is also useful to turn to a large Trust hospital, Midlands City Hospital Trust (MCHT), well outside London to consider the place of the internal market there and discover how its influence changes. In fact, the mini case study will only be presented in enough detail to show how much less important the internal market is on this site than the previous three.

Business as usual

Geography is not the only difference MCHT has with respect to the London sites. It is a large teaching hospital which became a Trust in 1992. It is an acute unit but has no A&E facilities. These are all provided for by another even larger, nearby teaching hospital. This agreement with respect to A&E symbolizes the more 'comfortable' circumstances at MCHT.

In the run-up to becoming a Trust in April 1992, management initiated a modest cost-cutting programme which mainly involved the temporary halt on promotions and an appointments freeze. This enabled the hospital to enter Trust status with a balanced budget.

Other changes have certainly occurred but these have mainly been due to the alterations of a management and organizational nature which, in all probability, would have occurred with or without the internal market. This is not to say these are necessarily small changes. For instance, there are actually three hospitals in MCHT's area. The third will be absorbed by MCHT and its larger neighbour on the basis of a quite amicable sharing out of the extra work load. However, in common with the ILT, the MCHT also felt that the much advertised freedoms of Trust status were 'probably oversold'.

One of the more important changes for the MCHT is the creation of GPFHs. This they share with SLTH and LDH if not ILT. But again, like SLTH, they only represent a few per cent of their work load. Again this is set to expand in the next year and will continue to grow for the next few years. In the short to medium term the GPFHs' share of the health spend is likely to be less than the DHAs but it will be none the less critical to the viability of MCHT. The Trust has made significant efforts to court local GPFHs by keeping them well supplied with information and inviting them to express their views to the managers and consultants of the Trust. Even now, if GPFHs were to switch to the other nearby provider, MCHT would notice the loss.

In the main, even for our London hospitals, where competition did arise it was limited and only 'at the margins'. MCHT's area does not have the 'over-provision' London experiences and, if the Tomlinson Report (1992) is significantly implemented, even this limited competition will markedly reduce. As Lilford (1989: 1190) says, 'Only in London can we expect significant (and overdue) rationalisation.'

As has been mentioned already, there are other health providers in MCHT's area who, in principle, could act as competitors of MCHT. MCHT's large neighbouring teaching hospital in particular is held in high regard both locally and nationally. To date these two hospitals have decided implicitly, if not explicitly, to create a relationship based on cooperation, not competition. Both hospital managements recognize that each Unit should play to its strengths and the management at the MCHT told us that these rarely overlapped. Confrontation over shares of 'business' in the area seems quite unlikely. For the forseeable future there is no real pressure – internal market or otherwise – that could create this. The only uncertainty in the system is GPFH and the build-up of this will be steady enough that it probably will not seriously disrupt existing patterns.

The internal market is thus only a minor change element for the MCHT within a range of local factors. There is much evidence from this site that, in comparison to the other case studies, the changes introduced by the internal market have been to do with enhancing the power of local GPs, particularly to influence hospital policy – with respect, say, to waiting lists for acute referrals and to quality issues. It is not enough in itself to ground the conclusion that 'managed competition' declines as one moves away from the capital. However, it is consistent with such a view and the national studies also suggest this is the case.[20]

CONCLUSION

We now wish to draw conclusions about our material in the context of the wider NHS. In particular, we will:

(1)   consider some of the implications of 'competition' and 'protectionism' at the individual provider level for the overall NHS and the need for explicit regulation of purchasers – DHAs and GPFHs – and providers;

(2)   look briefly at the consistency, or otherwise, between the findings in our mini case studies and those in the wider survey reported in Chapter 7 as a way of gaining some indication of in what respects we need our Unit-based work to be representative of the NHS generally and where this is helpful to a study like ours;

(3)   review the mini case studies in terms of our basic research questions[21] which revolved around the place of the internal market in the strategic response of our four Units and, linked to that, decide whether it is indeed possible to make meaningful generalizations about the impact of the internal market on the NHS as a whole;

(4)   remind readers that the short period over which 'managed competition', and research into it, have existed and uncertainties about the degree of implementation the Tomlinson Report (1992) will receive exist as two significant caveats that surround our conclusions.

Sub-optimization and the need for regulation

In its original formulation Government policy was probably presented with competition between providers as likely to be widespread and expected to produce greater efficiency and effectiveness. Although policy-makers would now acknowledge that such competition is only likely in London and large cities, the question arises as to whether the efficiency and effectiveness gains of individual providers automatically translate themselves into equivalent gains for the system overall.

As Chapter 12 makes clear,[22] *at the Unit level*, whether actions of purchasers and providers are best dubbed as 'competition' or 'protectionism' depends on where one is standing. This is true, for example, of SLTH's desire to 'compete' with neighbouring DGHs and its worry these same neighbouring DHAs will be 'protectionist'. A retort to this could be that SLTH's main commissioning body may have 'protected' it from 'competition' by placing contracts with SLTH, not with providers outside the area. Such a policy could be depicted as a way 'to keep a strong "home market"; to establish a good "export" base' (Crump *et al.* 1990: 552).

It is not always clear whether this 'competition' and 'protectionism' as seen at the level of individual Units is beneficial or detrimental to the wider NHS and its patients. There is as yet no effective regulator publicly charged with taking this wider view and ensuring, in particular cases, purchasers' and providers' actions enhance overall and nationally defined norms of efficiency and effectiveness. This is not just a London or big city problem as the rising number of GPFHs makes the need for ensuring they are accountable an acute one.

On the representativeness of our findings

There are no major inconsistencies between conclusions reported in the large-scale survey in Chapter 7 and the findings in our four mini case studies. For example, in Chapter 7 it was reported that most DGMs rejected the idea that they were 'protecting' their own provider Units[23] but the case study material in Chapters 7 and 8 suggests that this is not always the case. In their different ways both chapters found evidence of providers being worried about the impact of GPFHs, even though they still constitute a low percentage of purchasing power. A final similarity worth noting is that both chapters point to a lack of adequate information systems as an important problem arising from the rapid implementation of the Reforms.

But there are some important differences in approach that ought to be highlighted. For instance, Chapter 7 finds some evidence of the internal market 'biting' in the inner city. Chapter 8 could be seen largely as an elaboration of that general point. But, as this occurs, even our shorter case studies begin to move into the particular circumstances of a given provider. Whilst common themes could be extracted, we think it is not these that are of real interest but rather the specific, and thence unrepresentative, details uncovered about particular cases.

Thus ours is a study centred mainly on such specific details; we do not expect or need them to be representative of the NHS as a whole beyond establishing, as we already have, the broad concurrence between large-scale studies like Chapter 7 and our own intentionally narrower, more detailed piece of work. This becomes an important point in the next subsection too as, right from the outset, it speaks against the likelihood of the place of the internal market in the Reformed NHS being meaningfully captured in broad generalizations about its role throughout the whole system.

The place of the internal market in the four strategic responses

Starting with the key environmental circumstances, they relate to the internal market in three different ways in our mini case studies. First, some of these environmental circumstances are directly created by the internal market: for example, the withdrawal of contracts (chiefly for routine work) by purchasers nearby to ILT and LDH to their own local hospitals. Second, there are instances where the underlying cause is the Government health Reforms but not the internal market directly which is simply the mechanism for effecting changes in another part of the Reform package. For instance, SLTH and LDH are significant losers under the change in the method of allocating funds within the NHS. A lower level of contracts is how this is expressed in the new system. Third are problems which are not to do with the current Reforms and may even predate them, for instance the 'over-provision' of acute services in London, which may be resolved by the Tomlinson Report (1992). In lieu of that occurring, over-provision remains a significant factor but again the internal market and contracting are merely the mechanisms, not the source of the change. Overall then the internal market is directly and indirectly *an* 'engine of change' and *a* way in which other changes – some to do with the Reforms, some not – are effected.

When introducing what we have called the enabling/limiting factors, a plethora of intra- and inter-professional, administrative, cultural, historical and economic matters enter the picture which have nothing in themselves to do with the internal market.

'Managed competition' emerges from our material as one major factor amongst a host of influences that together shape these strategic responses. Studying this complexity demands an 'eclectic' approach from researchers (Pettigrew *et al.* 1992: 8). Our simplified model in Figure 8.1 is of use here as it is possible and desirable to link its main elements with the degree of complexity the subject matter requires. Although we have been able to offer here only four brief case studies, and thence simply been able to begin to show this complexity, hopefully enough has emerged to indicate the usefulness of our simple framework.

Metaphors, 'master statements' and over-generalizations which purport to say something about the operation of the internal market throughout the entire NHS function stand more in the way of real knowledge rather than constituting it in a powerful, compressed form. This is true whether the depiction of the internal market is of a market in the common and strong sense of that term as the irresistible 'engine of change', the 'driving force', propelling everything else. If the internal market is a market, it is a market like no other.[24] The converse is equally unhelpful: to ignore the effects it clearly is having on ILT, SLTH, LDH and other NHS Units. No unqualified global statements about how 'managed competition' works can really aid comprehension. That only comes through the very details such statements suppress.

Two concluding caveats

Even the detailed findings in this chapter may need further qualification. First, no research into any aspect of the Reforms in the acute sector can have been data gathering for more than a few years and this is a very short time-span on which to base solid conclusions.[25]

Second, a key factor in the first two mini case studies, and probably the third as well, is the over-provision of hospital services in central London. Clearly, the extent of implementation of the Tomlinson Report will affect the conclusions of our individual London case studies.

To date, the politicians, the ultimate arbiters here, have been quite ineffective. For example, the Winner Report of 1972 or the findings of the London Health Planning Consortium (1979, 1980, 1981) could lead one to expect the Tomlinson Report, the 1990s re-examination of this vexed question, to be as ignored as its predecessors were. Although writing as we are in the immediate aftermath of the release of the Tomlinson Report, predictions are still not easy to make. However, it does seem possible that this time at least a partial implementation may occur.

NOTES

1 Refer to p. 102.
2 This chapter, in common with most chapters of the book, is concerned only with the changes as they affect the so-called acute services provided in NHS hospitals. This is done because, although the community sector is becoming relatively more important, the main changes in that sector are yet to occur.
3 Further, our thanks go to these managers and other NHS personnel on whose cooperation and time our data-gathering efforts depend. Regretfully our acknowledgements cannot be precise if names are to remain hidden.
4 An effective review of many of the main issues raised by the idea of a strategy is contained in a recent debate about it (Crow 1989; Morgan 1989; Shaw 1990; Knights and Morgan 1990; Watson 1990).
5 For more on the internal factors, though not linked to the notion of a strategic response, see Tilley *et al.* (1991).
6 See pp. 118–9.
7 Refer to p. 118.
8 Cf. p. 120.
9 As expressed in such NHS documents as DoH (1991). See also Chapter 12 below.
10 See p. 187 which presents this scenario from the standpoint of the suburban District that is 'intruded' upon.
11 Refer to p. 149 for an elucidation of the important distinction between fixed and variable costs.
12 They are not alone in taking such a view. See, for example, p. 219 for another acute-services manager in an inner London teaching hospital on the feasibility of winning new business in that way and pp. 197–9 on how capital charging, depreciation, work load and a variety of other factors affect price competitiveness.

13 That 'bullet' has clearly been more substantially and widely raised for the London Health Service by the Tomlinson Inquiry (1992) which could well be implemented in part, if not necessarily in all respects.

14 Cf. p. 124.

15 Another significant factor here is that ILT, unlike the Guy's Trust, lacked the dubious honour of being dubbed the 'flagship' of the NHSTs and thence finding itself at the centre of intense media interest. Refer to pp. 230–1.

16 Cf. p. 215.

17 Refer to pp. 218–9 for another acute manager's comments on the rapidity of the introduction of the Reforms, including the internal market, and the problems generally of trying to plan when knowledge of the behaviour of the Unit's costs is 'rudimentary'.

18 Refer to Chapter 11 for a detailed account of the industrial relations side.

19 Cf. pp. 193–4 where the DHA has undertaken a similar survery of GPs.

20 Refer to pp. 122–3.

21 See p. 123.

22 See pp. 185–6.

23 Refer to p. 105.

24 Cf. Chapter 5.

25 Refer, for instance, to Pettigrew (1985) which argues strenuously for, and delivers, a longitudinal study of change at ICI and his recent study of the NHS itself (Pettigrew *et al.* 1992).

REFERENCES

Agnew, T. (1992) Managers' verdict: internal market does not yet exist, *Health Service Journal*, 5 November, 8.

Crow, G. (1989) The use of the concept of 'strategy' in recent sociological literature, *Sociology*, February, 1–24.

Crump, B. *et al.* (1990) The DGM's Dilemma, *Health Service Journal*, 12 April, 552–3.

DoH (Department of Health) (1989) *Working for Patients*. London: HMSO.

DoH (Department of Health) (1990) *National Health Service and Community Care Act*. London: HMSO.

DoH (Department of Health) (1991) *The Health of the Nation*. London: HMSO.

Dobson, J. (1992a) London Lifeline Fund, *Health Service Journal*, 23 July, 5.

Dobson, J. (1992b) Statement on Trusts could disqualify twenty applicants, *Health Service Journal*, 3 September, 5.

Griffiths, R. (1983) *NHS Management Inquiry Report*. London: Department of Health and Social Security.

Ham, C. (1992) Revisiting the internal market, *British Medical Journal*, 2 February, 250–1.

Knights, D. and Morgan, G. (1990) The concept of strategy in sociology: a note of dissent, *Sociology*, August, 475–83.

Lilford, R. (1989) Looking to a better future, *Health Service Journal*, 28 September, 1190–1.

London Health Planning Consortium (1979) *Acute Hospital Services in London*. London: HMSO.

London Health Planning Consortium (1980) *Towards a Balanced Framework Reconciling Service with Teaching Needs*. London: HMSO.

London Health Planning Consortium (1981) *Primary Health Care in London*. London: HMSO.

Mintzberg, H. (1988) Opening up the definition of strategy, in J. B. Quinn *et al.* (eds.) *The Strategy Process: Concepts, Contexts, and Cases*. (eds.) Englewood Cliffs, NJ: Prentice-Hall, 13–20.

Morgan, D.H.J. (1989) Strategies and sociologists: A comment on Crow, *Sociology*, February, 25–9.

Pettigrew, A. M. (1985) *The Awakening Giant: Continuity and Change in Imperial Chemical Industries.* Oxford: Basil Blackwell.

Pettigrew, A. M. *et al.* (1992) *Shaping Strategic Change: Making Change in Large Organizations – The Case of the National Health Service.* London: Sage.

Shaw, M. (1990) Strategy and social process: military context and socio-logical analysis, *Sociology*, August, 465–74.

Tilley, I. *et al.* (1991) Hospital organization and intra-hospital interest groups: a preliminary look at change perspectives in an NHS hospital. Paper presented to the British Sociological Association Annual Conference, March, University of Manchester.

Tomlinson, B. (1992) *Report of the Inquiry into London's Health Service, Medical Education and Research.* London: HMSO

Watson, W. (1990) Strategy, rationality and inference: the possibility of symbolic performances, *Sociology*, August, 485–98.

Willcocks, L. and Harrow, J. (eds.) (1992) *Rediscovering Public Services Management.* London: McGraw-Hill.

9

Contracting and the Quality of Medical Care

Susan Kerrison

QUALITY, ITS DIFFERENT CONTEXTS AND DIFFERENT MEANINGS

'Quality' may be emerging from the NHS Reforms as one of the central notions in contracting but, in practice, it is a slippery notion and its measurement is even more vexed. The word 'quality' has now permeated all aspects of the work of the NHS and a survey (Dalley 1990) of 'quality initiatives' in the Health Service revealed that the term is applied to a whole range of developments, from the planting of spring bulbs around hospitals to the enhancement of communication skills with patients or a proposed system of managing the NHS along TQM (total quality management) lines (Pfeffer and Coote 1991). For the medical profession an important development in 'quality management' has been the introduction of a system to monitor quality of medical care: medical audit.[1]

But let's for the moment concentrate on one NHS setting where quality is important, the contracting process in the internal market. Even in this one context two not necessarily compatible views of 'quality' coexist. First, commissioners are being encouraged to use their purchasing power to buy services which are cost-effective. Since cost-effectiveness here means purchasing services which produce maximum health benefit for the money spent, DHA commissioners are concerned with the outcomes of health care and the factors which are already known to affect this. Implicit in this view is the notion that resources currently deployed and largely controlled by the medical profession could be better spent if medicine were open to market discipline and competition for 'quality', in the sense of cost-effective services, occurred.

Second, commissioners are being encouraged to insist that the services they purchase meet definable 'quality' standards. In this case 'quality' may not refer to outcomes or health gain but to process measures which specify acceptable practice to which providers should conform. The commissioners' insistence on this is thought to guard against declining standards which could occur if competition were based on cost alone. In this case the commissioners' views of what constitutes a quality standard may be influenced by factors other than a desire to maximize health gain. Political pressure to produce an equitable service or consumer preference such as setting standards for waiting time in out-patient clinics may be seen as being of equal or greater importance. On the other hand, standards based on these values may not necessarily be the most cost-effective way of doing things.

So commissioners may set a variety of standards for providers, sometimes based on different notions of quality, and providers may adopt their own standards to be used in the internal management of provider organizations. What is unclear at the moment is how the differing processes of adopting standards by providers and commissioners are developing and how, if at all, the standards emerging within these different contexts are related to one another. And, of real importance in terms of Government policy, how can the commissioners influence the providers' standards? The answer which emerges from the White Paper (DoH 1989) and subsequent documents is to see the relationship between commissioner and provider as one which can be entirely embodied within a contract where the quality of the health-care product is specified or defined. Defining the relationship between commissioner and provider in this way means that the construction, production, and control of information about quality which places obligations on the provider becomes central to the relationship between the two and assumes great importance. Furthermore, as we investigated the issue it became apparent that one key group of providers, the medical profession, in particular doctors in provider Units, will have key role at all stages in defining, shaping and manufacturing the information required by purchasers to monitor the process.[2] This somewhat paradoxical situation means that, although in theory a distinction can be made between the internal standards in provider Units and those used in contracting, in practice they may turn out to be very similar. Consequently, the initial aim of the internal market to produce cost-effective medical care by subjecting care to market mechanisms controlled by a contract starts to look distinctly problematic.

THE COMMISSIONER, THE PROVIDER AND THE MEDICAL PROFESSION: REPLACING SOCIAL VACUUM WITH SOCIAL RELATION

The neat and tidy version of the relation between DHA commissioner and provider in Government thinking depends on somewhat atomized, disconnected commissioners conjuring up and deploying quality standards on to the supplying Unit. To leave this one-way street of influence and begin to replace social vacuum with social interaction this chapter draws upon the insights gained from our fieldwork at Brunel into provider Units on the introduction of a system to monitor quality in medicine, that is, medical audit. It explores the links between this type of quality monitoring and its other setting, quality monitoring in NHS purchase contracts, the centre of interest in this chapter. Further, it considers both the practical problems of obtaining information needed for 'quality' monitoring in contracts and the influence that the medical profession may exert on this process.

Put simply, the attempts to obtain information to define and monitor quality in contracts are dependent on the following:

- the availability of 'yardsticks' to measure quality – these may be either standards or outcome measures;
- the legitimacy of the standard or outcome measure chosen (will influential players accept the chosen measure as a yardstick?);
- the ease with which information can be collected to assess whether the standard has been met.

An important point to note is all these areas must be negotiated with the medical profession – so let's start our deliberation with a brief look at quality monitoring of doctors, medical audit, and how it relates to setting quality standards for contracting.

Setting the standards

The production of standards against which to measure medical practice was resisted for many years as explicit standards were thought to inhibit clinical freedom (O'Dowd and Wilson 1991). Consequently, as the development of standards is a relatively new phenomenon, the range available is far from comprehensive, but over the last few years developments have proceeded a pace. These include the organization of a series of consensus conferences by the King's Fund, the setting-up of working parties by the Royal Colleges and the start of work on the production of standards by many other *ad hoc* professional bodies (Smith 1991). The Government has also instituted its own Clinical Standards Advisory Group to monitor and legitimate the standards in use. With the exception of the King's Fund, which used a pluralistic model of consensus development including non-experts from many different interest groups, all the other standard-setting bodies have been made up almost entirely of medical experts. Furthermore, the King's Fund has now ceased running its consensus conferences, leaving the field of standard setting to professional groups and organizations.

As Harrison (1992) points out, in a market where standard setting is heavily professionally dominated, fundamental conflicts of value are likely to occur. The values of the medical profession which underpin these standards may be fundamentally different from those which purchasers may wish to adopt. For example, at a King's Fund consensus conference on diabetic care where the panel consisted almost exclusively of expert members of the medical profession, a standard was proposed from the floor that all newly diagnosed diabetics should see a dietician. This was initially objected to by many members of the panel on the grounds that it was undesirable, impractical and inefficient as dietary advice could easily be given by both nurses and doctors. After some debate it was decided that the standard should, in fact, remain as the panel wanted to increase the number of dieticians available in provider Units and did not want to undermine the situation of existing dieticians. In this case, it might be argued that the commissioners' interest is at odds with professional values but, in other circumstances, professional values may be legitimated by public concern and not be so easy to dismiss. For example, values such as equity in terms of access to and the distribution of care, while having considerable professional and public legitimacy, may conflict with efficiency of the service. None the less, their inclusion could be seen as performing the role envisaged for them of counterbalancing the undesirable effects of a market that might otherwise be governed by economic and efficiency factors.

Yet despite this potential of professions to undermine the notion of quality as a means of producing greater efficiency, the involvement of professional providers in contract specification appears inevitable. Even the first volume of a new *British Medical Journal* publication, *Quality in Health Care*, announced a series of articles on providers' view of quality where experts from a wide range of medical specialties would be asked to 'wear the purchasers' hat' and set out what quality standards they would require if they were purchasing services (Adam 1992).

While standards have been formulated at a national level to aid contract specification, it is clear that negotiation with providers over quality standards must also take place at a local level. At present the standards formulated nationally are only available to cover a small range of health care. Local commissioners may possess or have access to (e.g. via their Directors of Public Health) insufficient expertise to cover the whole range of health care and, in the absence of all-emcompassing national standards, the expertise of local providers may need to be sought. But, more fundamentally, even if available nationally, or Regionally, formulated standards may be inapplicable to local settings and inefficient to operate within a local context. One Region in our study set standards for the treatment of upper gastrointestinal haemorrhage, but the shortage of endoscopists and the fact that some hospitals were on split sites meant that the Region's standards were impossible for all units to fulfil. In this situation it is unclear whether local providers would argue for more resources or ignore these standards if accommodation with purchasers could be reached on other issues. In practice, as Day and Klein (1987) pointed out in their study of accountability in public services, it is impossible to enforce standards which are not acceptable to both parties. In the local situation standards may prove highly negotiable; the effect of these negotiations on the efficiency and effectiveness of care has yet to be revealed.

Difficulties in monitoring standards

While the difficulties of standard setting are becoming well known, the problems of monitoring such standards are not so widely appreciated. At present the IT infrastructure for monitoring standards is largely absent. Although computerization has proceeded rapidly in recent years, the existing systems and those currently being planned predate the general use of standards in medical care and the extent to which such databases can be used to monitor standards is unknown. The fact that in many places clinicians were not involved in the development of these systems (Packwood *et al.* 1991) meant that their primary purpose was seen as a means of collecting activity data.

This does not augur well for the use of such systems to monitor the quality of medical care. In fact, a nationwide survey of medical audit support staff that our research team undertook revealed that the use of such systems for audit is low. Only 10% of these staff had ever used an RM or case-mix database in an audit and 20% elaborate HISS (Hospital Information Support System).

Furthermore, should such systems prove unsatisfactory for the monitoring of the quality of medical care, they may be difficult and costly to change. The systems are in effect controlled by managers in provider Units and financed and run by these institutions. The extent to which they may be willing to adapt them to the requirement of commissioners is unknown. Indeed it may be very difficult to adapt such systems while the standards to be used are still being contested.

For the monitoring of outcomes even greater development is needed as this requires the long-term follow-up of patients, either in out-patient departments or outside the hospital. Unlike the USA where some have suggested that an individual's dealings with the medical insurance companies mean that outcome data can be collected with ease – almost as a by-product of the administration of medical insurance (Ellwood 1988) – very few Districts in the UK can follow up patients through, for example, links between GP and hospital records. Furthermore, if the decision to commission a service is based on outcomes produced by particular providers, changes of contract will take a very long while to work through the system. It may take a number of years to assess whether the outcome of a particular intervention is successful, so commissioning for quality in the form of outcomes will contribute to making the internal market static.

The lack of any routinely collected computerized data for the purposes of monitoring quality in the initial stages of contract development means that commissioners will have to rely heavily on data from other sources. The most fundamental and important of these is the medical record. With the introduction of the internal market the medical record has assumed even greater importance in the management of health care. Apart from its obvious role in documenting activity which can be costed, in the absence of computerized records it is the only comprehensive data source which can be used to monitor quality of care. But at present the structure, organization, completeness and availability of medical records appear to be very variable. Concern over this issue has prompted leaders of the medical profession (e.g. Hopkins 1991) to argue that the first objective in improving the quality of medical care should be to improve the medical record. Without accurate comprehensive records little quality monitoring or purchasing for quality can occur. For example, research into outcomes from surgery for colorectal cancer reveals large variations in mortality. Without any supporting data on the many variables which may determine this outcome, it is not possible to understand the cause of such variations. In the context of the internal market this makes it impossible for purchasers to exercise choice about the best buy on the information available. If this type of information is absent then the temptation may be to concentrate on factors where data are more easily available. A study of quality of care and competition in the USA health-care market (Robinson 1988) suggests that, despite powerful pressure from insurers, the competition is over structural factors such as the availability of medical technology or the ratio of qualified staff to patients. Should these input factors become considered as quality standards in this country then the use of 'quality' as a mechanism for increasing efficiency, that is outputs, may become severely weakened.

But there is another aspect to the process which further muddies the waters for monitoring standards of care. Assessing quality in medical care for contracting has been described here in terms of setting and monitoring standards. In a different context this exact same process which in most cases would use the same standards and the same data source, the medical record, is called medical audit. But for the medical profession, audit is clearly defined as peer-group review (Shaw 1992): a process entirely internal and confidential to the medical profession where doctors assess the quality of their own work. These different views of the purposes of audit lead to ambiguity about whether audit is meant to serve the needs of the internal market for information about quality or the internal control of the profession. From our research it seems that in practice the way audit has been implemented would suggest that it is the view of audit as a professional tool which has prevailed. This leaves unanswered the question of where the data for monitoring quality contracts will come from.

Audit has been implemented as a confidential process encapsulated within the medical profession. The professional control of the process has been enhanced by the administrative mechanism for allocation of resources. Audit funds have been allocated through Regional and local audit committees which are constituted almost entirely from the profession. Although the intention was to allow aggregate data to be made available to managers to supply them with information about the quality of care being provided in the institution they managed, the priorities of clinicians for monitoring their work and collecting data may not be the same as the requirements of the institution for contract monitoring. In fact, in our survey of medical audit support staff, only 8% of respondents report being involved in formulating criteria or standards for use in contracting and 17% have been involved in providing audit information for monitoring contracts.

CONCLUSION

These problems are further compounded by the fact that, in the absence of any large-scale computerized data sets, the only comprehensive source of information for monitoring quality of medical care is the medical record and this remains confidential to the clinician. The fact that setting standards requires the expertise of medical providers coupled with the profession's current practical control of the primary data source means that the original notion of quality in contracts as a means of influencing the direction and work of the medical profession and purchasing for efficiency is severely weakened. Thus, it would appear that those who wish to use contracts as a means of judging performance are inevitably drawn into discussions with the performers, that is the doctors, themselves not only about what rules should be used in their judgement but also who can legitimately have access to the data required for monitoring performance. The process of specifying quality in contracting, which initially appears as a mechanism for influencing and controlling contractors, in practice requires subtle complex negotiations between the two parties.

The use of the notion of 'quality' to represent cost-effective care may have been one of the central planks of the White Paper but the current preoccupation of managers with implementing the Reforms and trying to get good cost data, coupled with the issues highlighted here, may push the process of monitoring quality in contracting away from concentrating on the production and control of information towards other types of relationship. Some see this in terms of providers developing long-term relationships with purchasers (Hughes and Dingwall 1990); others argue for strengthening the peer-review process while, at the same time, making it more transparent (Day and Klein 1987). Whatever the advantages and disadvantages of these other mechanisms, the practicalities, the costs of data collection and the power of the medical profession to resist external scrutiny exerted through everyday interaction with managers of institutions and purchasers all conspire to push the process of quality monitoring away from clearly definable quantitative standards.

NOTES

1 For two clinicians' view on medical audit, see pp.247–8.
2 See pp.192–4 and p.215–6 below for practitioner accounts of the medical profession's role in monitoring.

REFERENCES

Adam, S. (1992) Purchasing for quality: the provider's view, *Quality in Health Care*, 65.

Dalley, G. (1990) Quality management initiatives in the NHS: strategic approaches to improving quality. Unpublished paper 18. Centre for Health Economics, University of York.

Day, R. and Klein, R. (1987) *Accountabilities: Five Public Services*. London: Tavistock.

DoH (Department of Health) (1989) *Working for Patients*. London: HMSO.

Ellwood, P. (1988) A technology of patient experience, *New England Journal of Medicine*, 1549.

Harrison, A. (1992) Auditing audit, in A. Harrison and S. Bruscine (eds.) *Health Care in UK, 1991*. London: King's Fund Institute.

Hopkins, A. (1991) Approaches to medical audit, *Journal of Epidemiology and Community Health*, 1.

Hughes, D. and Dingwall, R. (1990) Sir Henry Maine, Joseph Stalin and the reorganisation of the NHS. Paper presented to the Medical Sociology Group conference of the British Sociological Association, September, Edinburgh.

O'Dowd, T. and Wilson, A. (1991) Set menus and clinical freedom, *British Medical Journal*, 450.

Packwood, T. *et al.* (1991) *Hospitals in Transition: The Resource Management Experiment.* Milton Keynes: Open University Press.

Pfeffer, R. and Coote, A. (1991) *Is Quality Good for You? A Critical Review of Quality Assurance in Welfare Services.* London: Institute of Public Policy Research.

Robinson, R. (1988) Hospital quality competition and the economics of imperfect information, *The Milbank Quarterly*, 465.

Shaw, C. (1992) The background, in R. Smith (ed.) *Audit in Action.* London: British Medical Journal.

Smith, T. (1991) In search of consensus, *British Medical Journal*, 800.

10
Contract Pricing: A Management Opportunity*

David K.D. MacKerrell

The aim of this chapter is to place the problems of arriving at prices for treatments into the context of current commercial practice. This process indicates a number of interesting subjects and we will examine three particular areas in more detail in order to highlight the opportunities inherent in the changes rather than the problems which are all too obvious to anyone who has to implement the directives.

The introduction of an internal market based on prices determined by cost has imposed enormous responsibilities on those managers charged with the calculation of these figures as well as setting in train a significant change in the culture of the whole Service. The existing method of financial control was based entirely on restricting total expenditure. This is now being replaced by a system incorporating an element of 'managed competition' which should allow providing institutions actually to increase expenditure if they can attract sufficient extra paid work. The effectiveness of this approach depends, however, on the production of accurate costs for medical procedures. What happens to those institutions which fail to attract sufficient business is not made clear but the inference must be that they will shrink in order to match their expenditure to their income.

The new method of financial control has necessitated a change in the type of financial information required. Previously information was required to operate controls with a historical focus: 'How much have we spent? How much do we have left?' Now the need is for additional forecasts of future activity: 'How many treatments are we going to contract for next year? At what price? How much money will that give us to spend?'

The enormous increase in the amount of detailed information required to operate successfully in the internal market will clearly involve much effort and cost to produce. However, it also carries with it unique opportunities for managers to influence three very important apects of business management:

* I wish to acknowledge the considerable help I have received from Ian Tilley in the form of a detailed reading and valuable suggestions to improve the first draft of this chapter.

- the enthusiasm of customers, by the level of prices set;
- the behaviour of colleagues, by the method of apportioning indirect costs for pricing purposes;
- the structure of the organization, by the design of the internal-control systems.

These opportunities are not covert operations designed to increase the influence of financial managers; they are the possibly unplanned by-products of decisions which have to be made in order to implement the changes mandated by the NHS Management Executive (NHSME). In order to delineate these opportunities it is necessary to examine problems associated with costing and pricing contracts.

PROBLEMS FACING PROVIDERS

This section considers some of the particular problems encountered in NHS acute Units which are establishing costs and prices and relates them to developments in management accounting in the private sector. These developments will be of considerable interest to managers who find themselves operating in a competitive environment for the first time.

The fundamental principles set out by the NHSME (1990: 1) for the establishment of service costs and prices are:

- Prices should be based on costs.
- Costs should generally be arrived at on a full-cost basis.
- There should be no planned cross-subsidization between contracts.

The second principle referring to 'full cost' requires some explanation. Figure 10.1 compares current manufacturing terminology with its NHS equivalent.

Although there are no real problems of terminology, differences emerge when we look at how these figure are calculated following the recommendation of the NHSME (1990: 2) to use 'average specialty costs'.

Prime cost versus specialty cost

In industry the prime cost of a product is calculated by taking the cost of the raw material needed for the production of one unit and adding the labour required to produce that unit. The NHS equivalent is derived by adding up the total costs allocated to that specialty in a year and dividing this total by the number of finished consultant episodes (FCEs), thus arriving at a cost per consultant episode. The current absence of adequate case-mix information[1] for the majority, if not all, providers means that the cost per consultant episode is a rather crude approximation. Indeed commentators have expressed the view that 'specialty costs offer little if any contribution to the contracting process' (Prowle *et al.* 1989: 51). This view is supported by the interim findings of a research study, commissioned by the Chartered Institute of Management Accountants, into the prices and costing approaches adopted

MANUFACTURING Unit cost:		NHS Procedure cost:	
Direct: Materials	**		
Labour	**		
Prime cost	**	Specialty cost	**
Manufacturing overhead	**	General services	**
Manufacturing cost	**		
Admin. and selling overhead	**	District and Regional costs	**
FULL COST	**	FULL COST	**

Figure 10.1 A comparison of costing terminology in manufacturing and the NHS

by hospitals in the West Midlands: 'The data base revealed vast variations in the specialty prices . . . a consultant episode can cost from £350 to £1,353 in obstetrics and from £469 to £3,417 in dermatology and so on' (Ellwood 1991: 27).

This problem of a lack of detailed reliable information is continued when we come to consider the methods used to apportion overheads/general services.

Manufacturing overheads versus general services

In industry, manufacturing cost, which is used for the valuation of manufactured stocks and work in progress, 'will include all related production overheads' (Statement of Standard Accounting Practice No.9 1975: 2). The usual method for arriving at this figure in an organization which has a number of different departments and a range of different products is to take each production department and allocate indirect manufacturing overhead costs (for example, storekeeper's wages, factory rent) to that department. Next these total costs are reallocated over the actual items produced or operations performed. The use of a single basis for apportioning all overheads, a blanket rate, is only recommended where all products are identical.

Bearing in mind that approximately 40% of hospital costs are indirect, the apportionment of this cost is clearly important. Furthermore, given the fact that 'the vast majority of hospitals included such costs by an arbitrary addition to in-patient and out-patient contracts' (Ellwood 1991: 28) coupled with the imprecision of specialty costs noted earlier it is perhaps not surprising that procedure costs varied to an even greater extent than consultant episodes. Ellwood (1991: 27) found variations of up to 1,280% and observes 'such variations could be due to the crude nature of the costing approaches rather than true variations in treatment patterns and the cost of resource inputs'.

From a practical point of view the NHSME guidelines have produced extraordinarily different results in different hospitals. The solution is clearly that more detailed information is required and it makes obvious sense to make as much use as possible of the experience of industry in dealing with these considerable problems. In order to appreciate the current thinking in industry it will be necessary to refer, albeit sketchily, to the history of costing as this will shed some light on how techniques were developed to solve problems as they occurred and the range of options available to the NHS. Throughout the chapter I rely on the high-profile account by Johnson and Kaplan (1987).

The development of costing

Essentially the first time that a need for costing was recorded occurred during the Industrial Revolution. The concept of conversion cost was devised in order to control the activities of workers in the new factories. This concept was used to analyse the expenses incurred in converting raw materials into manufactured products in order to control those operations and increase efficiency. One important point is that these calculations only incorporated variable costs.

The distinction between variable and fixed costs is fundamental to an understanding of the whole story and current developments both in industry and in the NHS, so it is important to establish a definition. Variable costs are those that vary in direct proportion to the level of manufacturing activity (for example, raw materials, piece-work wages). Fixed costs are those which do not change, in the short term, with increases or reductions in production (for example, factory rent, fixed salaries paid to factory supervisors, depreciation of machinery). Thus in an electricity bill the units consumed are a variable cost and the standing charge is a fixed cost.

To restate, conversion costing at a single location needed to take into account only variable costs in order to control the activities of the employees. The expansion of these enterprises on to different manufacturing sites obliged the proprietors to take into account the fixed costs of the different sites in order to compare and control the performance of the managers in charge of the various locations. Larger industrial and commercial organizations devised performance measures which could be used to compare efficiency between a number of different, although comparable, production or service centres. An excellent example of these performance measures is the 'cost per ton-mile' developed by the US railways in the late nineteenth century. These performance measures incorporated direct fixed costs (for example depreciation of production machinery) as well as direct variable costs (e.g. raw materials) but not indirect costs (e.g. head office rent). The last category was not included because it was not deemed relevant, for control purposes, to load each separate unit with a share of such centrally incurred costs and then to attempt to compare their performance. The formulation of performance measures for hospitals is a pressing need since, from the above evidence, a 'consultant episode' does not seem to be sufficiently precise.

However, returning to our brief history, the inclusion of indirect overhead costs into the calculations finally occurred in the USA in the early years of the twentieth century, with the development of conglomerates where proprietors needed to compare the return on their investments in different industries operating in quite separate divisions.

Johnson and Kaplan in their background history argue that all the main techniques in current use had been established as early as the start of the First World War. This version has not been universally accepted by accounting historians but the fierceness of the ensuing debate indicates that there must be some truth in their contentions. What has occupied accountants since 1914 is the search for more effective ways of applying these techniques, the incorporation of computers into the systems for performing the calculations and different ways of apportioning indirect costs to products or services. We shall be referring to some of these recent developments later, namely activity-based costing (ABC), just-in-time manufacturing (JIT), and total quality management (TQM), but all the reader need be aware of at this stage is the diversity of approach available to meet particular situations, always bearing in mind the distinction between variable and fixed costs. Our major concern, now that we have looked at the types of cost brought into consideration by proprietors in order to manage their businesses, is to look at what methods are used by the private sector to set prices for their goods and services.

Methods of pricing

In a purely competitive market the pricing mechanism operates in order to balance supply and demand, with prices constantly changing in order to achieve that balance. The internal market in the NHS is a long way from the economists' concept of a purely competitive market.[2] None the less it is clear that price is intended to have some effect on the contracting strategies of the purchasing authorities. The insistence of the NHSME that prices should be based on full cost – including all direct and indirect fixed and variable costs – is at odds with the way that industry usually goes about setting prices. In non-monopoly situations when there is considerable demand and a significant number of producers and purchasers, the price is determined by the market for all participants. Where there is no such established price a producer would tend to use a variable cost basis, that is, ignoring fixed costs, as a first step to establishing a selling price. This approach uses the concept of contribution as the first step in establishing a selling price. The contribution is the difference between the selling price of a product and its variable cost. This amount is regarded as a contribution towards fixed costs and profit. The important division is between variable costs and fixed costs (see above).

The procedure used to arrive at a selling price might be as follows. First the variable costs are established. Next a standard mark-up is added to arrive at a provisional selling price. The sales department then forecasts how many items are likely to be sold at that price. From this information the accountants then calculate the total contribution (contribution per unit times number of units sold) in order to establish if this total contribution is large enough to pay all expected fixed costs, leaving enough to provide a reasonable profit margin. If the first attempt does not provide a satisfactory return then different selling prices with their associated likely volumes and total contributions are considered in order to find the combination which will maximize contribution, in order to pay all fixed costs and provide the required profit.[3] With this information on a number of options the manufacturer can then decide which products to produce, and in what order of priority. This approach to setting a selling price relies on an accurate split between fully fixed and truly variable costs which in practice is extremely difficult to achieve. However, this textbook approach does not begin to exhaust the actual methods used in the private sector to set selling prices. For example, several extremely successful Japanese producers are believed to start from the other end of the equation: the selling price, rather than likely costs, of a new product. The marketing department decides on the selling price and the production engineers then design it down to an acceptable variable cost. Or manufacturers can rely on what the sales department says is the market price and wait until the end of the year and the final audit in order to find out whether they are making a profit. Each organization will have its own approach to setting a selling price and this brief account is merely intended to convey the diversity of approaches used by the private sector and hence potentially available to providing institutions in the NHS. We are now ready to consider our first area of opportunity for NHS managers in the internal market: the possibility, in theory at least, of influencing the throughput of their Unit by the level of prices they set.

THE FIRST MANAGEMENT OPPORTUNITY: INFLUENCING THE ENTHUSIASM OF CUSTOMERS BY THE LEVEL OF PRICES SET

The first point is that in commerce prices are not usually based on full cost, the way in which NHS managers have been directed to proceed (NHSME 1990: 1). They are normally determined by the market-place. Second, private-sector decisions concerning prices are not infrequently taken using a marginal basis, not a full-cost basis, at least in the short term. It is likely, as the internal market develops, that prices will have an increasing effect on the referral choices of purchasing bodies, especially where a particular NHS Unit faces at least a contestable market-place.[4] But how can a manager affect the result of a calculation when the method of calculation has been predetermined? Simply the manager must select an appropriate basis for allocating indirect costs to individual procedures in order to arrive at a 'full cost'. The following simple illustration demonstrates how the selection of different bases of allocation of general service overheads can affect a procedure price significantly.

A specialty has an allocation of general service (indirect) costs of £200,000;

400 procedures were carried out last year taking an average time of 30 minutes each, at a total direct cost of £400,000.

We are looking for a suitable basis to spread these costs over individual procedures. The details for two of the many procedures offered by the specialty are as follows:

Procedure A: Complex, requiring sophisticated equipment and expensive personnel; direct cost £1,000; takes 1 hour.

Procedure B: Straightforward; direct cost £600; but takes 2 hours.

All three bases for allocating costs to Procedures A and B in Table 10.1 – per procedure, per hour, or per £ of direct cost – are perfectly reasonable but give very different prices. Therefore the selection of the allocation base can significantly affect prices. This is not the only point where the selection of a cost-allocation basis can have a profound effect on the total cost of a procedure. Let's go one step back from the allocations in Table 10.1. How was it decided in the first place, that the sum of £200,000 was the correct proportion of the total general service overhead to charge to the specialty in our illustration? The answer is: on an arbitrary basis, chosen from a number of alternatives, using what information was available when the choice was made. Thus NHS managers are forced to decide from a number of alternatives which bases should be used at each stage of a complex series of allocations and reallocations. Each decision will affect the 'full cost' of a procedure and the cumulative effect can be profound. Each individual basis has its pros and cons. None represents a theoretical ideal and each NHS Unit must make its own combination of choices unfettered and unguided by the NHSME. Such ambiguity exists in the published accounts of the private sector since stocks of manufactured goods and work-in-progress are valued including manufacturing overheads. But industry has learned that the variable basis is infinitely more valuable for decision-making, such as setting prices. The cost-allocation decisions of NHS finance directors and chief executives will have a profound effect on their Unit's prices while conforming exactly to the

Table 10.1 The allocation of general service costs

	Per procedure* (£)	Per hour† (£)	Per direct cost‡ (£)
Procedure A	500	1,000	500
Procedure B	500	2,000	300

* Per procedure equals total indirect costs (£200,000) divided by the number of procedures performed (400) or £500 per treatment for both Procedures A and B.
† Per hour equals indirect costs (£200,000) divided by the total hours (400 procedures at an average of 30 minutes per procedure throughout the specialty) or 200 hours giving a rate of £1,000 per hour or £1,000 and £2,000 for Procedures A and B respectively.
‡Per direct cost, that is, procedures should bear indirect costs (£200,000) in the proportion of their direct costs (£400,000) or an allocation of 50p per £1 of direct costs or £500 and £300 for Procedures A and B respectively.

NHSME directive that 'There should be no planned cross-subsidies' (NHSME 1990: 1)

It must be emphasized that these decisions do not affect the total level of overhead expenses, they merely change the way those expenses are reflected in the prices of individual treatments. Imagine a providing institution which has a very close relationship with one or two particular purchasers who require a relatively stable suite of treatments. The first attempt at pricing the level of service provided last year as a basis for next year's block contracts is found to be too expensive. Then the selection of another, equally defensible basis of allocating indirect costs to treatments may allow the provision of the same number of treatments or perhaps even more! For those NHS Units which face a degreee of competition in the internal market this 'flexibility' should prove invaluable.

This first opportunity is concerned with a Unit's relationship with its external customers, and is essentially one of decision-making on a once-a-year basis since price lists remain effective for 12 months. The second area of opportunity for managers also concerns the allocation of overhead costs but in a quite different context, the month-to-month internal management of the Unit. It is specifically about influencing the behaviour of colleagues from other professions by seeking ways of allocating overheads in internal reporting which give much more meaningful information than the arbitrary methods described above. The aim is to reflect more accurately the total cost consequences of individual decisions and choices. The third area of opportunity also concerns the internal management of a Unit but occurs in the search for a creative solution to the problem of selecting a system of internal control. However, let us continue with the theme of overhead allocation and look at the second opportunity.

THE SECOND OPPORTUNITY: INFLUENCING THE BEHAVIOUR OF COLLEAGUES BY THE METHOD OF APPORTIONING INDIRECT COSTS

The second area of opportunity is the possibility of influencing the actions of individuals in the organization through the method of allocation of overhead costs. As a by-product of this exercise you will also view the operation of your organization from an entirely different perspective. We have just seen how, in order to calculate the 'full cost' of a treatment, an element of overhead expense has to be added to the direct costs of a procedure. This is done by allocating a share of the total overheads to a department and then reallocating those costs to the procedures performed by that department. We have also seen that this process is arbitrary and imprecise and also that if 40% of the average NHS Unit expenditure falls into this category then these are important items. At this stage we should attempt a definition of direct and indirect costs. Direct costs are those which can be directly traced to the individual procedure (for example, consumables and direct labour). Indirect costs are all the rest, those items or classes of expenditure which cover a number of different procedures. In this section we are mainly concerned with the apportionment of general service costs and we will be using the pharmacy as an example because there is an immediate parallel in industry, that of the stores. In order to demonstrate how the method of allocating indirect costs can influence the behaviour of colleagues we must first look at the traditional method of allocating service department expenditure.

The textbooks describe how the cost of running a service department is first collected in a cost centre. That cost centre is charged with all the expenses, salaries, premises costs, light and heat, etc. That total is then reallocated to the production departments on a suitable basis. The stores is a close equivalent to the pharmacy, and the probable basis of reallocation would be the number of stores requisitions issued in the previous period by all the production departments. When it came to allocating production overheads to individual products for stock valuation purposes then all the indirect costs, in the absence of better information, would be apportioned to those products using the most reasonable basis, probably the amount of time spent by direct labour on making those products.[5] This method provided a reasonable basis for valuing stock when the majority of service departments were linked to the amount of direct labour (for example, personnel, wages, canteen). But manufacturing is becoming increasingly automated and the direct labour cost as a proportion of total cost can shrink to 5% or lower. So the use of the direct labour basis for apportioning overheads is not sufficiently precise for internal decision-making in such areas as pricing and product mix. The search by manufacturing industry for a solution to this problem has led to the development of activity-based costing which seeks to link all costs to cost drivers, those actions which require money to be spent. In the particular case we will be looking at there was a problem with the steadily increasing cost of running the stores. The stores manager was unable to contain costs because the designers required an ever-increasing number of different parts which meant that the stores had more goods in them which meant more money was needed to finance the increased stock. The stores also needed more space to house the increased stock and more employees to control the stock. Management experienced great difficulty in trying to convince the designers to use standard parts instead of new slightly different parts. This may have been because the cost calculations charged products only with the bought-in price of the components. The cost of running the stores was lost in a charge for general overheads over which the designers had no control. This case demonstrates that by improving the quality of information provided to colleagues it is possible to effect a change in their approach to their jobs. This approach is particularly relevant to the NHS in that a method has to be devised to base prices on full costs, and it makes obvious sense to take advantage of the latest developments in industry when seeking to implement a system originally devised by industry.[6]

An example of ABC in use

An excellent example of the problems of apportioning the cost of running the stores in a manufacturing environment is contained in a case study on

Tektronix: Portable Instruments Division (B) (Cooper and Turney 1988). This case concerns a manufacturer of portable electronic instruments who allocated the costs of running the stores, along with other service departments, on the basis of direct labour.

However, with the development of manufacturing processes the company had reduced labour costs to only 4% of total costs. There was a widespread belief that the system of overhead allocation did not reflect the true cost drivers. Management also believed that the increasing costs of the stores operation were due to a proliferation in the number of different types of part held. Management decided that a new basis had to be found which would accurately reflect the cost drivers and help reduce the proliferation of parts.

Four cost drivers were identified:

(1) costs due to the value of parts (interest on the total value of stock held);
(2) costs due to the absolute number of parts (space occupied by the stores);
(3) costs due to the maintenance and handling of each different part number (maintaining separate specifications and separate ordering/ reordering quantities);
(4) costs due to each use of a different part number (costs of stores issues).

They found that (3) was easily the most significant of the four, and therefore decided to allocate the costs of maintaining the stores on a two-stage basis. First, the total cost of running the stores was divided by the number of separate part numbers in order to arrive at a cost for maintaining a part number. Second, this annual cost was divided by the annual usage, in units of that particular part, thus arriving at an overhead rate for each part. These costs would be added to the buying-in price for each part and designers would be made aware of the substantial cost savings which could be made by using standard parts.

ABC's potential usefulness

The important point here is that management was looking for a way to reduce the number of separate parts carried in the stores, and by selecting a basis of overhead apportionment which reflected the main cost driver they hoped that cost-concious designers would react by using standard parts. These were much cheaper than special orders for the company as a whole, a fact that the original allocation system did not reveal.

The parallel between this problem and inefficient resource use in the NHS is clear enough. It is important to note that there are additional costs involved when changing an existing system, but these can be minimal where there is no existing system. Indeed Bromwich and Bhimani (1989: 5) emphasize that 'there is no doubt that where activity-caused costs can be measured in a meaningful way, activity-based costing can be expected to yield substantial benefits but the cost of the process needs to be considered'.

This case study also illustrates that technical accounting procedures can have clear organizational effects. This theme is continued by our consideration of the third area of opportunity which explores the interrelationship of accounting control systems and the formal structure of organizations.

THE THIRD OPPORTUNITY: INFLUENCING THE STRUCTURE OF THE ORGANIZATION BY THE DESIGN OF THE INTERNAL-CONTROL SYSTEM

The third area of management opportunity facilitated by the introduction of treatment pricing is the organizational aspect of how an enterprise views itself and controls its activities. The example taken to illustrate this is to contrast an older approach, standard costing, with the more group-focused JIT production methods successfully pioneered by large Japanese companies.

The decision to introduce commercial practices on a significant scale into the NHS inevitably brings a different viewpoint from which to judge an institution. There are many pitfalls in this process, but there is the chance to incorporate the best of current commercial practice without the necessity of suffering the trauma of evolving through all the stages that have so far marked this process for the private sector. There are currently a number of developments in management theory being applied to the manufacturing sector. Concepts such as JIT manufacturing or total quality management (TQM) are both aimed at changing the way management views, controls and organizes the operations for which it is responsible. I will be concentrating on JIT which has clear implications for quality.

The history of how traditional control principles evolved in the West demonstrates how those methods came to concentrate on individual rather than group performance and a hierarchy of responsibility also focused on individuals.

Continuing our history of accounting control systems

Again turning to Johnson and Kaplan's (1987) historical sketch, the first concepts of costing were basically developed during the Industrial Revolution in order to control the efficiency of the conversion processes in the factories of the new vertically integrated industries, such as textiles. The owners of factories needed information on the internal operations of their factories which now took in wool and produced finished cloth. Arising out of this conglomeration of different processes was a need for information on which departments were most proficient in particular processes, and the cost breakdown of the overall operation, not only to take advantage of any efficiencies but also to control the activities of the workforce. It is worth remembering that these factories commonly produced only a single product so that the measurement of output was straightforward. Expenses were charged to specific departments and the output of those departments was compared with the costs thus producing a measure of efficiency and a basis for control.

During the late nineteenth century there emerged a new group of specialist businesses with processes which could be applied to produce a huge variety of different products. For example, an engineering company expert in drilling, boring and grinding would perform these three basic functions on a variety of different parts. The emergence of this variety of products meant that there was no one simple measure of output which could be applied to all products. Some castings could be both bulky and very heavy but require little skilled machining; others could be small and light yet need considerable amounts of intricate work. Weight, for instance, was not a sufficiently sensitive measure of output to be useful in both cases.

Such firms therefore developed the idea of a predetermined 'standard' for the amount of work required to complete a single operation. Breaking down the production process to individual operations allowed an accurate assessment of how long each process would take and therefore cost. More importantly it allowed the efficiency of operators to be controlled by comparing their hours worked with the standard time they should have taken to achieve their output.

Standard costing is an effective method of control where activities can be broken down into individual operations which are repetitive and identical. It becomes impossible to use where activities are not identical as each operation has to have a different standard, and the expense of calculation of these standards is unwarranted if these operations are only performed occasionally.

Standard costing emerged clearly as the preferred method of controlling mass production. It is still the current norm in the industrialized West even though it requires a vast number of records to be collected, weekly records of each productive employee's performance, a separate standard for each operation, and huge numbers of comparisons to be made and variances investigated by very many skilled and therefore expensive staff.

During the 1970s, while standard costing remained supreme in Western manufacturing circles, the Japanese producers were devising entirely new control concepts which have been increasingly studied in Western countries because of the success of Japanese manufacturing organizations.

Developments in Japanese industry

While Western manufacturers were frequently basing production on big batches in order to spread the fixed costs of setting up the machines over a large number of items, the Japanese with JIT manufacturing were striving to achieve a continuous stream of products, all being worked on at the same time, proceeding through the production line in unbroken succession with components arriving just as required, reducing stock levels towards zero. Further finished goods would be delivered to waiting customers as they emerged from the factory.

Figure 10.2 is not intended to be a summary of all the differences between the two production cultures; it merely highlights some of the major contrasts between the opposing approaches.

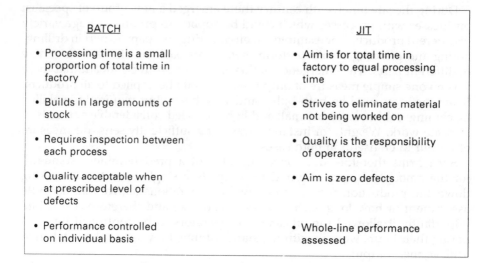

BATCH	JIT
• Processing time is a small proportion of total time in factory	• Aim is for total time in factory to equal processing time
• Builds in large amounts of stock	• Strives to eliminate material not being worked on
• Requires inspection between each process	• Quality is the responsibility of operators
• Quality acceptable when at prescribed level of defects	• Aim is zero defects
• Performance controlled on individual basis	• Whole-line performance assessed

Figure 10.2　Batch and JIT: contrasting elements of production control. *Source*: Johnson and Kaplan (1987)

The benefits of the Japanese approach to production organization are much too numerous to mention here as are the difficulties which have to be overcome before the benefits are realized. It must be remembered also that these techniques were developed in a high-volume production environment rather than a purely service operation.

The two main benefits to the NHS manager are: first, the considerable saving in internal documentation by controlling an entire production facility rather than each individual working in that facility; and, second, the real improvement in the quality of production and considerable potential savings in the cost of quality control that often occur as a result of acknowledging the dependence of each member of a team on the people before and after them in the line and relying on the self-discipline of team responsibility.

The real basis of Japanese manufacturing success is not confined to one area: their current production techniques using robots and computer control; the relationships between banks and manufacturers, between the big producers and their component suppliers; the climate of industrial relations; their cultural or religious legacy; or whatever. The true source of their success in Japan or that of Japanese manufacturers operating in the West itself is their capacity for adapting constantly to changing circumstances and their enthusiasm for continuous learning and improvement.

The challenge for the NHS manager is to avoid what may seem the natural path to follow: standard costing, at a time when its dysfunctional effects have never been more loudly voiced and private-sector firms are engaged in considerable debate and experiment with the new control principles and organization structures.

The opportunity here is for the NHS manager to take advantage of these new developments like JIT and avoid the pitfalls of trying to adapt standard costing to a hospital environment, to select a system of control which utilizes the self-discipline of teamwork by being based on group performance, with the promise of considerable cost savings and quality enhancements.

CONCLUSION

We have looked at three areas where, by making a particular selection from the many alternatives available, management can steer the organization towards – rather than away from – enhanced efficiency and effectiveness. There is enough latitude in the guidelines presented by the NHSME to enable the manager making the selection to contribute significantly to the direction, the behaviour and the structure of their Unit.

Some warnings ought to be posted along the way. First, decisions made now will assume a momentum of their own and may be difficult to redirect or reverse at a later stage. Consequently it is important to take these decisions with the future in mind, rather than the past. Second, in the words of the NHSME (1990: 2), 'The benefits from more detailed cost analysis should always exceed the cost of producing it.' This should perhaps be put on a large sign on the desk of every person producing management information. Management information systems can be extremely expensive to create and there is no one correct way, no magic formula for producing information. There is a constant temptation to invest in the next stage – the latest piece of hardware, the most up-to-date piece of software – but, if the outcome is not a different, better decision, then the effort may well be wasted. The final thought is that, although requiring large amounts of hard work in a subtly changed environment, the process of setting prices does provide the manager responsible for calculating the numbers with a large, powerful lever which, certainly for those Units facing 'managed competition', must be used effectively.

NOTES

1 For some details about case mix see pp. 92–4.
2 For an examination of this notion and its usefulness in considering the internal market in the NHS, see pp. 70–2.
3 In the case of the NHS internal market Units are limited to a return on assets employed of 6%. Refer to p. 61.
4 For a brief explanation of this idea, see p. 71.
5 This was, you will recall, the third method used for pricing purposes in Table 10.1.
6 ABC is sufficiently new that considerable controversy and a large literature surrounds its use in the private sector, with prominent writers like Johnson and Kaplan (1987) seeing it as something of a panacea for all the ills of management accounting. For a more cautious appraisal by prominent UK academic accountants refer to Bromwich and Bhimani (1989).

REFERENCES

Bromwich, M. and Bhimani, A. (1989) *Management Accounting: Evolution not Revolution.* London: Chartered Institute of Management Accountants.

Cooper, R. and Turney, P.B.B. (1988) *Tektronix: Portable Instruments Division (B) 9–188–143.* Boston, Mass: Harvard Business School.

Ellwood, S. M. (1991) Costing and pricing healthcare, *Management Accounting* [UK], November, 26–8.

Johnson, H.T. and Kaplan, R.S. (1987) *Relevance Lost.* Boston, Mass: Harvard Business School.

NHSME (National Health Service Management Executive) (1990) *Costing and Pricing Contracts.* London: HMSO.

Prowle, M. *et al.* (1989) *Working for Patients: The Financial Agenda.* London: Certified Accountants Publications.

Statement of Standard Accounting Practice No. 9 (1975) *Stocks and Work in Progress.* London: HMSO.

11

Industrial Relations under 'Managed Competition'

Roger V. Seifert

INTRODUCTION

As yet there is little hard evidence as to the impact of the internal market on industrial relations in hospitals. There is some information about developments in single-employer Trusts, but at this time it is difficult to distinguish between changes caused by various aspects of the 1990 Reforms and those attributable to more general movements in the Health Service.

This paper sets out a few of the main features of current industrial relations and provides examples of recent issues. The two major concerns for the management of the providers of health care are the total costs of employing any given mix of labour (pay, employers' on-costs and conditions of service), and the managerial controls over the workforce required to secure highest levels of performance at least possible cost. Competition between providers for contracts within the internal market will result in pressures to reduce total and unit costs of labour, and in increased competition for scarce labour which will push up some labour costs.

What follows is a brief summary of the traditional approach to industrial relations in the NHS and some comments on the mechanisms and issues associated with hospital-level pay bargaining. It ends with a few points about managerial controls through the introduction of human resource management, flexibility, reduction in the role of trade unions and the use of procedural agreements to enforce the right to manage. It is based on the preliminary findings from our current research project at the Centre for Industrial Relations, University of Keele, into hospital-level industrial relations.

TRADITIONAL METHODS OF SETTLING THE TOTAL REMUNERATION PACKAGE FOR HEALTH SERVICE STAFF

Between 1948 and 1984 the pay and conditions of service for the vast majority of NHS staff were determined through Whitley Councils in which national agreements set effective rates. In such a collective bargaining system staff were divided into functional units, such as nurses and ancillary, and most negotiations were multi-union/multi-employer. The main NHS employers, the health authorities/boards, agreed a common set of propositions with which to bargain against whatever group of trade unions represented the Staff Side. For example, nurses, midwives and health visitors are represented on their Whitley Council by 12 organizations of which the largest are the RCN, NUPE, COHSE, RCM, NALGO and the HVA.

For both sides such a representative system meant that there were often bitter divisions amongst the parties on each side which delayed settlements and made it easier for the DoH to frustrate negotiations by intervening on behalf of government. This aspect of Whitley has been analysed in terms of the problems of intra-organizational bargaining (Walton and McKersie 1965), and has been subject to frequent reports and calls for reform (McCarthy 1976).

Three salient features of this system were that:

(1) it allowed little scope for local variation;
(2) increasingly it led to settlements only after industrial action and/or pay inquiries;
(3) it encouraged trade union recognition and high levels of membership.
                            (Clay 1929; Clegg and Chester 1957)

A combination of interrelated factors caused the breakdown in this traditional system of which the current developments form a part. As Table 11.1 shows, in the 1960s and 1970s levels of employment in the NHS expanded rapidly and the balance of staff composition changed. For example, while the numbers of hospital doctors rose by 285% between 1951 and 1985, professional and technical staff numbers increased by 530%, but ancillary grades went up by a mere 35%. At the same time the latter's pay tended to fall behind other groups as a result of the uneven impact of incomes policies and also due to public expenditure squeezes (Mailly *et al.* 1989). It became increasingly difficult to manage the Service effectively, and both managers and staff were worried and frustrated by the lack of action and reform (Edwards 1979).

There was an emergent revolt from below, caused by three main factors within the NHS:

(1) larger hospitals with the associated problems of large employment units (Carpenter 1988)
(2) relatively poor pay and conditions (Halsbury 1974; Clegg 1980);
(3) the implementation of modern management techniques (Griffiths 1983).

The first response of staff was to join trade unions in large numbers, and for an important minority to become active in them (Taylor 1978; Carpenter 1982). There was an expansion of stewards among both the traditional TUC-affiliated general unions (NUPE, COHSE, NALGO and MSF) and the single-profession associations (BMA, RCN and CSP) which developed their own stewards' networks in the mid-1970s when they became more like trade unions (Seifert 1992). This expansion of trade union activity fed into, and gained strength from, increased levels of industrial action. Between 1972 and 1982 there

Table 11.1 Numbers of staff employed in NHS hospitals by category

Year (at 31 Dec.)	Medical and dental staff (whole-time)	Nurses and midwifery staff*	Professional and technical staff†	A&C staff†	Domestic and ancillary staff‡	Total
1951	11,375	188,580	14,110	29,021	163,666	406,752
1952	11,894	194,861	14,844	29,101	171,077	421,777
1953	12,036	201,564	17,061	31,429	151,700	413,790
1954	12,510	204,485	18,331	32,795	155,774	423,895
1955	12,866	206,567	19,404	33,421	157,917	430,175
1956	13,240	212,917	19,941	34,593	160,463	441,154
1957	13,523	218,331	20,383	35,904	163,548	451,689
1958	13,575	226,770	20,879	36,643	171,077	468,944
1959	19,198	236,717	22,970	37,212	201,624	517,721
1960	19,853	242,164	24,002	38,450	202,968	527,437
1961	20,345	249,571	27,460	40,877	210,308	548,561
1962	21,095	264,657	28,555	42,675	215,528	572,510
1963	21,684	267,725	29,850	44,075	215,245	578,579
1964	22,147	275,537	31,060	45,667	217,410	591,821
1965	22,939	290,338	32,720	47,872	218,191	612,060
1966	23,605	303,338	34,353	50,110	224,005	635,411
1967	24,652	315,896	36,112	51,902	229,596	658,158
1968	25,680	320,142	36,929	51,434	227,039	661,224
1969	26,604	330,684	38,763	54,097	227,461	667,609
1970	27,398	343,664	41,696	56,877	229,313	698,948
1971	28,852	361,980	43,089	60,050	235,642	729,613
1972	30,379	382,652	45,343	64,551	236,940	759,865
1973	31,670	392,387	47,785	69,184	231,050	772,076
1974	33,026	408,146	47,015	89,999	230,944	809,130
1975	34,817	445,720	57,011	106,454	235,209	879,211
1976	35,759	452,882	65,204	113,637	242,212	909,694
1977	36,796	452,258	65,357	114,206	241,823	910,440
1978	37,981	450,042	69,024	116,080	241,047	914,174
1979	39,525	460,683	72,390	118,691	239,419	930,708
1980	40,618	476,182	74,558	121,528	240,791	953,677
1981	41,465	502,581	78,269	125,275	241,718	989,308
1982	42,159	509,454	80,543	125,483	239,865	997,504
1983	43,006	509,656	82,505	126,914	239,565	1,001,646
1984	43,315	509,708	86,893	127,522	239,319	1,006,575
1985	43,799	514,962	88,872	128,567	221,429	997,629

* Whole-time and part-time.
† Excluding part-time staff in Scotland.
‡ Including works, maintenance, ancillary, ambulance and transport staff.

Source: Office of Health Economics (1987) *Compendium of Health Statistics*. London: Office of Health Economics, 23.

was widespread industrial action, including some notable national strikes of ancillary workers in 1972, nurses in 1974, doctors in 1975 (Iliffe and Gordon 1977), ancillary and technical staff in 1979, nurses and others again in 1982 (Morris 1986).

Industrial action, trade union growth and management reorganizations, as well as the increased size of hospitals, combined to create a situation in which government ministers needed to control discontent and to reduce public concern over underfunding and poor management. Pay inquiries were the chosen method. In 1974 the Halsbury report (Halsbury 1974) was the response to strikes by nurses and Professions Allied to Medicine (PAMs), and in 1979/80 the Clegg Commission came after action by ancillary and ambulance staff (Clegg 1980). There had been several other less well-known inquiries into the pay of staff such as those for administrative and clerical (A&C) (Hall 1957) grades and electricians (Davison 1973). The point is that government ministers and senior civil servants have tended to prefer arbitration through pay inquiries rather than be faced with industrial action. In 1984 that preference was translated into a Pay Review Body (PRB) for nurses and PAMs as a form of standing arbitration. This was derived from the Doctors' and Dentists' Review Body which had been operating for the pay of doctors and dentists since the early 1960s. At present 60% of NHS staff have their pay determined through a PRB, the rest through Whitley (Seifert 1992). The internal market and the NHSTs represent a challenge to this policy initiative, and the refusal to allow ambulance staff a pay formula/PRB after their 1989 industrial action (Kerr and Sachdev 1991) indicates the changing attitudes towards arbitration by government and employers under 'managed competition'.

There are three main conclusions from a study of recent history of NHS industrial relations which are relevant for the internal market and Trusts:

(1) When local bargaining was introduced in the 1970s for ancillary workers through the National Board for Prices and Incomes recommendations (1971) there was an increase in trade union membership, activity and industrial action.

(2) NHS staff have a deep commitment to felt-fair comparability in the determination of their pay as shown in previous pay inquiries. Such a profound belief in comparability is partly acknowledged in PRB and Whitley deliberations, but it will be sharply challenged with local pay bargaining and with the introduction of job evaluation and performance-related pay.

(3) Industrial action has an important impact on the attitudes and behaviour of the parties and some groups of NHS staff will be better placed in the Reformed system to take such action.

LOCAL BARGAINING: THE MECHANISMS

For collective bargaining to proceed at NHST level, and in particular in hospitals as providers of contracted services,[1] there has to be some formal mechanism. Collective bargaining assumes trade union recognition for pay-bargaining purposes as opposed to recognition just for representational purposes. Normally workplace-level bargaining contains three elements:

(1) bargaining formally over pay and conditions, over issues of interest;

(2) bargaining within agreed procedures about the implementation of national agreements and/or local agreements and bargaining over rights such as with grievances and discipline;

(3) informal bargaining and/or custom and practice.

Elements of all three have existed in the NHS since the early 1960s, but by the end of the 1980s it was awash with large numbers of grievances and custom and practice were substantial factors (Seifert 1992). The requirements of the internal market mean that pay and conditions need to be, from a business perspective, closely associated with the nature of contracts and the imperatives of the market. Of course, any such financial logic is mediated through the traditional and institutional features of NHS industrial relations, and hence the muddle and hesitancy exhibited by most NHSTs in their first year of operation (Seifert 1990).

The institutional and legal position is that DMUs cannot break away from nationally determined pay and conditions except when flexibility is built into national agreements and when staff are not covered by such agreements. In contrast Trusts can and have moved away from national agreements since they are not bound by either Pay Review or Whitley.[2] However, in this section I proceed from the assumption that trade unions are being recognized for collective-bargaining purposes since this is the case for all DMUs and for most NHSTs (Industrial Relations Service 1991). Also continuing in this fashion seems to be the policy intention of most future Trusts.

There is a wide diversity of representative bodies for NHS staff, and this reflects divisions within and between staff groups. Overall NHS union density remains high at about 75% which suggests there are about 750,000 whole-time equivalent (wte) trade unionists within the NHS. In practice there are more union members since part-timers belong to unions and many staff on a break from work retain membership. This means that NHS staff belong to some of the largest unions in Britain. The unions have normally been divided into two camps. The 'open' general unions are associated with TUC affiliation, traditional shop-steward networks, and they mainly organize workers across industries and occupations. These unions tend to recruit most members from the local labour market and utilize traditional trade union defence methods such as collective bargaining and industrial action. The largest of such unions within the NHS are NUPE, COHSE, NALGO, MSF, GMB and TGWU.

In contrast there are the 'closed' single-profession associations which tend to recruit exclusively from within the NHS, are not affiliated to the TUC, tend to oppose strike action, and favour legal enactment and pressure-group politics to defend their members' interests (Turner 1962).[3] While the largest of these – the RCN – is very large by any standards, as Table 11.2 reveals, only three others – the BMA, RCM and CSP – have more than 20,000 members. Their strength derives from having nearly all of the profession in membership and from controls over the labour supply. In the mid-1970s many developed their trade union functions for the first time by establishing stewards' networks and increasing the number of their industrial relations officers.

These divisions between the 'open', general trade unions and 'closed' single-profession associations are important for the new, single-employer bargaining that is to accompany the emergence of NHSTs and the internal market, but the divisions have somewhat blurred in the last few years. For example, the EETPU was expelled from the TUC while the SOR has become affiliated. In addition, the larger general unions have lost members through privatization of services, while most of the professional organizations have increased their membership. The HVA recently merged with MSF, and the whole nature of NHS trade unionism is undergoing immense internal upheaval. The most important development is the nearly completed merger of NUPE, COHSE and NALGO.

When single-employer NHSTs decide on the best format for hospital-level or Trust-wide bargaining the changes within the trade unions will be important. So far only one or two Trusts have decided to 'de-recognize' existing trade unions and move to more or less unilateral determination of pay and conditions (Industrial Relations Service 1991; COHSE 1991). For example, Northumbria Ambulance Service was one of the first NHSTs to move radically away from national agreements in order to reduce pay and conditions (NUPE 1992: 5). Most have adopted one of two models: the so-called 'mini-Whitley' because it allows for bargaining on a functional basis with staff groups, and single-table bargaining where all staff organizations are represented on a small negotiating committee (the Pay and Conditions Executive) and then report back to a larger Staff Side Joint Shop Stewards Committee. In the latter case some bilateral negotiations take place over specific issues.

For example, the Walsall Trust recognizes 16 organizations on its Joint Staff

Table 11.2 Estimated trade union membership of main health unions in 1990

Single-profession associations:

Association of Clinical Biochemists (ACB)	2,600
British Association of Occupational Therapists (BAOT)	10,500
British Dental Association (BDA)	14,200
British Dietetic Association (BDA)	2,300
British Medical Association (BMA)	86,000
British Orthoptic Society (BOS)	1,400
Chartered Society of Physiotherapists (CSP)	26,500
Health Visitors' Association (HVA)*†	16,500
Hospital Physicists' Association (HPA)	1,600
Royal College of Midwives (RCM)	35,000
Royal College of Nursing (RCN)	285,000
Society of Chiropodists (SOC)	5,000
Society of Radiographers (SOR)*	12,500

General unions (NHS membership only)

Confederation of Health Service Employees (COHSE)*	210,000
Electrical, Electronic, Telecommunication and Plumbing Union (EETPU)	10,000
General and Municipal Boilermakers (GMB)*	40,000
Manufacturing, Science, Finance (MSF)*	50,000
National and Local Government Officers' Association (NALGO)*	65,000
National Union of Public Employees (NUPE)*	230,000
Transport and General Workers' Union (TGWU)*	30,000
Union of Construction Allied Trades and Technicians (UCATT)*	7,000

* TUC affiliated.
† Merged with MSF.

Source: Seifert, R. (1992) *Industrial Relations in the NHS*. London: Chapman & Hall, 51, 116.

Committee. Some single-union deals have been considered by NHSTS but Freeman Group in Newcastle rejected such a notion after union objections. East Gloucestershire Trust has reduced the number of unions sitting on the relevant negotiating bodies as compared with the original Whitley list, but such a move tends to reflect the restricted nature of the business, and local strengths and weaknesses in union organization. Manchester Central has formed single-table bargaining with functional subcommittees.

Our research at Keele has shown that the nature of the bargaining mechanism will tend to reflect three forces at work:

(1) the strength and preferences of the Staff Side;
(2) the local traditions;
(3) the preferences of the managers.

The more important issue is not the mechanism as such but which of the original Whitley unions are recognized. Again this depends on the type of Trust and agreements between unions and managers. So if it is a large London teaching Trust then more unions would be involved than with a small community or mental health Trust. The part of the country is also relevant, with NHSTs in large cities and towns more likely to face stronger union and community pressure for bargaining than those isolated in the south west or north east. Thus, recognition for bargaining purposes has been an issue resolved at local level between the management and representatives of existing strong unions. Exceptions have been limited to either single-activity NHSTs or those in more isolated areas and traditionally with weak unions. There is no business reason for NHSTs under pressure from market competition to abandon collective bargaining, and much of the debate has been a political smokescreen rather than a serious consideration of management options.

Pay determination: performance, labour markets and the needs of the business

In a sense the formal mechanisms adopted are a result of the creation of single employers, while the outcome from the bargaining process in terms of pay and conditions reflects the business pressures generated from the internal market. At present the earnings of NHS staff tend to be determined nationally, although variations in earnings at local level partly reflect the make-up of earnings of different staff groups. As Table 11.3 shows for nurses, for most professional staff the bulk of their earnings is from basic pay awards from the PRB. Extras tend to depend on London weighting, and allowances such as for student training, psychiatric leads and acting-up. For nurses shift allowances are important as is on-call for radiographers. The rates of these extras are determined nationally, but the amount of overtime is decided locally. Other groups such as ambulance, ancillary and technical staff have much of their pay made up of overtime, shift payments and bonus awards (Table 11.4).

If such a system were maintained then there would already exist within

Table 11.3 The nurse paybill: the breakdown of the estimated* paybill† for Great Britain

	Cost	
	Cash(£)	As percentage of paybill‡§
Basic pay	5,601.3	84.89
Special duty payments	644.3	9.77
Overtime	67.2	1.02
London allowance	128.9	1.95
Geriatric lead	10.5	0.16
Psychiatric lead	50.4	0.76
Regional secure unit allowance	1.7	0.03
On-call allowance	6.0	0.09
Standby allowance	1.4	0.02
Redundancy and maternity pay	38.1	0.58
Other pay-related items‖	28.8	0.44
Other non-pay related allowances¶	8.7	0.13
Flexible pay pilot scheme	10.8	0.16
Sub-total‡§	6,598.0	100.00
Employers' costs**	744.7	—
Agency staff costs	120.8	—
Total‡	7,463.5	—

* Estimates are based on estimated out-turn figures for Great Britain for the first quarter of 1991–2 adjusted to take into account the staging of the Review Body's recommendations for 1 April 1991, and the provisional staff total at March 1991. NHS Trusts are included. The flexible pay estimate is based on details supplied by Districts in respect of their successful bids.
† Excludes students on Project 2000 courses, and senior nurses and midwives.
‡ Totals may not equal the sum of components because of rounding, and percentages have been calculated from unrounded figures.
§ Excluding employers' national insurance contributions and superannuation, agency staff, students on Project 2000 courses and senior nurses and midwives.
‖ Includes arrears of pay items such as protection and notice payments.
¶ Includes such items as uniform and initial expenses allowances.
** Employers' national insurance contributions and superannuation.

Source: Bett, M. (1992) *Review Body for Nursing Staff, Midwives, Health Visitors and Professions Allied to Medicine. Ninth Report on Nursing Staff, Midwives and Health Visitors 1992.* London: HMSO, 24.

Table 11.4 The make-up of earnings for selected NHS occupations in 1991

Occupation	Average gross weekly pay including allowances (£)	Overtime (£)	Bonus (£)	Shift payments (£)
Nurse (F)	265.10	2.90	0.20	19.80
Administrative and clerical (F)	190.00	2.50	0.50	0.90
Ancillary (F)	142.80	8.60	8.40	11.10
Care assistant (F)	158.80	5.30	0.20	11.00
Administrative and clerical (M)	308.50	6.30	1.00	1.70
Ambulance (M)	263.90	26.40	0.10	3.30
Ancillary (M)	175.40	25.80	11.60	15.50
Hospital porter (M)	179.40	27.00	11.10	17.50

F = Female, M = Male.   *Source:* New Earnings Survey 1991 it some scope for local variation for performance and labour-market supplements. Many hospital managers, senior NHS executives and Conservative politicians believe much more local flexibility is needed. Three major devices – Whitley-plus agreements, job evaluation and performance-related pay – have been developed to meet these demands.

The Whitley-plus agreements for ancillary, technical and A&C staff, the first way of achieving greater pay flexibility, are national minimum rate agreements which include local flexibility on pay and conditions explicitly to reward performance or to resolve labour-market problems of recruitment and retention. Early evidence is that these are quite successful. Discretionary payments were first introduced through national agreements in 1989 for nurses and for A&C staff. Similar agreements have been reached for medical laboratory scientific officers (MLSOs), works staff and ancillary grades (Income Data Service 1991). Such local flexibility within national frameworks also applies to some conditions of service such as a recent agreement on career breaks. Unions such as COHSE and MSF favour this type of bargaining arrangement.

Job evaluation structures are being introduced by many NHSTs and constitute a second way of securing more pay flexibility. In Central Manchester they are pioneering a structure developed by the management consultants KPMG, while in East Somerset they prefer the system of Hay MSL. The main issues are how is it being introduced and how will it alter current payment

Table 11.5 Flexibilities available at 1 December 1991, Whitley-plus

Staff group	Starting salary	Promotional increases	Local supplement	Geographical allowance	Job content	Efficiency incentive bonus schemes
Administrative and clerical	Yes	Yes	Yes	No	No	No
Ancillary Staff Council	No	No	Yes	No	Yes	Yes
Ambulance staff	No	No	No	No	No	Yes
Ambulance officers	No	No	Yes	No	No	Yes
The Professional and Technical 'B' Council of Whitley	Yes	No	Yes	No	Yes	No
Scientific and Professional Management Advisory	Some	Some	Some	No	Some	No
Panel for maintenance staff	No	No	No	No	No	No
Professions Allied to Medicine	Some	No	No	No	No	No
Nurses and Midwives*	Yes	No	No	No	No	No
Doctors and dentists	Some	No	No	No	No	No
Senior managers	Some	No	No	Some	No	No

* Excluding senior nurse managers.
Yes: flexibility is available.
Some: flexibility is available in some cases.
No: no flexibility.

Source: C. Shepherdson *et al.* (1992) *What's the Use of Whitley?* London: North West Thames RHA Human Resources Directorate.

structures and grades. In Manchester its introduction is being accompanied by widespread consultation and negotiation with Staff Side organizations. This means that the factors themselves and their weightings are subject to bargaining. Once the structure is agreed then the NHST can decide how to implement it. In particular, the normal bargaining issues are the protection of individuals whose jobs have been downgraded (red circling) and the appeals mechanisms. As important will be whether the new structure significantly improves upon and upsets the old. The management are looking for a simpler grading structure, and one in which there are fewer appeals and less conflict. It hopes to link the payment structure to a single salary spine system. In this case it is not yet clear whether grades on the spine will be overlapping, or how movement will take place within grades.

A central question is whether the job evaluation structure reflects labour-market strengths and weaknesses. It should do so and it should create a job hierarchy in line with business needs. If it does both these things, there is a strong chance that traditional felt-fair comparisons will be outraged, and this could lead to further staff problems. Other related issues include where health-care assistants will be slotted into the new hierarchy; they will become an increasingly large group as Project 2000, the new more college-based approach to nurse education, takes effect and health-care assistants replace student nurses on wards.[4] Finally, there is some talk of the end of automatic incremental rises and their replacement with performance-related increments as suggested by St Helens and Knowsley Community Health Trust. Indeed job evaluation may be part of a wider management initiative to deskill certain jobs and to introduce new grades into the pay spine without any agreement with the trade unions.

Performance-related pay (PRP) is indeed sufficiently important to emerge as the third device to introduce pay flexibility into the Service. It was originally mooted as a major method for motivating managers and senior professionals within the NHS (Trent RHA 1989), but has recently been treated with greater scepticism. Some of the reasons for both the enthusiasm and the doubt are familiar in all work settings and others are NHS specific. Familiar problems, frequently voiced by the Arbitration and Conciliation Advisory Service (ACAS), are, first, that PRP may motivate those who receive it, but not those who fail to get the bonus; second, managers might compete with each other in ways detrimental to the organization's business plan; third, managers may engage in target hitting; and, finally, it may prove very expensive if incentives are to be worthwhile. In addition, what is often being rewarded is effort and not performance, and this increases worries over measurement and the fair distribution of incentive bonuses.

As far as the NHS-specific problems are concerned, the two major criticisms have also been about measurement and teamwork. The first goes to the very heart of professional objections over management controls of the quality of their treatment of patients. The use of Health Service Indicators has been controversial even with the better quality of information coming to management from the Körner statistics (Körner Reports 1982–4). But for many aspects of NHS work HSIs cannot be used to decide performance payments to targeted workers. The NHS operates very much on a team basis in terms of the treatment of patients. Individual reward systems may further fragment and undermine that important element of the overall performance of the service. A recent article makes the point that 'arguments raging about the suitability of performance-related pay in the NHS have now extended into the medical field' (Limb 1992: 10).

The 1992 PRB report on nurses (Bett 1992) noted that the decisive change in pay determination was the way in which the internal market is forcing managers to emphasize the management of labour costs. With 57 Trusts in operation and another 102 about to start, decentralized bargaining is the future for most staff. The PRB members have heard the tolling of their death knell: 'the Health Department's drive for decentralisation of pay determination and other management issues, their continuing emphasis on achieving pay flexibility, and their wish to see pay related to performance have, however, impinged on this review' (Bett 1992: 2).

The key issue is that PRB takes serious note of Staff Side arguments based on comparability and the cost of living while the Government and employers are anxious to secure pay agreements based on affordability and productivity (Wootton 1962). The Citizen's Charter apparently requires a closer link of pay with performance. The interim position outlined by the DoH is for future PRB reports to set a 'target average percentage pay increase' (TAPPI) with a basic amount for all staff and the remainder available for local flexibility. The propaganda point is that NHSTs would use the TAPPI as a benchmark for their own pay settlements, although there is no good reason for believing such a proposition.

As the PRB reported on the Department's evidence,

> because NHS Trusts were free to make new contracts with their staff, they were likely to break away from the national Negotiating Council rates . . . the Department said that on present plans about 85% of NHS staff could be in Trusts in two years time, and that between now and then Trusts would increasingly be using the Review Body recommendations as a benchmark from which to set their own pay rates.

> (Bett 1992: 6)

The benefits of PRP seem not to be directly related to the performance of staff nor indeed the immediate reduction in labour costs. The two most obvious reasons for the pursuit of PRP are that, first, in the case of managers, it separates them in terms of pay and activity from the rest of the staff and their trade unions and, second, it weakens collective bargaining in general and eventually undermines the trade unions. These policies coincide with the management-control arguments dealt with in the next section.

Other reasons for introducing extra rewards for some staff are linked to the labour market and business needs. Labour markets are tricky to assess and it is even harder to know with any precision how much more an employer needs to pay in order to recruit and retain staff. Some staff are very much part of a local labour market such as ancillary, lower clerical and married women part-timers amongst professional staff. What does this mean? In large urban areas many of them can, in some circumstances, leave to find work in another hospital or industry. In contrast those in geographically isolated regions with little alternative work are stuck with their current employer. Other groups such as doctors, nurses and PAMs, and scientific and technical staff may be part of a Regional and national labour market. With nearly 160 Trusts after April 1992 and a variety of employers within the DMUs, the competition for staff amongst providers will intensify.

The end of multi-employer national bargaining means that each employer has to enter the various labour markets in order to secure the optimal labour mix for themselves. This will provide scope for three developments:

(1) stronger unions representing those staff in the strongest labour markets;
(2) greater turnover and less commitment from staff poorly represented by their unions and underpaid by management;
(3) a major increase in internal relativities as between Health Service work in terms of NHST, geography and occupation.

A fragmented workforce, fragmented bargaining and insecure employment may favour the short-term business plans of some employers some of the time, but it will mitigate against any national training, promotion and career planning, mobility and loyalty of staff.

It is possible that short-term labour market supplements conflict with performance rewards and that both are out of line with business needs (Brown and Rowthorn 1990). For example, technical grades in short supply may command better salaries than high-performing professional workers locked into their current employers. In addition, local managers will be tempted to indulge in the classic roundabout of golden handcuffs and golden hellos for staff in temporary shortage, staff hoarding and poaching, and this will undermine both PRP systems and job evaluation pay structures. This will generate the necessary conditions for leap-frogging pay claims for some groups of staff.

MANAGERIAL CONTROLS

In order to secure business objectives, especially when they are short-term market-determined ones, managers must control the essential activities of their workforce. This is often not only difficult but the main cause of lack of business success. Therefore the new single-employer Trusts must put the establishment of managerial control at the top of their agenda. A great deal of what passes for serious studies of management and worker motivation concentrate on two main elements: the carrot and the stick. Both are aimed at maintaining the ability of the employer to receive maximum production for minimum cost. This is partly achieved by factors outside the control of single employers such as the legal inventions surrounding the contract of employment and rights and duties of the parties under such a contract.

The starting point for any discussion of control is threefold: the carrot and the stick already referred to, and the ideology to obscure the use of either as a control mechanism. This latter is often known as the management ideology of unitarism, and that certainly describes the attitudes and behaviour of increasing numbers of senior managers within NHS employer Units. The importance of this aspect of management has been the introduction of human resource management (HRM) as the substitute for traditional personnel management.

There is a problem in being clear minded about HRM since most of its promoters and practitioners have as yet failed to define what it exactly is and does. For our purposes it can be treated as a symbol of political change leading to some specific shifts in management behaviour:

(1) a more anti-union approach;
(2) the subordination of the personnel and industrial-relations functions to tighter corporate policies;
(3) the utilization of a range of employee-participation measures aimed at securing staff acceptance on the substantive changes wanted.

The importance of ideology is immense in current attempts to redefine the nature of NHS employment from management by consensus to management by contractual obligation. Ideology, remember, is not just thinking which is incorrect, 'but which is systematically deflected from truth because of its conformity to the limited vision and sectional interests of a particular social class' (Cohen 1988: 238). This is well illustrated by the case of a disadvantaged worker taking on, being 'forced' to take on, a poorly paid hazardous job. The key issue is that such are the wider pressures on low-paid and poorly qualified workers that they are in a real sense 'forced' to enter into a contract of employment which is necessarily unfair to them.

If this is the case then NHS workers who are forced to apply for their own jobs from a private contractor, and/or for a lower-paid job with an in-house bidder, and/or become non-core workers will all tend to have their pay and conditions reduced. As part of this process they will have their individual rights and their trade union representation systematically eroded. The logic of this is clearly shown below in the debate on skill mix, but the debate is inconclusive since it fails to address this most important underlying feature of employment: the uneven balance of power between employer and individual worker in the labour market which creates an essentially exploitative contract of employment for the least skilled and lowest-paid health staff.

Of equal importance are concrete manifestations emerging today of this unequal contract, and these include greater flexibility in pay and conditions, an emphasis on productivity and the related matter of alterations in skill mix. Ever since the failures of the 1974 reorganization that sought to streamline bureaucratic command from the centre downwards, and the Griffiths (1983) reforms which sought to streamline management from the centre downwards, NHS management concern has been towards greater staff controls through the generic notion of flexibility: flexible working hours, contracts, conditions and payment systems (Warlow 1989). The flexibility is designed to reflect the day-to-day operational changes in the needs of the business and the local market conditions. It is associated, however, with more bureaucratic management as personnel has to individualize and maintain thousands of contracts.

The skill-mix option has received much attention and has been adopted in some NHSTs and DMUs. It was always the case that managers had some freedom over the staff mix necessary to deliver the service, but that freedom is now complete within legal and contractual constraints. The most favoured change is the substitution of less skilled labour in place of the skilled workforce – hence the use under Project 2000 of health-care assistants and generic helpers in place of qualified nurses and PAMs. It is also the case that subcontracted services – in catering or cleaning for example – use less well qualified staff on lower pay and conditions of service than before (Privatisation Unit 1990).

Much of the skill-mix debate has been centred on poorly developed labour-economic concepts of a core and peripheral workforce in which the business bestows its blessings on core groups and pushes the costs of change and failure on to the non-core staff. The extent to which managers are worried about the public face of this message comes with the euphemistically entitled 'reprofiling' exercises and labour-utilization experiments. The most famous recent case was the paper prepared by Dyson in which he rightly attests that 'with the increasingly competitive nature of purchaser–provider contracting this reduction in unit labour costs will be vital to the success of many Trusts' (NHSME 1991: 6). The section in the report which won it instant publicity was:

> effective case mix analysis on the wards will allow for a much more carefully planned and targeted skills mix related to differing degrees of clinical need and Trusts will be tempted to avoid bed-blocking in surgical wards by separating those patients who do not achieve discharge for social reasons into wards that may be managed without the benefit of nursing staff and may even be managed in other locations, such as hotels.
>
> (NHSME 1991: 8)

The unions reacted with some ferocity, and NUPE pointed out that some NHSTs were already applying the core/non-core treatment to staff such as in the South East Staffordshire Community Health Trust and the North Middlesex Trust. NUPE suggests that such schemes led to immediate redundancies such as at Guy's and Lewisham Trust and Bradford Trust in 1991 (NUPE 1992: 9).[5] The issues are twofold: one, the use of new grades of staff such as health-care assistants outside traditional trade unions and bargaining in order to establish management control over such grades and to use them to undermine other staff; and, two, the return to health employers as 'hire and fire' employers for sections of the staff in the posts most easily replaced and least involved with public awareness of patient care.

However, other control mechanisms not directly linked to core and non-core labour markets are important to achieve the likely business goals for Trusts: reduction in the influence of the trade unions, and greater emphasis on the control aspect of procedures.

To begin with, the question of trade union recognition has thrown up a series of competing options for managers. These include:

(1) total absence of all trade unions;
(2) recognition of some larger and/or more relevant unions and de-recognition of others;
(3) recognition given to all unions but for representation rather than bargaining.

All three options and several more have been debated by management and the politicians. Figure 11.1 and Table 11.6 provide a summary of some of the management advice in this area.

Much of the debate, however, has been based on widespread misunderstanding of the nature and functions of trade unions. The evidence from our research at the Centre for Industrial Relations at Keele has been that most managers have accepted what they have inherited. Where unions are strong, they have been recognized. Where they are weak, they have been effectively ignored. The evidence from the NHS and other industries about this type of control mechanism – the weakening of trade unions – is that it has only a variable success and is often risky and unpredictable. Certain factors seem to emerge:

(1) The unions tend to merge and therefore the employer is left with fewer larger and stronger unions with which to deal.
(2) There tends to be an increase in local steward activity and this alters the balance of power within the union downwards, a development that often makes it less easy to control and more likely to experience some form of local industrial action.
(3) Where successful control of staff through union de-recognition occurs, the result can well be increased staff turnover, reduced staff loyalty, and it is likely to make the management of labour costs less rather than more, as assumed, controllable.

All this may well explain why NHSTs by and large still abide by what they inherited in terms of trade union recognition. None the less, other changes, with control implications, have occurred. For instance, prior to the present health Reforms discipline, appraisal and redundancy/redeployment procedures functioned so as to create fair treatment in order to reduce the conflict potential in these workplace issues. The NHS procedures on discipline, for example, allowed appeals beyond the employer, the DHA. In both NHSTs and DMUs the move is to end the appeal process at the level of the employer, although individual workers can still use industrial tribunals. Nearly all NHST employers have now abandoned the national appeals machinery embodied in Section 32 of the General Whitley Council and, as COHSE believe, 'it has been made clear that as far as the Trust is concerned, its decisions are final' (COHSE 1991: 3).

This represents a shift in the use of procedures by managers towards a more overtly oppressive policy. For example, some NHSTs have introduced

STRENGTHS	WEAKNESSES
• Helps improve industrial relations	• Removes some of managers' freedom of manoeuvre
• Helps improve communication between staff and managers	• Can be time consuming
• Provides a safety valve by preventing dissatisfaction and unrest building up to bursting point. Collective bargaining has been called the management of conflict	• Requires additional managerial skills, which may be in short supply
	• Inexperienced or unskilled bargainers on either side can cause major problems
• Channels over-optimistic aspirations of staff into more realistic areas	• Some managers are vehemently opposed to unions, whilst others favour them, so there may be inter-managerial conflict
OPPORTUNITIES	**THREATS**
• By initiating recognition procedures, managers may have more freedom to design a system which best suits their situation	• Deciding which unions to recognize can be problematic, and inter-organizational rivalry may occur
• By taking the initiative, management is likely to win respect from the trade unions that they recognize which may well create a good atmosphere for the start of local bargaining	• Over-hasty initiation of recognition procedures may result in managers being faced with situations for which they are not prepared
• By taking the initiative, managers may present a better image to staff	• Managers in some localities may never be faced by a demand for recognition from unions; so by instigating recognition procedures, they may cause themselves work which might otherwise have been avoided

Figure 11.1 Recognizing trade unions: strengths and weaknesses, opportunities and threats. *Source*: N. Harding (1991) *Recognizing Trade Unions*. London: North West Thames RHA Pay Unit: 5

Table 11.6 The tests for recognition options to meet

Options		Three tests		
		Feasibility	Represent-ativeness	Workability
(1)	Recognize all Whitley unions and include all in negotiations	Difficult	Good	Cumbersome
(2)	Recognize only all unions currently with members on site	Difficult	Good	Cumbersome
(3)	Recognize all but negotiate with a few bargaining committees where different unions are represented	Reasonable	Quite good	Practical
(4)	Recognize only a few unions	Difficult	Poor	Possible
(5)	Establish broadly based committees	Possible	Quite good	Practical
(6)	Single union	Most	Poor, unlikely	Impossible
(7)	Staff Council/Association	Unlikely	Probably poor	Difficult
(8)	Negotiate with employees individually with no union recognition	Most unlikely	Self-represent-ation	Cumbersome
(9)	Ballot all staff	Problematic	Good	Cumbersome

Source: N. Harding (1991) *Recognising Trade Unions*. London: North West Thames RHA Pay Unit, 20.

new clauses into their disciplinary procedures, the most famous of which are about whistle blowers. Confidentiality clauses now exist in many NHSTs such as South Devon Healthcare Trust and, in early 1991 when a consultant went to the press over the treatment of a cancer patient at the Christie Hospital in Manchester, the employer ordered an inquiry under Professor Orme in which the clear conflict of interest between market-driven health services and professional-driven health care emerged (Orme 1991).

Some NHSTs have downgraded the trade union representative function within such procedures. Epsom Health Care Trust, for example, does not refer to trade unions in its new disciplinary procedure. Other changes to discipline include the overt reference in the St Helens and Knowsley Community Health Trust to dismissal being the appropriate penalty for staff taking industrial action. In general there is a management mood in some NHSTs and DMUs to use discipline to promote both compliance with the Reforms and to gain staff obedience to the new methods of pay determination. Hence, 'there also needs to be a link with performance and appraisal criteria if the SGT [Self-Governing Trust, the original name for what became NHSTs] is determined to reinforce, encourage, reward and punish certain behaviours' (Trent RHA 1989: Para. 3.12).

In all such cases disciplinary codes and related activities are aimed at frightening the entire staff into obedience. Our prediction is that there will be an increase in performance-related disciplinary cases and the introduction of performance criteria in deciding redundancies.

Other areas that ostensibly allow staff to bargain over specific issues in a formal and orderly manner (Fewtrell 1983; Swabe *et al.* 1986) – grievance/

dispute procedures, equal opportunity policies and health and safety policies – could from another angle be mechanisms to avoid conflict based on collective bargaining at the workplace. However, these issues may not have produced much current change as in the case of grievances and health and safety this more individualistic approach has developed within the NHS over the years and, as a recent report on the workings of equal opportunities policies within the NHS found, managers tended to pay only lip service to such agreements (Equal Opportunities Commission 1991).

More importantly, with the advent of Whitley-plus, there will be scope for bargaining over the 'plus' element of agreements. Some NHSTs have done this and others intend to reduce these bargaining opportunities and restrict trade union involvement. In some cases alternatives are being used such as quality circles, team briefings and 'meet the managers' sessions. Early reports are that such practices are not successful, although they will increase as managers seek to gain control through bypassing traditional trade union and individual worker rights to bargain over specific issues of right and of interest.

CONCLUSION

The internal market creates pressures for the single-employer Trusts and their managers that are concise and inescapable. They mimic, in business terms, some of the typical issues confronting private-sector employers in medium-sized labour-intensive service industries. The immediate need is to endeavour to gain control over total labour costs through the remuneration package, and over unit labour costs through managerial controls of performance.

In order to achieve these aims managers have to come to terms with the main obstacles, as they see them, to the glittering prize of flexibility. These are trade union opposition and private-sector encroachment. Most of the NHS trade unions have made their opposition to Trusts and the internal market plain. The RCN considered that Reforms would 'threaten the principles and effectiveness of the NHS' and the main risks included 'the threat to continuity of care, reduced consumer and community access to a comprehensive range of local health facilities . . . and distortions to the labour market and the worsening of regional skill shortages' (RCN 1990: 1,6). NALGO voiced the frustrations of many trade unionists when it stated that 'we have never been told why it is better for the ambulance service to opt-out, why a trading agency is better than a supplies department, why a private firm is better than a cheaper profit-making estates division' (NALGO 1990: 16).

Private health companies are constantly assessing the benefits of taking over aspects of current NHS activity. This is sometimes done in collaboration with senior managers and management consultants, and often with the approval of Government ministers. Further privatization and subcontracting is inevitable under the combination of the internal market and modern management concerns such as with total quality management (TQM) and just-in-time (JIT) inventory controls. TQM and JIT alone would push most NHSTs to contract out more and more services.[6] Such private-sector take-overs are a threat to both management and staff because the former will lose control over services and the latter are likely to suffer a reduction in terms and conditions of employment.

The internal market, therefore, forces NHS managers to target total and unit labour costs as prime business areas for control and reduction. Single-employer pay bargaining and increased managerial controls over performance will be the established norm in the future Health Service, and the traditional concerns of NHS staff and their trade unions will turn increasingly towards the traditional concerns of all workers and unions in the private sector. NHS industrial relations will be dragged into mainstream industrial relations of the 1990s with all that entails in terms of union mergers, increased local industrial action and constant fights over redundancies and deskilling.

NOTES

1 For a provider manager's view on the question of contracting and employment policies in a shadow Trust, refer to p. 225.
2 Refer to the Introduction for more on the differences between DMUs and NHSTs.
3 Cf. p. 124, an instance of doctors taking unusual protest action in opposition to local management.
4 See p. 277 for more on the industrial relations implications for nursing of the internal market and the Reforms.
5 Cf. p. 230 for another view on industrial relations at the Guy's and Lewisham NHS Trust.
6 See Chapter 10 for further explanation of total quality management and just-in-time inventory controls.

REFERENCES

Bett, M. (1992) *Ninth Report of the Review Body of Nursing Staff, Midwives and Health Visitors 1992*. London: HMSO.

Brown, W. and Rowthorn, R. (1990) *A Public Services Pay Policy*. Tract 542. London: Fabian Society.

Carpenter, M. (1982) The labour movement in the NHS: UK, in A. Sethi and S. Dimmock (eds.) *Industrial Relations and Health Services*. London: Croom Helm, 74–90.

Carpenter, M. (1988) *Working for Health: The History of COHSE*. London: Lawrence & Wishart.

Clay, H. (1929) *The Problem of Industrial Relations*. London: Macmillan.

Clegg, H. (1980) *Standing Commission on Pay and Comparability*. London: HMSO.

Clegg, H. and Chester, T. (1957) *Wage Policy and the Health Service*. Oxford: Basil Blackwell.

Cohen, G. (1988) *History, Labour and Freedom*. Oxford: Clarendon Press.

COHSE (Confederation of Health Service Employees) (1991) *Trusts in Trouble*. Banstead, Surrey: COHSE.

Davison, W. (1973) *Report of the Inquiry into the Remuneration of Electricians Employed in the NHS*. London: HMSO.

DoH (Department of Health) (1989) *Working for Patients*. London: HMSO.

Edwards, B. (1979) Managers and industrial relations, in N. Bosanquet (ed.) *Industrial Relations in the NHS*. London: King Edward's Hospital Fund for London, 125–43.

Equal Opportunities Commission (1991) *Equality Management: Women's Employment in the NHS*. Manchester: EOC.

Fewtrell, C. (1983) *The Management of Industrial Relations in the NHS*. London: IHSA.

Griffiths, R. (1983) *National Health Service Management Inquiry*. London: Department of Health and Social Security.

Hall, N. (1957) *Report on the Grading Structure of the A & C Staff in the Hospital Service*. London: HMSO.

Halsbury, J.A.H. (1974) *Committee of Inquiry into the Pay and Relevant Conditions of Nurses and Midwives*. London: Department of Health and Social Security.

Iliffe, S. and Gordon, H. (1977) *Pickets in White: The Junior Doctors' Dispute*. London: MPU.

Income Data Service (1991) *Pay in the Public Sector: Current Patterns and Trends*. London: IDS.

Industrial Relations Service (1991) NHS Trusts: employment terms and bargaining survey, July, No. 491.

Kerr, A. and Sachdev, S. (1991) Third among equals: an analysis of the 1989 Ambulance Dispute, *British Journal of Industrial Relations*, 127–43.

Körner Reports (1982–4) *Steering Group on Health Services Information*. London: HMSO.

Limb, M. (1992) Divided over dividends, *Health Services Journal*, 13 February, 10.

McCarthy, W. (1976) *Making Whitley Work: A Review of the Operation of the NHS Whitley Council system*. London: HMSO.

Mailly, R. *et al.* (1989) Industrial relations in the NHS since 1979, in R. Mailly *et al.* (eds.) *Industrial Relations in the Public Services*. London: Routledge, 114–55.

Morris, G. (1986) *Strikes in Essential Services*. London: Mansell.

NALGO (National Association of Local Government Officers) (1990) *Patients before Profits: A Positive Agenda for the NHS*. London: NALGO.

NHSME (National Health Service Management Executive) (1991) *Trust Network*. London: NHSME.

NUPE (National Union of Public Employees) (1992) *NUPE's Evidence to the Health Select Committee's Inquiry into 'NHS Trusts'*. London: NUPE.

Orme, M. (1991) *Report on the Events at Christie Hospital in the Week Commencing 4 February 1991 Concerning Interleukin-2*. Manchester: Christie Hospital.

Privatisation Unit (1990) *The Privatisation Experience: Competitive Tendering for NHS Services*. London: Joint NHS Privatisation Research Unit.

RCN (Royal College of Nursing) (1990) *RCN Response: Working for Patients*. London: RCN.

Seifert, R. (1990) Prognosis for local bargaining in health and education, *Personnel Management*, June, 54–7.

Seifert, R. (1992) *Industrial Relations in the NHS*. London: Chapman & Hall.

Swabe, A. *et al.* (1986) The resolution of disputes in the NHS, *Health Services Manpower Review*, 3–5.

Taylor, R. (1978) *The Fifth Estate: Britain's Unions in the Seventies*. London: Routledge & Kegan Paul.

Trent RHA (Regional Health Authority) (1989) Paper for general managers on Self-Governing Hospital Trusts: *Personnel Policy and Practice – The Challenges of the SGTs*. Trent RHA.

Turner, H. (1962) *Trade Union Growth, Structure and Policy*. London: George Allen & Unwin.

Walton, R. and McKersie, R. (1965) *A Behavioral Theory of Labor Negotiations*. New York: McGraw-Hill.

Warlow, D. (1989) *Report on the Conditions of Employment of Staff Employed in the NHS*. London: DoH.

Wootton, B. (1962) *The Social Foundation of Wage Policy*. London: Unwin.

Part 2

PRACTITIONER ACCOUNTS

12

The District and the Reforms: New Roles in the Changing World of Health Care

Michael Kerin

Q: Can you tell me about your post and the main responsibilities it involves?

A: I am the Director of Commissioning for Greenwich Health Authority.[1] That basically involves:

- obtaining information from needs assessments and service evaluations;
- building up a strategic vision of where we, as a District purchaser, are going;
- developing a health strategy for the District;
- creating our purchasing plans in consultation with a wide group of interested parties – the FHSA, the Community Health Council, social service departments, hospitals and the like;
- negotiating contracts with providers to secure those plans;
- monitoring the contracts when they are in place and, where necessary, adjusting them;
- starting the whole cycle over again.

Q: That is helpful as clearly your role as a DHA purchaser of health-care services is a newly defined one, even if it had a 'prehistory', as it were, in the old District planning department.[2] All significant aspects of your role will doubtless emerge in the interview; however, I particularly wish to ask you about the following:

(1) *the policy context* in which you operate, stressing *the pros and cons of the Reforms for Districts*, with particular reference to the internal market;

(2) *some organizational implications of current health policy*, including the current shake-up, the almost 'merger mania' among DHAs, which is beginning to involve FHSAs as well;

(3) *the contracting process*, such matters as the way in which you define the health needs of your residents and, from this, construct a health strategy; how a commissioning plan is produced; and how the contracts work – the type you sign; how you deal with the problem of price

variability between providers; the relative importance of price and non-price factors; and so forth.

And, by way of a conclusion to the interview, I wish to return to your role in the light of our discussion, with you pulling out its central characteristics.

To give immediate focus to our discussion, where, very briefly, do you see commissioning going in its medium- to longer-term future? One thing I do expect is that you are unlikely to focus as much on hospital health care as most other contributors have found appropriate. Am I right in thinking your brief is becoming one which is centrally about the whole range of health provision in Greenwich, not just hospital-based medicine?

A: You are correct in suggesting it would make no real sense for me to discuss DHA commissioning and my part in it only in terms of what hospitals supply. The long-term position is still to develop but some dimensions of the role for the District are, none the less, beginning to emerge. Key elements seem likely to include that purchasing will have primary and community health care at its very heart, partly due to the general direction of Government policy and partly due to the merger, in some form or other, of DHAs and FHSAs. But whether we retain the full secondary, hospital-focused dimension depends on how important GPFHs become.

Q: Let's start with how you view health policy in Britain today, in particular the functioning of the internal market. This is of significance to us providing as it does the essential framework, the policy context, in which the DHA operates and is involved, along with other institutions, in actively constructing that policy in the sense of influencing how policy pronouncements actually work on the ground and thence what effects they have.

THE POLICY CONTEXT: THE PROS AND CONS
OF THE REFORMS FOR DISTRICTS

Q: I would like to start by hearing your views on the Reforms and the internal market, their advantages and disadvantages.

A: A key advantage is simply the establishment of the purchaser/provider split. It has created the possibility for DHAs to look at health-care needs rather than having virtually all their energies engaged in overseeing and managing the hospitals in their District. We are now free to look at a much wider segment of health care, beyond what is the immediate responsibility of Greenwich Health Authority – the DMUs as they are now called. In being able to think about health care in the round, we are able to draw in primary health-care workers, the GPs particularly, far more effectively than ever before. It has also focused our minds on the balance between health-care services provided for Greenwich residents from inside and outside of the District and to review that balance.

The internal market has forced us to be more outward looking in our orientation, to consider more alternatives to the traditional way of running things in this District. This is certainly good not only in terms of planning the service but also in delivering it to patients. It is also encouraging the hospitals themselves to think more carefully about the service they provide for these patients and, additionally, what information and interchange of ideas they give to GPs. Previously a recurring complaint of GPs had been that they never even knew when their patients were admitted or discharged from hospital. Responding to this is now more of an issue to all hospitals as, ultimately, the GP has the power of referral and can say 'I don't think much of the service I'm getting from that hospital.' Due to the nature of London's health-care provision, there are likely to be alternative hospitals nearby. This means the pressure is on for hospitals to be far more integrated with the GPs and provide a better service in terms of information about what they are doing and when.

The speed of implementation has created some problems. Here I am not referring to whether the changes should have been piloted but simply that they are coming on-stream very quickly. There is a certain inevitability about that because, even though the policy has been to let off the brakes in stages, the whole thing is now gaining its own momentum. This has meant, however, that it is very new to everybody and we are all having to learn as we go along.

The risk is that we become obsessed with the changes rather than the services that are being delivered within these changes. One of the ways things were kept under control at the crucial initial stages was through the DoH's decision to maintain a 'steady state' in 1990–1. The risk with steady state is, of course, that it could slow up beneficial changes that were already planned to happen.

With respect to NHSTs, the third wave will certainly be very large. There is no doubt that Trusts have proved highly controversial inside and outside the Service. They have, for example, evoked considerable discussion about whether and to whom they are accountable. But in terms of the Reforms leading to change in the system, we see GPFHs as likely to introduce far more unpredictability than NHSTs. One hears them described as 'the joker in the pack', 'the wild card', even 'the genies that have been let out of the bottle'. All these images indicate that the very concept of Fundholding was introduced to shake up the system, to galvanize some of the changes.

Currently in our area we have only three Fundholding practices representing a bit over 10% of the population in the District. However, Fundholding is gaining much momentum with extensions to the eligibility criteria and number of practices that can apply for GPFH status. There is less clarity than in the case of the Trusts about the GPFHs' accountability. They are given a level of resource. They are meant to work alongside the DHAs and FHSAs. Yet, for perfectly good and justifiable ethical reasons, which can benefit their patients, GPFHs could make decisions that disturb the viability of a range of services for other patients of a whole host of other GPs.

The essential point is that each of the different components of the current policy contains within it both risks and opportunities depending on where one is standing. They certainly don't all point in the same direction. But no one is yet clear how to use all these various levers to best effect or even what the overall effect will be when they're all pulled at the same time.

Let's consider this important point at a different level. Decisions taken by individual NHS purchasers and providers may contain an opportunity for one decision-maker and likely threats for others. The best way to explain this is to give concrete examples. First, a small case study relating to the multi-District alcohol and drug service organized by a neighbouring provider, Bexley Hospital. It only needed one of the purchasing agents, in this case the South East London Commissioning Agency (SELCA), to say they were withdrawing from Bexley's alcohol service in order to develop their own – something that makes perfectly good sense from SELCA's standpoint – and the Bexley service is suddenly not viable. That meant we in Greenwich, who were also using the service, had a problem that required solving very quickly.

Another example, but one where Greenwich can secure an advantage, concerns the ophthalmology service at Greenwich District Hospital which has had long waiting lists. Consequently, large numbers of Greenwich residents were referred to Moorfields, the famous eye hospital in central London. Having greater control over our resources now, we can put more funds into ophthalmology locally to improve the service. From our standpoint this is a good move as our residents don't have to go to Moorfields for procedures that can be done perfectly well in their own area.

It is important to remember that the internal market operates in different ways in different parts of the country. The local hospital in suburban towns and rural areas usually serves a clearly defined population. There the internal market tends to be more about power than trading, more about how the Service operates and is managed; about how GPs and consumers, both of whom have been made more influential by the Reforms, obtain more from their local hospital.

In the larger towns and cities, certainly London, there are usually one or more credible alternatives to the local hospital that DHAs and GPFHs could consider. Our two small case studies, the Bexley alcohol service and the ophthalmology referrals, indicate what can happen where such alternatives exist. They also demonstrate that what poses a problem for one part of the system may well constitute an opportunity for another part.

We have particular issues surrounding the local Greenwich hospitals, one of which runs specialist units for cardiothoracic services and neuro sciences as well as local acute services. Their costs are relatively high due to the London weighting impact on payroll, the largest expense hospitals incur. What they have to address is being squeezed between hospitals in the shires who, with their lower expense ratios, could become more aggressive, and the London teaching hospitals, trading on their reputation and expertise, who might also target that Greenwich market.

This by no means exhausts the possibilities. My last case study in this section concerns my DHA and a contiguous one, Bexley, and the three acute hospitals serving these two areas. The first hospital involved is Greenwich

District Hospital which largely serves Greenwich people plus smaller numbers from nearby Lewisham and northern Bexley. The second hospital is the Brook General Hospital, well known for the Regional specialties mentioned above.[3] However, its District functions are currently distributed approximately 50/50 between Greenwich and Bexley residents. The third hospital, Queen Mary's Hospital in Sidcup, the only NHS acute hospital within Bexley Health Authority, serves Bexley people and significant numbers in south Greenwich and Bromley.

The first point to make is that the previous health-funding regime caused the issue explored in this case study. Queen Mary's is a relatively new, but under-used, hospital. This arose because under the old system DHAs were allocated money according to the historic use made of their hospitals. Queen Mary's and Bexley DHA were in a catch-22 situation: they could only obtain extra funding when they got the patients in but they couldn't get them in till they had the money to do the work!

The new system can free this up due to the change to funding on a weighted capitation basis for one's residents rather than on the use made of one's hospitals. As Bexley Health Authority is controlling the pot of money for its Bexley residents, there is now the means of transferring work into Queen Mary's.

But again there is another side to this. Resources are finite and there are limits to the extent one can make efficiency improvements. So where is this hospital getting its extra patients from? The answer clearly is they're going to be taking in patients from other Units. The main one affected in this case is the Brook Hospital. In other words, the market creates challenges and they have to be managed.

In this case you have DHAs that, in simple terms, have resources to finance two general hospitals but can't manage to maintain three. Under the old planning model people at least knew what they would have done next. Under the new system there is a tension between the DHAs and GPFHs as commissioners and the providers, all the more so if they're NHSTs vigorously pursuing their own particular ends. The result is that the hospital service in my part of the world has become a far more volatile and less controlled mechanism than before.

In our last case study, if work starts transferring from the Brook to Queen Mary's the latter may get ever cheaper than the former as its fixed costs are spread over a larger work load. For the opposite reason, the Brook is going to become more expensive.

It is possible to envisage DHAs, as presently configured, in their purchasing role acting almost like GPFHs, each looking after their own corner. There is a need for regulators who could exert some wider influence and restrict decisions that may be optimal in economic terms for one part of the NHS but sub-optimal in various ways for the whole Service. This will require action from the Secretary of State for Health; she could, for example, assign this task to the RHAs.[4] None of the direct parties in the market can establish such controls themselves. In fact, most are still none too clear about their own individual roles. We still need to learn what lies below the market language and market behaviour and what it really means to be entrepreneurial or business-like, if we are to serve our patients and our residents well.

Q: I would now like to move from the policy setting created by Government and the DoH and its pros and cons from your standpoint as a DHA commissioner to exploring some of the organizational implications at District level of the changes.

SOME ORGANIZATIONAL IMPLICATIONS OF CURRENT HEALTH POLICY

Q: The issues I would like to cover are:

(1) What are the changes that had to be made in Greenwich Health Authority in order that it could function effectively in its newly defined commissioning role?

(2) How separate is the District purchaser from the local provider Units and will that change over time?

(3) Looking at the wider picture, there have been many recent mergers, amalgamations and other, looser agreements between adjoining DHAs, something now extending to include FHSAs. Why is this occurring in the NHS generally? What's happening in your area?

(4) What role remains for Region given all the changes at the District and Unit levels that we have been discussing?

From District planning to health-care commissioning

Q: How is your District reorganizing and changing itself in order to be able to operate as a purchaser of health care?

A: I am glad you asked just about my District as the wider view is varied and complex. Different pictures emerge in different parts of the country. How particular Districts reorganize is very much affected by local circumstances, past history and the like.

We have had real stability in Greenwich. The old planning department at District headquarters was reorganized as the focus for the new commissioning role. Nearly everyone who was part of that department moved over into the new structure.

Since the Reforms there has been a small, but balanced, amount of movement of administrative personnel between District and the two acute provider Units at Greenwich.[5] This is useful; it would be extremely unfortunate if a divide were to emerge between the two functions. A degree of circulation of staff both aids the employees' personal career development plans and encourages a full and adequate knowledge of the new system to emerge and spread relatively quickly. Otherwise commissioners and their staffs would know little about how hospitals currently work and Unit managements and administrative personnel would not know enough about how DHAs make decisions about resources and health needs.

It is important to prevent the 'over-glamorizing' of jobs with the providers relative to commissioning. We have achieved this to date, perhaps because there are not yet any NHSTs in our area. In some other parts of the Health Service the Districts have lost too many of their most capable staff to newly forming Trusts and just at the very time when the District is itself experiencing changes equally substantial, if different from those in the Trusts.[6]

Q: The Reforms have sometimes been identified with large increases in managerial and administrative staff. Did your DHA hire new staff, at least in the short term?

A: Yes, a few. That is equally true of the providers as well.

Q: The NHS has a long history of using external management consultants. In the reorganization of the District has that proved to be a useful option?

A: There can be advantages in technical areas, for example IT. But it is important to recall that, especially in the early stages, such outsiders were likely to know even less than us about the detailed local changes we needed to make. Further, some Districts had some bad experiences of management consultants generally and in relation to their commissioning role. Perhaps the Districts hoped for too much; the management consultants promised too much and delivered too little. That made us cautious.

In the event we used one particular management consultant who had undertaken a lot of work for our Region and for SELCA in organization development. As we move towards joint commissioning with the neighbouring DHA and the FHSA, we will need to buy in some management consultancy expertise around the development of this new organization, both its technical aspects and team building.

Exploring the purchaser/provider split

Q: The genuine separation of the District as a commissioner and the local hospitals as some of its likely providers is a centre piece of current health policy. Given a long history presumably of substantial links between Greenwich Health Authority and the two acute hospitals in the area, how, and to what degree, can an adequate degree of distancing begin to occur?

A: Greenwich has always been a centrally driven District. Owing to historical funding and provision problems, District headquarters has maintained a strong hand in regulating the finances and keeping things under control in the Units.

With the introduction of a purchaser/provider split, there was a danger, initially, of going to one extreme or the other. The first extreme is to push this split to the ultimate: the providers very quickly run themselves; the District stands back entirely. From our past history the rapid creation of the separation was an unlikely option if only because the controls District managers were endeavouring to get firmly in place to regulate overspends and other problems at the provider level were not then secure enough. So it simply did not seem feasible to let a thousand flowers bloom suddenly all over the District.

The opposite extreme would be to ignore the purchaser/provider split entirely. For a while at least some Districts tried to do that. They, in effect, endeavoured to change the hats but not the substance and perhaps hoped the Reforms would go away. We chose a middle path based on organizational distinctions at District headquarters. In particular, two distinct posts were created: my own as Director of Commissioning and another as Director of Development dealing with provider issues.[7] This forced the split as high up the District organization as possible. It also worked to keep the transitional period as short as possible. These were the basic premises of a policy designed to steer us between the two extreme options of sudden break or trying to stop any meaningful separation of functions. This course seemed both realistic and in tune with our past history.

Q: Have there been significant changes in your area at the Unit level linked to the Reforms?

A: Most of the Greenwich Units are likely to apply to be third-wave NHSTs.[8] Given current health policy, obviously Trust status is the preferred option. That application will cover both acute Units in the Greenwich District because the mainstream acute services at both the Brook and Greenwich Hospitals are now under one UGM who has a manager at each site reporting to him.

There have been other important changes that have integrated the hospital and community services, something of real importance given the changes in our role. Geriatric hospital services have been organizationally linked to community provision, with both now inside our Community Care Unit. Similarly paediatric medicine is now part of the integrated Child Health Unit.

We are working to create over time a more client-focused organizational and management structure. The changes to our Community Care and Child Health Units were part of this in that the hospital/community division was eliminated in these areas. The NHS Reforms have speeded up all these developments although they were likely to have occurred anyway.

Mergers, joint commissioning and a changing mission for the DHA

Q: The impression I frequently gained, certainly in the early days of *Working for Patients* and the new NHS Act (DoH 1989, 1990), was that not infrequently the new providers, the NHSTs, were perceived as the glamorous, exciting part of the new system and much less was said about purchasing. Am I right here? Is it changing? In creating and extending the role of commissioning of health-care services into new spheres like the community, what role did the centre and Region play?

A: Originally nobody really knew what commissioning involved. We couldn't go and buy in 'commissioning' 'off the peg'. Some of the Health Service think-tanks were, however, working hard on the new role of purchasing.[9] Region put on various seminars but they were having their own problems with redefining their own place in the rapidly changing world of British health-care delivery.[10] Finally, as you say, commissioning nationally had a low profile. All the initial impetus was indeed on developing Trusts. The then Secretary of State for Health gave priority to that aspect. However, over time, purchasing has been accorded a greater focus.

But the initial lack of emphasis to commissioning perhaps partly explains why an opportunity was also lost in this same early period of the Reforms for the role of FHSAs and DHAs, especially in relation to one another, to be really thought through at the central policy level.

The underlying philosophy behind the Government health initiatives meant that DHAs would withdraw from managing hospitals and concentrate on developing the health of their local population, to be the champion of the people. The FHSAs grew out of the old Executive Committees who held GP contracts. Over a number of years the FHSAs have broadened out from this a great deal into primary health care across the board. They now have a commissioning role, equivalent to that of DHAs.

It makes sense to contemplate an integration of these commissioning roles. But serious steps towards integration were difficult to start with, partly because this had a lower priority nationally and partly as, on the ground, there were personal and organizational blocks to such integration even though much else encouraged a serious look at the matter.

Things have changed a good deal now. The Government's policy of increasingly developing primary and community care relative to hospital provision[11] supports closer coordination between DHAs and FHSAs. Similarly, a clear implication of the Reforms for DHAs is to become more involved in these primary and community spheres, to forge effective links with GPs, and connect with local authorities on community care. Our involvement with hospitals will fit in around these new commitments. As a result, new associations are being considered not only between us and our neighbouring DHA in Bexley but also with the local FHSA which already covers both boroughs.

Additionally, there are organizational issues around scarce skills. You can get more than twice the value in terms of management skills if we come together; the same applies to more effective links with the FHSA.

Much of what DHAs and FHSAs are engaged in will increasingly require working closely with local authorities' social services departments as well as in the provision of community care or on wider issues like environmental health, housing or whatever. To forge these links twice over seems costly and cumbersome, and, if a spirit of cooperation can be fostered, a better service will emerge after April 1993 when the community part of the NHS and Community Care Act 1990 (DoH 1990) becomes operational.

Of course, there are obstacles to overcome but the upshot of all this is that we are trying to develop a joint health strategy between the two DHAs and our FHSA which draws in staff and information from the three authorities. At the same time we're looking at what are the organizational issues both around working together and developing that joint health strategy. Increasingly links are also being forged with the social services departments in both boroughs.

Under the current timetable, our RHA expects us to have a closer working relationship with Bexley Health Authority by April 1993. That will be the first step in formalizing the various inter-agency links I have mentioned.[12]

What role for Region?

Q: You mentioned South East Thames RHA and its catalytic role in terms of the reorganization at the District and FHSA levels. What about Region itself: how do you see its role in the changing world of health care?

A: At the time of this interview, they have a confused role nationally because there is no clear vision from the DoH yet about the RHA's new place in the changing NHS. There seem to be conflicting assessments: on the one hand, RHAs are important as they are required to manage the internal market. On the other hand, NHSTs are not accountable to them. Similarly, the whole management of capital may or may not be under their control. Periodically rumours fly round the system about precisely what will be the reduced number of Regions (and Districts for that matter) that will emerge. For the moment working at Region must certainly be more difficult than in other parts of the Service.

Despite this ambivalence and the lack of clarity about the role of Regions, the DHAs and Units have had to proceed and implement the new policy so they are learning as they go along what the Reforms mean in different parts of the NHS. But the Regions are at arm's length from this and often can't actually learn much unless purchasers and providers share with Regions what they are doing. That doesn't add much to their credibility. Given this distance from what the DHAs and Units are doing, inevitably the sort of guidance Region puts out has to be tentative, sometimes rather vague.

Q: I would now like to move to a different aspect of your job, to the contracting process: first, specifying the health needs of your residents and creating a local health policy; second, and still part of your planning role, how a commissioning plan is formulated; and, finally, focusing on the contracts underlying that plan.

THE CONTRACTING PROCESS

From health needs to health policy

Q: How well equipped are you and your staff to carry out a health audit of your population?

A: We are certainly at an early stage with this part of commissioning – the 'we' meaning us here at Greenwich Health Authority, but also nationally.

There is one local point I should make: just at the moment I am somewhat hampered as our Director of Public Health post is unfilled. This Director is normally very much involved in needs assessment and related work. Until that vacancy is filled, I have to rely on assistance from such quarters as the Public Health Director in the neighbouring Bexley Health Authority and the South East Thames Institute of Public Health.

Two problems we Directors of Commissioning have to face at present are: one, a lack of staff generally with skills appropriate to the many tasks commissioning involves; and, two, the difficulty of quantifying in order to obtain relevant targets for evaluation purposes – and the fact that there is scant agreement on the few measures that do currently exist. The Department has funded various projects to date on needs assessment. However, the results so far are fairly basic and still open to debate.

In the face of such limited material on needs assessment, our approach has to be eclectic. For example, rather than worrying about researching priorities, if we identify a particular health problem in our area and have a capable clinician who wants to become involved, our current approach is simply to attack it forthwith.

Q: You just mentioned working with local doctors. Does their involvement cover other areas – for example, helping you develop your strategy or simply contributing some of the details required in your formal specification of the health services you want to buy?

A: Initially the specifications were really just descriptions of the service most recently provided and so we did look to our local hospital doctors for help. As we move on from that, we can draw in doctors from a whole variety of Units. That is one of the advantages of London; it is relatively easy to obtain advice from a wide field. We are also developing closer links with local GPs, so that their needs and perspectives are fully heard.

Q: The internal market has been welcomed by some consultants but is causing anxiety to others, for example those working in the so-called Cinderella specialisms like psychiatry, care of the elderly and care of the mentally handicapped.[13] Are there any grounds for their fears, now or in the future? How is the commissioning cake divided up between these and the more mainstream, often more high-tech, specialties?

A: One of the changing features of the Reformed NHS is the rising primacy of the GPs, be they GPFHs or not. Many factors explain this, including the expectation that the majority of GP practices will become Fundholders.[14] Along with other constituencies,[15] their preoccupations are extremely important to us. We have conducted a survey of all our GPs using techniques not unlike this interview. A clear conclusion is that a key concern remains waiting times for elective secondary, that is acute hospital, referrals. Referrals for psychiatric acute services and to care-of-the-elderly beds are not such a concern as usually they will be emergency admissions at a point of crisis for the patients and their relatives.[16] Certainly we are not planning to cut services for these areas of need. As the likely role of GPFHs increases, the GPs' concerns will then directly affect the relative size of contracts placed with differing hospital special-ties.

Q: In your areas of contracting what happens in the case of what one might call 'competing services'? For instance, clinical psychologists and occupational therapists (OTs) appear to be, or might be in the future competing to provide a number of similar services. I have certainly heard fears expressed by clinical psychologists that they might be seen by buyers of health care as simply more expensive than OTs and clinical psychology may shrink in numbers under 'managed competition'.

A: Basically there are two situations that can occur nowadays. Let me use examples to convey them. The first case of your 'competing services' could involve a powerful clinician, often in particular specialties; cardiothoracic surgery and other high-tech, high-profile work would be likely cases. Such a clinician could be expected to be vigorously pressing for as much work as possible. With a finite resource, if this person obtains more, clearly others get less. Our approach to date is, if the managers of one of our hospitals can't properly control their clinicians to the contracts we set them, the hospital has got to cover the extra costs this creates. In that way we can endeavour to stop contract monies being sucked in from community, or what we have specified as priority-care areas in the hospitals themselves. But part of this story will also need to involve a power battle being fought out within the hospital, between the various clinicians.

The second aspect of my response to your question is that the internal market arrangements are going to force us to think rather more carefully about why we buy certain procedures and whether they're actually worth buying. There are a whole host of different types of situation requiring exami-nation. Some are like your example of clinical psychology and occupational therapy; others are concerned with particular surgical specialties: varicose veins is one that is always mentioned, plus the 'trail-blazing' treatments like *in vitro* fertilization (IVF) that are done on research monies or have grown out of a particular evaluation. All such procedures need to come under some form of scrutiny and, in theory at least, there will be a large number of medics and other health-care professionals who are going to have to justify much more carefully what they're doing and why they're doing it.

Regrettably there are many procedures within the clinical field which have not been evaluated in this way. None the less, the painful process of appraisal needs to occur. It will take a great deal of time and effort.

Who should conduct such evaluations is another hard problem to face up to. My view is that, if we have a national health service, they need to be decided nationally. If, say, IVF is going to be provided within the NHS, it should be available to residents of all Districts.

Arguing for national evaluations does not cut across the view that the level of funding should reflect local priorities. Greenwich has a relatively young population; higher than average incidence of cardiac illness, lung disease and asthma; there are issues around perinatal mortality and the care of physically disabled people; and so forth. Those conditions are clearly issues for us and we would like to focus our attention on them, identifying why they are health problems here and see what we can do about them. The preventive focus of British health policy of today (DoH 1991) requires such an approach. However, we might rely on national assessments of other conditions, if we know there is nothing exceptional about them in Greenwich.

Developing the commissioning plan

Q: What is involved in developing a purchasing or commissioning plan for your District? What is its purpose?

A: I have spoken at some length already of our emerging links with Bexley Health Authority and the Greenwich and Bexley FHSA.[17] Producing a commissioning plan has formed part of that developing collaboration. The first plan we produced involved simply the bringing together of the health work that had already been going on in the area.

Before the Reforms, Greenwich Health Authority had acquired a good reputation for joint care planning with the FHSA, local authorities (particularly their social services departments) and the voluntary sector. Over a considerable number of years a range of joint strategies had been produced and implemented. This means now that, as those same organizations participate in, for example, developing the commissioning plan, they feel comfortable with this approach. In working on this plan, what we, in effect, said was: this is where we have come from; now, given the new measures, where do we have to get to?

The annual reports written by the previous Director of Public Health in Greenwich[18] and one we recently had written for us by the Institute of Public Health were other inputs for constructing the purchasing plan. These reports constituted our broad vision. We then developed that through joint planning with providers. The Community Health Council also gave us information that we particularly wanted to home in on. We ended up producing a document which goes through what commissioning is, how we are proposing to develop such matters as quality assurance and needs assessment and then presenting the plans that we have for contracts. Between being prepared and being cleared by the RHA, the draft plan had been seen by various outside interests, especially those represented on the joint care planning teams.

Why do we need to produce such a commissioning plan? First, to demonstrate how we would implement national and Regional objectives. Locally we wanted to use this opportunity to set out our own thoughts on how we would develop commissioning and various Greenwich issues that were not in the Regional objectives. Our formal document drew together all the relevant threads and that amounted to nailing our colours to the mast: this is what we are going to do for the coming year.

Q: Can we now turn our attention to the contracts themselves, such matters as the type of contract involved; the way you deal with ECRs; the relative importance of price and non-price factors like quality; and whether price variability between potential providers creates problems for you at District?

How contracts work

Q: First, how many provider Units do you sign agreements with?

A: More than 20, ranging from our 4 in-District Units through to teaching hospitals like University College Hospital and Guy's.

Q: Your life as a purchaser could well be simpler if there was a standard classification system – Körner or diagnostic-related groups (DRGs) or whatever – used in negotiations and in actually writing the service agreements. Is there anything like this?

A: No, not quite! The individual Units normally break things down by specialty and that information is likely to be Körner based at least. The specialist hospitals like the Royal National Orthopaedic Hospital use more detailed analyses because, in effect, they deal with one specialty so will break this down further. There is no real uniformity across the system.

Q: There seems to be pressure in quite a few parts of the NHS to move from block contracts to ones of the cost-and-volume and per-case variety. Is that your experience at Greenwich?

A: Presently they are still largely block contracts but they're becoming more hybrid in that they may have trigger points. This may mean no more than stating, 'Once you have delivered *x* quantity of episodes, we'll talk again.' There are a couple of smaller specialist contracts, like one with the Royal National Orthopaedic Hospital, that are more cost-and-volume in nature. Obviously we have some per-case agreements for, say, Greenwich residents who are in long-stay accommodation. We would then write a contract for just one individual at one residential home. However, in terms of resources, the great majority of our contracts remain of the block variety.

Q: What about ECRs? They seem likely to make your planning activities rather more difficult.

A: ECRs are just over 1% of our total spend but more than 5% of our administrative costs. They are a complication because they're costly to administer as well as making our planning more complex.

My impression is that, for most DHAs in the first year of contracts, ECRs were a bit of a lottery in as much as the information we had about the previous year's experience was obviously going to be limited. Nevertheless, from that information we had planned for around two-thirds of our ECRs being emergency cases. That meant they would be carried out and we would simply be told about them afterwards. All we had to do was make sure that the invoice was for a Greenwich resident and pay up. In the case of elective ECRs the Unit expecting to do the work needs to contact us, obtain our agreement first before they do the work, thus giving us much more control over things, including price, than for the emergency cases.

In the event our elective ECRs were slightly down compared with the previous year and the emergency ones were significantly up. Given our lack of control over such referrals, we faced a significant overspend.

Why that is so, we are still not fully clear about. We have, however, some leads. First, when we made our estimates, no provision was made for ECRs from Scotland and Wales. In reality we faced a steady trickle of these cases plus one major car crash in Scotland involving a Greenwich family.

People's travel patterns are important for ECR costs. If our residents holiday in this country and become ill, they are a charge on Greenwich Health Authority. If they become ill whilst abroad, the charge is on the DoH under international reciprocal arrangements. The Gulf War occurred over the period concerned and that might be why we had a large number of ECRs from UK tourist areas. It seems fewer people took foreign holidays. That's a speculation but one thing is clear: planning for ECRs is complex and for the moment we lack adequate models and data.

Q: How important is price in deciding who gets the contract? And, when you have made that choice, how do you persuade the GPs, whom you write contracts for, to accept your decision and refer there?[19]

A: Price is certainly a consideration but it isn't the only one, and that's a major point in my opinion. We have to carry the GPs; they make the referrals.

In situations where our GPs don't want to refer to a particular provider, we are led in these circumstances into a debate with them as to why they don't want to refer there. It might well be the GPs have no idea of the detailed costs of various procedures and, when they are told, are likely to be responsive. Previously they had never known how much it costs to refer a patient to Unit A as opposed to Unit B. If quality of care is comparable at the two Units, most seem willing to support the cheaper option as they can clearly see how much that will benefit the generality of the population, including their own patients. It might also encourage the higher-priced supplier to regulate its costs better.

Q: Certainly in the early days of the internal market, the one thing journalists reported was a good deal about price variability between different providers for similar services. How do you respond to this? Is the problem reducing?

A: Yes, there is an issue here although, as you suggest, it is lessening as we all gain experience of operating in the internal market. We do receive prices from a number of hospitals and we can question the ones that seem particularly out of line.

I'll give you an instance of this variability – oral surgery, which is doubly interesting as exactly one of the key clinicians was involved at both sites, Greenwich District Hospital and the Guy's Trust. In Year One of contracts Guy's prices were nearly five times that of Greenwich. In Year Two, surprise, surprise, the prices are rather more similar.

Each of our providers needs to give us a price for each specialty they offer. This reflects their particular cost structure, their fixed, variable and semi-variable costs.[20] Now the first cause for substantial price variation can arise because of the assumptions each Unit is making about the level of contracts they will secure in the coming year. Naturally enough, if they overestimate work load, the fixed component of their costs – itself a high percentage of overall costs – will eventually be spread over the lower-than-expected contract throughput, and cost per episode, and thence the price, could well rise dramatically. The opposite is true if they underestimate.

A second major reason for variability is the location of the hospital, the age of its fabric and the type of hospital. Greenwich District Hospital has a cost advantage over Guy's or St Thomas's as, being on the fringes of London, it isn't going to attract as high a London weighting for staff as do those two inner London hospitals. But Greenwich will be at a cost disadvantage to other possible providers, in Dartford or Medway, say.

In relation to buildings and other large capital assets, Greenwich District Hospital is relatively new. It may have lower costs than a Unit whose fabric is much newer – and therefore more highly valued and thereby attracting larger capital charges – or a Unit whose buildings are older and less well planned, so that they have to employ more staff. But to indicate the complexity of the actual cost structures of hospitals and why some degree of price variability is inevitable, Greenwich Hospital also has higher costs in some areas due to the type of hospital building it has. The particular heating system in the hospital made good sense in the early 1970s when it was built but is now relatively expensive to operate.

A third source of Unit cost and price dispersion relates to the vagaries of management accounting, the ease with which accountants can assign various costs in different ways.[21] This arises because they are able to use different cost-allocation principles and this can produce wide variation in the figures. This is particularly obvious with ECR prices. Particular specialties, often the smaller specialties, are extremely expensive in one Unit and very cheap in another. The difference is usually a mixture of the factors we have been talking about, one of which could well be the ways in which overhead costs have been assigned.

Within the Finance Department at Greenwich Health Authority one of our two Deputy District Finance Managers has a commissioning remit. He is involved in looking at the details of the costings of the various Units. In the first year of contracts we had to take these figures with a pinch of salt. The NHS was in 'steady state' which in this area essentially meant agreeing, in the form of contracts, customary work loads with our traditional suppliers. The often considerable price variability between the various providers did complicate that exercise. I expect the prices we receive for the second year of contracting will be rather different for some Units from their previous year's figures and more in line with those of other Units.

Technically it is easy for them to become aware of such differences and adjust their own prices. The first way is via ECR prices which all Units must publish. From that, Unit managers can get an idea very quickly what other

Units are likely to be charging on their main contracts. The second route is to infer other providers' prices from discussions with various prospective purchasers who will tell them, for instance, with which prices they are happy and with which ones they are not. It is not difficult to draw conclusions from that.

Overall two points about price variability seem really significant. First, it is important to remember that, for reasons already outlined, price dispersion can't be entirely eliminated. But it will reduce as we all get a better handle on financial planning under the new regime. Second, 'steady state' is now off on most things. Units have to look more carefully at questions of work load, cost behaviour and contract prices.

Q: How do you deal with the non-price aspects of contracts – quality or waiting times, for example?

A: We have set up a quality assurance task team which covers Greenwich and Bexley Health Authorities and the FHSA. These non-price aspects are fully operationalized in our purchasing specifications. The specifications are then discussed with the providers. Essentially the first year was about describing what the provider had previously offered. We then used that as the basis for improving various target areas like waiting times and quality. In the meantime the Patient's Charter has come with further imperatives in these areas. They too have been fed in.

Next our Quality Assurance Officer makes regular visits to the local hospitals to monitor their performance. She links in with quality assurance people in all the neighbouring Districts. Further, the non-executive board members of our DHA and the Community Health Council are visiting too. All this information is pooled.

Earlier on I mentioned our survey of local GPs.[22] Quality was part of that – such matters as how GPs defined quality and what information they get from their patients about quality. We plan to extend this survey to include local hospital doctors in order to find out what's happening in the different specialties on the quality question. Our aim is to build up a comprehensive picture on quality. From there we have gone on to other key issues like waiting lists. The 'non-price factors' are a crucial part of DHA commissioning.

Your job and its chief characteristics

Q: I would like to end our conversation by coming back to the role of commissioner which you defined in your very first answer. What, in a few sentences, are your most important tasks as Director of Commissioning for Greenwich Health Authority?

A: First, to ensure that the debate on the internal market for health-care services is about more than just economic matters and price. Quality of care and access need also to be fully integrated into this market.

Second, I am a facilitator. A number of interest groups – GPs, community groups, providers – need to be involved in commissioning and I am in the centre of that.

NOTES

1 The coming together in an agency of the commissioning functions of Bexley DHA, Greenwich DHA and Greenwich and Bexley FHSA discussed on p. 191 occurred in September 1992 and Michael Kerin emerged as the Chief Executive of Greenwich and Bexley Joint Commissioning for Health.
2 For further discussion of this 'prehistory', see p. 188.
3 Refer to p. 186.
4 For a similar view expressed from the provider management side, refer to p. 211.
5 Cf. pp. 186–7 for some details about these two Units.
6 For one reason for these 'unbalanced' staff movements, see pp. 190–1.
7 For another way of dealing with this dimension of the separation process, refer to pp. 212–3.
8 Subsequent to this interview the Greenwich Healthcare NHS Trust was approved in the third wave and comes into effect in April 1993. It consists of all the District's provider Units apart from the mental handicap services.
9 For example, Ham (1990) and Ham and Heginbotham (1991).
10 For an elaboration of this, see p. 192.
11 Refer, for instance, to DoH (1991).
12 In September 1992 Greenwich and Bexley Joint Commissioning for Health was established by the three Health Authorities, Bexley DHA, Greenwich DHA, and Greenwich and Bexley FHSA.
13 See Chapters 16–18 for accounts of these specialities in the internal market plus one from a surgeon.
14 Cf. p. 116 for a similar prediction.
15 For example, p. 195.
16 Further, there are statutory requirements about this. See, for instance, p. 252.
17 Especially on pp. 190–1.
18 As previously indicated (p. 192), Greenwich Health Authority had no incumbent in post at the time of this interview.
19 As Opit makes clear this is a potentially significant problem especially for the NHS as a whole. See p. 85.
20 See p. 169 for definitions and examples of these terms.
21 Refer to Chapter 10 for a full account of this aspect of price variability that its author presents somewhat provocatively perhaps as offering 'opportunities' for management.
22 Cf. p. 193.

REFERENCES

DoH (Department of Health) (1989) *Working for Patients*. London: HMSO.
DoH (Department of Health) (1990) *The National Health Service and Community Care Act 1990*. London: HMSO.
DoH (Department of Health) (1991) *The Health of the Nation: A Consultative Document for Health in England*. London: HMSO.
Ham, C. (1990) *Holding on while Letting Go: A Report of the Relationship between Directly Managed Units and DHAs*. London: King's Fund College.
Ham, C. and Heginbotham, C. (1991) *Purchasing Together*. London: King's Fund College.

13

General Practitioners and the Market

Raymond Pietroni

INTRODUCTION

The Government's Reforms to the NHS were formally introduced on 1 April 1990 (the new GP contract) and 1 April 1991 (the introduction of the internal market into the hospital service). They have been widely seen as inaugurating the most far-reaching changes since the inception of the Service itself in 1948. GPs have thus been faced with major changes, both in the way in which they do their own work and in the complementary work of the hospital service.

The reforms have been presented as springing both from a need to improve efficiency and from a need to introduce more responsiveness to the requirements of the patient. Another view is that they are primarily a mechanism for keeping costs down. The truth is that probably both factors (efficiency and cost containment) have played their part.

GPs will readily understand the changes in their contract, which is more one of directing their work into various areas and changing the method of remuneration. The changes in the hospital service are primarily based on a change in ethos towards that of the businessman that is, purchasers and providers and the operation of the market-place. As such the language or jargon is unfamiliar and difficult, but it is essential for GPs to understand the workings of this new system if they are to continue to operate effectively on behalf of their patients. In any case it is only a matter of time before the ideas of the market-place spread to the organization of primary care. Then the FHSAs will be seen as 'purchasers' and the GP as the 'provider'.

More specifically, this chapter will consider:

(1) What is the meaning of the 'internal market' and how does it operate?
(2) What are the changes in management structure of health-care units, e.g. hospitals and GP practices, needed to achieve an effective market and the contracting process itself?
(3) How has the internal market impacted upon GPs, their patients and the District?
    (a) the new GP contract;
    (b) Fundholder status – its pros and cons;

(c) the effects of Fundholding on District priorities and budgets and therefore the consequences for the clients of non-GPFHs;

(d) the information systems needed by GPFHs for the contracting process;

(e) the relationships of GPFHs with their clients and other non-Fundholding GPs;

(f) the positive aspects of DHA purchasing on GP input to the commissioning process;

(g) the need for there to be improved GP primary and community health-care services as needs assessment and resource allocation become more appropriate to public requirements.

(h) the problem of ECRs and the GPs' freedom of referral.

(4) What are the influences on the market from GPs themselves?

THE MARKET AND HOW IT WORKS

A market is a place where goods are bought and sold. In the case of the NHS the 'goods' are medical services which are bought on behalf of the patient by 'purchasers' and delivered to the patient by the 'providers'. The market is said to be 'internal' because it only operates within the health-care system of this country.

The purchasers of these services include patients themselves, DHAs, GPFHs, private institutions, FHSAs, employers and insurance companies. The providers of these services include DMUs, NHSTs and private hospitals. The agreement for the delivery of these services is reflected in the contract drawn up between purchaser and provider. These contracts may include reference to the numbers of patients entitled to receive the service, the nature of the service itself, the quality level of the service and the cost of the service. Contracts are generally set for a period of 3 years, subject to regular review.

The purchaser/provider separation is central to the working of the market. The belief enshrined in this model is that competition for contracts will act as a motor to improved efficiency, cost containment and improvement in the quality of the service delivered. Eventually it is hoped that 'money will follow the patient' – by which is meant that successful Units will attract more custom and hence more income. This will help them to continue with their service improvement. Unsuccessful Units will be spurred on to improve their performance or failing that to withdraw from the market. Implicit in the system is the idea that unsuccessful Units will have to close.

DEVELOPMENT OF TRUST HOSPITALS AND FUNDHOLDING GPs

In order for the market to work most effectively the Government has sought to change the management structure of the hospitals and, to a certain extent, that of GP practices. A central idea is that management structures need to be simplified in order to facilitate change in the range and methods of service delivery.

The Trust hospitals have been set up to operate outside the control of the DHA. This is to give them greater freedom in developing their services. They will thus be able to respond to the requirements of the market and develop new services which are profitable and cut back on old services which are unwanted or unremunerative. They are free to employ such staff as they require and to pay them the appropriate rate irrespective of national guidelines. For the moment non-Trust hospitals will continue to be administered by the DHA – hence directly managed hospitals. However, to achieve a true separation of purchaser from provider, the intention must be that eventually every hospital will be independent of health authority control.[1]

Similar principles underlie the development of the Fundholding GPs. They have been given a budget with which to buy drugs and appliances, paramedical services and some hospital services (out-patient attendance, elective surgery and investigations). These GPs will be free to negotiate their own contracts with individual providers and shop around to get the best value for money on behalf of their patients. Any money 'saved' by improved efficiency is to be ploughed back into the practice to further improve the quality of care delivered by the Fundholding practice.

CONTRACT SETTING

DHAs have been charged with purchasing or commissioning services on behalf of their resident populations. Where the local hospital(s) have opted for Trust status, the DHA will be able to concentrate on commissioning. It involves an assessment of need,[2] plus negotiating, setting and monitoring of contracts. By concentrating on the health requirements of their population it is hoped that the DHAs will become more effective in procuring appropriate services for the patients in their District. Those Districts which retain control of the directly managed hospitals will have a dual role: both purchasing services for patients and delivering services through the DMUs they will continue to control. Their new management structure, however, is designed to keep these two functions at 'arm's length'.

Contracts will be set by the commissioning authority for all services. The authority is free to encourage the development of those services which it deems necessary for its population, and free to purchase the services at the most advantageous terms – to include both cost and quality. District residents will generally only be able to receive services from those Units where a contract is already in place. An exception to this rule is emergency care, which is to be freely available wherever the patient happens to be. The cost for this care, however, is recoverable from the health authority where the patient is normally resident. Patients are able to receive non-emergency care where there is no pre-existing contract through the medium of the ECR.

Unlike 'intra-contractual referral', ECR care is not available as of right. The GP is required to justify such referral or even obtain prior permission before the patient can receive this care. In practice most Districts have devoted a very small part of their budget to ECRs. Usually this is of the order of 5%. This budget has to cover extra-contractual emergency care and extra-contractual tertiary care as well. These generally consume three-quarters of the extra-contractual budget. Hence little remains to cover 'elective' ECR.

DHAs are required to remain within their budget. Their allowance depends on the decisions of the RHA. There has been a move to capitation-based funding. This means that funds will be provided on the basis of population numbers taking into account morbidity and mortality but with little regard to social, economic or other factors which are known to affect the demand for health care. This type of funding will cause particular problems to those health authorities which operate in the inner cities and large conurbations which tend to have a concentration of residents with such adverse factors.[3]

IMPACT OF THE MARKET ON THE GENERAL PRACTITIONER

The new market will have a profound effect on GPs and their patients. It is as well to remember, however, that GPs are already trying to cope with the major changes brought about by the introduction of their new contracts. This placed considerable new burdens on GPs in the shape of reorganizing their practices to deal with increased requirements for information, the development of target payments as a system of reward and the greater range of services which they now have to deliver in order to survive.

The greatest impact of the internal market on the GP will be the decision to become a Fundholder. The qualifying list size for this has gradually been reduced. At the same time the practice is expected to be able to demonstrate management skills which would allow it to make a success of Fundholding. Fundholding for GPs is a new idea and the absence of pilot schemes makes it difficult for them to decide what exactly is involved. On the positive side is the opportunity to make one's own decisions about where contracts are placed; the greater access to hospital services, and hence enhanced freedom of referral; the possibility of making savings through prudent management which can be invested in other aspects of the practice; and ultimately the satisfaction of providing a better service for the patients.

The disadvantages of the scheme are more extensive. The budget for the practice will be taken from the total allocation of the DHA. This fragmentation will reduce the purchasing power of the District, especially in the face of a large provider. This may reduce the District's effectiveness in developing suitable contracts for all patients. If the GP fails to manage his or her budget successfully, the DHA is required to pick up the pieces. In addition, the District is required to pay the cost of hospital care over £5,000.

Such untoward events may have an important effect on a District's budget. The GPFHs may distort the priorities for care set by the District; this is particularly true if the Fundholders direct a disproportionate part of their budget into clearing waiting lists. Those waiting lists may have developed in consequence of the District setting a lower priority, say, on elective surgery than on the care of the elderly or disabled. A District with several Fundholding practices may find its strategic plans significantly affected in this way.

The budget allocated for the GP may be insufficient. This may be due to incorrect assessment of the level of referrals or because of unexpected calls on the budget. These may arise through taking on 'costly' patients or other unforeseen circumstances. Budget-holding GPs become supremely cost-conscious GPs and may refuse to accept 'costly' patients on to their lists. No doubt well-meaning attempts to make a success of the budget may result in reduced choice for ill patients locally.

Budget holding inevitably places considerable new burdens on a practice. The practice's information system will have to be developed. Systems will have to be in place to set contracts, to monitor and possibly change them over time and to manage the finances of the whole process of contracting for care. The practice will have to expand its managerial team, new personnel will be taken on and partners will have to devote much more time to this aspect of practice management. Such time will inevitably be taken from time spent with patients. The doctor/patient relationship will also be affected and patients may well query decisions about their care and wonder how far they are affected by monetary considerations.

The GPFHs can do what the District cannot do: they are the gatekeepers and can choose to limit referrals if they wish. While this may lead to developing skills and services within the practice, there will be occasions when patients are not referred to hospital who would otherwise have benefited from it. This may occur especially towards the end of the financial year or if the practice is concerned about overspending its budget.

Budget holding will also affect the Fundholding GP's relationship with other GP colleagues. Patients from Fundholding practices have on occasions seemed to receive a better service from hospitals. This is because the contract set by the GPFH is more stringent in some respects than that set by the District, or because the provider Units are keen to attract GPFHs' custom and make 'special offers' for their patients. The Government hopes that this will act as a spur for Districts to improve their contract setting. Unfortunately any benefits to patients from Fundholding practices are often seen as being bought at the expense of all other District patients. This two-tier system offends against the principle of equity within the Health Service and is unacceptable to many patients and doctors.

It further enhances the inequalities between practices – that is, between Fundholding practices, which are usually bigger and better organized, and those in the inner city which are often single-handed or small. Such divisions are inevitable as the market forces act on purchasers and providers to increase competition. It is important to remember that while market systems will produce 'winners' and high-performers, they will also produce 'losers'. No patient will wish to be treated by a loser, whether that be a GP or a hospital Unit.

Most GP will not become Fundholders. The purchasing on behalf of their patients will be done by the DHA. They are charged with commissioning services based on the health needs of their district. Thus for the first time the

Health Service has an opportunity to be driven by the needs of the consumer (the patient) rather than those of the providers (hospitals and doctors). This is a much welcomed aspect of the new Reforms and provides an opportunity for Districts to 'start from scratch', as it were, and provide a Health Service that truly reflects the needs of their residents.

It is this requirement for information about need which has led to Districts seeking closer links with their GPs. GPs are correctly seen as being those professionals closest to the patient and best placed to make an assessment of needs. At the same time they have close working knowledge of health services available and are able to identify good and bad service delivery. GPs are thus finding themselves 'courted' not only by the District but also by providers who are keen to develop services which will attract contracts. This central role for GPs, while obviously attractive in emphasizing the importance of their contribution, leads to frequent requests for information, questionnaire filling and attendance at meetings. Many GPs are finding themselves overwhelmed with such requests and are unable to respond as enthusiastically as they would like.

Because of the limitations of their own budgets, Districts have to establish priorities for care. This will inevitably lead to rationing of some services and the disappearance of others in some Districts. GPs are naturally very reluctant to become involved in this aspect of Health Service Reforms which seek to make 'explicit' what has so far been 'implicit'. Many patients who are put on waiting lists often do not receive the service for which they have been waiting. For them the service might as well not have existed.

The new Reforms will make much clearer to patients what their District is willing to fund and to what level that service will be available. Decisions about such priorities should be made by a much wider group than that represented by the District managers and the GPs. The Oregon experiment in the setting of such priorities has generated much debate. GPs will have to accept that their contribution to this debate is essential. Where services are rationed or difficult to obtain, the GP will be caught in the cross-fire between the District which makes the decisions and the patient in the consulting room who requires the service. Not only will GPs have to explain such decisions to their patients but they may also have to explain their own position on the matter. GPs should lose no opportunity to point out that much of the conflict about important areas of care arises from the major underfunding of the Health Service – underfunding which has become cumulative over years of financial neglect.

As Districts struggle to contain costs, they will look again at the patterns of service delivery and endeavours to change these so as to shift the responsibility from the hospital on to the GP. The closer liaison between District and FHSA[4] will lead to reconfiguring of many services whose effective result will be to increase further the responsibility of the GP.

Many GPs are able to improve and develop their services but will want to insist that the appropriate resources are redirected from secondary care to primary care. Some activity is already being shifted in this way *without* prior discussion and agreement. Most notable is the now common habit of hospitals to restrict their prescribing to out-patients. Despite repeated instructions from

District, Region and the DoH, many hospitals have been successful in this practice. This does not produce much of a cost saving to the Health Service at all because drug costs are lower for hospitals – with their opportunity to buy in bulk – than in the community. In addition, the GP is often uncertain of the indications, side-effects and monitoring requirements of some of these drugs and the responsibility for care of the patient is blurred.

The GP is most likely to come into conflict with the District over the question of ECRs.[5] Although the Government insists that all such referrals should be honoured, and that GPs' freedom of referral is sacrosanct, many Districts have already overspent their ECR budget. As indicated earlier,[6] this budget was purposely kept small in order to have greater resources for the setting of basic contracts. Many Districts are effectively refusing to sanction ECRs; GPs are left with the task of explaining such decisions to their patients.

HOW THE GP CAN AFFECT THE MARKET

It is now common to be told that GPs are very powerful and that the future shape of the Health Service is in their hands. Unfortunately one is less often told *how* the GP can influence the NHS in this way. Many GPs, struggling to cope with their contracts and to absorb the changes of the Reforms, feel anything but powerful. Further, a sense of powerlessness is heightened in the face of reductions in services and problems such as those with ECRs.

One method of influence open to GPs is through their FHSAs. This of course depends on the management of the FHSA being receptive to such influence. Unfortunately there seems to be a new breed of FHSA manager, often without direct Health Service experience, who have already succeeded in alienating their GPs through obsessive insistence on small detail in the GP contract. An example of this is the refusal to allow a Professor of General Practice with 25 years' experience of running a child welfare clinic (and indeed experience of running courses on this subject) to be admitted to the new Child Health Surveillance list.

Nevertheless, in many areas FHSAs are consulting with their GPs and communication channels are being forged. FHSAs will become even more important with time as they develop their own commissioning roles. Although such commissioning will usually extend only to primary care, in some areas FHSAs are being given the lead in commissioning community health services. They have also developed increasing links with local authorities with whom they may plan joint commissioning in the implementation of the NHS and Community Care Act (1990). Such commissioning will be of central importance to the GP who is the focus of much of the health care provided in the community.

CONCLUSION

GPs will also seek to influence their local DHAs. The whole process of contract setting depends on accurate assessment of need, appropriate commissioning of services and then their monitoring and subsequent refinement. This process cannot proceed without the involvement of GPs who, in a sense, stand 'proxy' for their patients, the ultimate consumers of the services. In many Districts collaborative arrangements are in place and GPs are organizing themselves into appropriate groups so as to impact on the commissioning process. In a sense such a collaborative approach is greatly to be preferred to that of competing GPs as envisaged by the Fundholding scheme. The larger the resident population and consequent budget, the more effective will the DHA be in ensuring best value for money in its contracts. GPs will also have an opportunity to suggest changes in service delivery and be influential in developing new services. They will have to become involved in establishing priorities for care and in suggesting effective ways of dealing with ECRs. Involvement in this process is very time consuming and appropriate resources will have to be deployed if it is to be successful.

The provider Units too have not been slow in consulting their GPs. They are beginning to appreciate that the Health Service is now driven to a larger extent by the needs of the patient than before. The person best able to assess and articulate that need is the GP. Many GPs have noticed that their hospital colleagues are now much more attentive and responsive to their requirements. Unfortunately the gross underfunding of the Health Service (in comparison with other European countries) has a severely limiting effect on what can be achieved. Nevertheless, these are important and timely changes in the basic relationship between GP and consultant which should eventually lead to a better direction of activity. Flowing out of this improved collaboration is the possibility of developing joint clinical protocols for common conditions, and ensuring that primary and secondary care are much better integrated than is the case at present.

All in all, the effect of the internal market Reforms on the Health Service can truly be said to be revolutionary. Although many GPs remain profoundly opposed to many aspects of the market, their basic pragmatism will help them to make the most of the system and seek to temper its 'commercial' thrust. GPs in the UK did not need the internal market; the internal market needs the cooperation of GPs if it is to be made to work.

NOTES

1 Whatever the policy intent, opinions are divided as to the extent this will be realized in practice. See, for example, p. 116 where it is predicted that in 5 years, not only will most NHS Units be Trusts but also that GPFH will be the normal mode for GPs.
2 Refer pp. 88–91 for an account of some of the complexities of needs assessment.
3 King's Healthcare is a good example of a 'loser' under the new funding formula. See pp. 213–4.
4 See pp. 190–2 for more on liaison and mergers between DHAs and FHSAs.
5 For elaboration of this point, see p. 85 above.
6 See pp. 203–4.

14

The Purchaser/Provider Split as seen by a Major Provider: The Case of King's Healthcare

Julian Nettel

Q: Can you tell me about your position in the management structure at King's?

A: There is a Chief Executive; he runs the entire provider organization. I operate below that level and am responsible to him for the bulk of acute services. I have an equivalent at the community level.

Q: Is King's a Trust yet?

A: No, not yet. The Tomlinson Inquiry has blocked that for the time being.

Q: The purpose of this interview is to focus on how King's is being affected by 'managed competition'. Specifically, I would like to ask you about:

(1) *senior management views on the Government's health Reforms* of which the internal market is a significant aspect;
(2) *the specifics of your 'market-place'*:
    (a) the amalgamation of your DHA with the two neighbouring DHAs to create one very large purchasing body, the South East London Commissioning Agency *(SELCA), and with three large teaching hospitals* – Guy's and Lewisham NHS Trust,[1] St Thomas's Hospital[2] and King's Healthcare – operating in the SELCA area;
    (b) the effects of the *change in the funding formula*[3] from RAWP to weighted capitation;
(3) *how the internal market works at the Unit level*, e.g. the contracting process, the back-up information including costings, etc.;
(4) *the reaction of the other health-care professionals*, especially the doctors, *to the Reforms*;
(5) *the changes in organizational structure and the training for new roles* in the world created by the implementation of 'managed competition' and the Government health policy generally at King's.

Let's start with your attitude to the current health policies.

SENIOR MANAGEMENT'S VIEWS OF THE HEALTH REFORMS

Q: I want to ask you, as a senior manager at King's Healthcare, your general reaction to the NHS Reforms?

A: Overall my feelings are positive. The separation of provision from purchase is an immensely powerful framework which generates all sorts of incentives to improve performance that frankly were just missing before and, to that extent, Trust status, GPFHs and all the rest are subordinate spin-offs from that fundamental step.

Operating in the internal market requires us to provide services under the auspices of a business plan and thus engage in far more extensive planning and control at the Unit level that this implies. The introduction of these internal disciplines has been welcomed by the King's managers as they force people to focus on fundamental issues, on those things that serve to clarify the hospital's objectives. This makes their managerial task much more focused and, in that sense, straightforward. Although the environment has become infinitely complex and difficult, the fact that we are running things ourselves in terms of generating an income stream as well as focusing on managing the expenditure side has been appreciated by managers.

That said, there is still a lot of worry and concern about whether we have the systems in place and the data available to be able to operate effectively in the new environment. In particular, there is a real anxiety that we don't have a sufficient handle on how our costs behave at different levels of output, something that we need to know to be able to manage and compete effectively.

Q: What, in your opinion, is the thinking behind the internal market in health care?

A: The Government has pursued a policy of trying to separate purchasing from the provision of public services generally. The Health Service was just one aspect of that broad policy stance. We have seen it in local authorities, for instance. To that extent it has been part of a wider thrust to improve accountability and clarify roles. It has created incentives throughout the system for people to do better. We have by no means moved to a free-for-all market which conceivably could have been created. Going that far would not have been the optimal way of proceeding.

Q: Even though the policy aim may indeed not have been an unregulated market, has implementation produced any unanticipated, even unwelcome, results, at this early stage and here in London?

A: Yes, the situation is becoming less regulated in some ways and often this doesn't make a great deal of sense from a strategic point of view. For instance, there aren't many unemployed cardiac surgeons in south east London at the moment: they are being employed like there is no tomorrow. In this part of the capital there have been three new cardiac surgery appointments at the three different cardiac centres, including our own, over the first few months of 1992.

Everybody is tooling up to do everybody out of business. This hardly makes a great deal of sense. The leverage and the wider planning capability that used to exist at Regional level are fragmenting as a result of the devolvement of purchasing responsibilities to DHAs and GPFHs.[4]

Frankly, this part of the new policy hasn't been fully thought through. What it has done is to create a climate where a shake-out is a possibility but this is likely to occur in a messy, rather than in a planned, manner. I cannot imagine in 10 years' time there will be three thriving cardiac surgery centres in south east London. And yet today each hospital concerned is absolutely determined that whoever gives up cardiac surgery it will not be the one. Each of us has rationalized, in our own terms, why it is absolutely justifiable for us to proceed in this way. That is just one example.

Q: You mentioned the prior planning and control functions undertaken by Region and the DoH. Do you agree with the view that Regions could become the regulators of the Reformed NHS? Another view is that the NHSME will enlarge and Regions will wither or disappear.

A: I can see the need for somebody formally to regulate the market. If we go on to see most providers becoming NHSTs and the GPFH system takes off, one could speculate that in 5 years' time, the NHS will essentially consist of a network of GPFHs and NHSTs trading between themselves.[5]

That surely would require a regulatory body to police a set of rules as to how that market needed to operate. Service planning and coordination across boundaries are required if you are going to have a high degree of 'atomization' within the system. A strategic framework to compensate for this will be essential and I would guess that's what Regions will be up to.

A number of NHS Regions have already been offering Units guidance in their emergence as separate providers, as separate businesses within the Health Service. This is a transitional step for Regions which, without wanting to be disloyal, are still trying hard to find new roles for themselves. As things stand at present, from the provider point of view, they appear more and more irrelevant.[6]

Q: What about the private sector? How do you see that developing within the internal market?

A: There is clearly a theoretical opportunity for it because contracts are up for grabs. There has even been the occasional GPFH signing a contract with the private sector. The fundamental problem with private-sector health care in the UK is it can't look after sick people! That's a pretty important inhibitor on what it can do. I firmly believe that, in the London context, we could blow the private sector out of the water if we bothered to.

Q: What about Trusts? Does the internal market require Trusts in order to work effectively?

A: I think being a Trust is becoming more and more inevitable. Apart from any deliberate political push in a particular direction, as the purchaser/provider split becomes more and more part of the culture of the Service as a whole, it's going to be very difficult indeed, within the compass of one organization, to reconcile those things.

Just as an aside, I think the further maturing of the internal market will require FHSAs to change quite fundamentally too. They cannot run with two horses forever. There is only one direction in which they can go: that's to become closely involved with their DHAs in commissioning and eventually to become one organization.[7] In the interim, joint commissioning between FHSAs and DHAs is likely. Eventually local authorities will have to be looked at very closely too.

Q: Is being in London a problem with its higher wage costs, capital charges and the like?

A: It is difficult to see many up-sides to it!

Q: Let's begin to explore the London factor and other issues in more depth as we look at some aspects of the environment you face.

SOME OF THE SPECIFICS OF YOUR 'MARKET-PLACE'

Q: I would like to concentrate on two main issues: first, the emergence of SELCA with its three large provider hospitals including King's and, second, the effect on your hospital of the change in the funding arrangements in the NHS from RAWP to weighted capitation.

SELCA and its three provider Units

Q: The most obvious place to start is with SELCA, the joint commissioning body for three DHAs: your own District of Camberwell, West Lambeth, and Lewisham and North Southwark, with its three large teaching hospitals: King's, St Thomas's and the Guy's and Lewisham Trust as its main providers. Why was SELCA set up?

A: There was a need, from the purchasing point of view, to bring together the three teaching Districts as this produced a critical mass of population which gave the amalgamated body real leverage to make changes, eventually including such things as being able to assess the health needs of this population more effectively than the separate DHAs could achieve. Further, there is no doubt that in south east London the system is very tight because there is a lot of hospital provision which needs sorting out one way or the other.

Q: A purchaser/provider split requires a real separation between the organizations representing each function. Let's explore how far that separation goes. For example, the District remains your employer, and you and the other senior managers are annually appraised by the DGM. Does that not limit the split?

A: No, not at all. The situation is not quite as you have described. To all intents and purposes our employing authority is King's Healthcare which, as I mentioned earlier,[8] is a Trust on hold till 1993, a quasi-Trust if you like. Although Camberwell Health Authority remains the statutory authority for employment purposes, from 1 April 1992 for all purchasing matters SELCA reports to Lewisham and North Southwark Health Authority as, with the formation of the Guy's and Lewisham NHS Trust and its separate Community Trust, it is the only one of the three DHAs in SELCA with no provider responsibilities. This means we have a mechanism for fully separating purchaser from provider. Culturally there really is no difficulty in having Camberwell in existence as the statutory authority to ensure we continue to be paid and employed.

Q: I would like to continue with this question of the degree of separateness of purchaser and provider but from a different angle. When SELCA is drawing up purchasing specifications as a prelude to placing contracts, are King's clinicians directly involved in helping them with the technical details that go in these specifications?

A: The purchaser specifications are drawn up by SELCA using their public-health specialists. They are then put out for comments and consultation. That's when our clinical directors and clinical specialists get involved, taking a view about whether what is being asked for is reasonable.

Q: Let's think about SELCA now in terms of the degree of competition within it. If the internal market you face is going to move beyond being largely a new set of administrative procedures – and quite expensive ones at that – and involve actual competition between provider Units, it will certainly happen in London,[9] particularly here in South London. Previously, you had a close relationship with Camberwell Health Authority and now you are in SELCA with Guy's and St Thomas's. Are you really in competition with those other two Units within the enlarged purchasing authority SELCA represents?

A: Oh yes. But let's go one step back from that. The key strategic issue for King's is more about the interpretation of the new funding formula, weighted capitation.

Change in the funding formula

A: In all four metropolitan Regions there has been a recognition that money needs to move out of central London, out into the shires. In a sense this is just consolidating a direction that had been determined right back to the RAWP days reflecting, as it does, major long-term demographic trends: the shift of the population out of the big cities like London and the age composition of those moving out of the cities.

South East Thames RHA has developed its reallocation policy more aggressively – involving both larger shifts of funds over shorter time scales – than the other three Regions. SELCA currently has a budget of £230 million and is due to lose 10% of that over the next 5 years.

The weighted capitation formula in South East Thames RHA is also different from the other Regions in that it does not explicitly take into account indexes of urban or social deprivation. At the moment it uses, as a proxy for these, standardized mortality ratios and thus funding is very much dependent upon the age profile of the population and is weighted heavily towards the elderly, very large numbers of whom reside within our RHA on the south coast of England.

All this has significant funding implications not only for SELCA as a whole but also within it. West Lambeth has some way to go towards its weighted capitation position; so too has Lewisham and North Southwark. But Camberwell is already there because we happen to have more urban deprivation and considerably higher standardized mortality ratios than anywhere else in the Region. Our argument has been that, as the major local provider to Camberwell, we should have less of the weighted capitation problem visited upon us as a provider than the other two teaching hospitals. SELCA, however, have not seen it that way. They've seen the exercise as about an equal sharing of the funding loss by each of the three providers. Consequently, this year they are proposing to subject each of the three hospitals to a 1.5% cost improvement factor which reduces the budget allocation for each Unit by that amount over the previous year.

At King's we say that is not fair as it takes no account of the fact that we are required to continue to provide a much higher level of health provision for our Camberwell residents than is true for Guy's and St Thomas's. If SELCA ignores the higher level of social deprivation in our area and applies the 1.5% across the board, they are hitting the Camberwell population twice. First, our residents are not being compensated for the fact that they are already at their weighted capitation point and, second, their local provider of health services is being impoverished. SELCA's 'purist' view has, in a sense, created a tension between King's and them. I don't know how it will eventually be resolved. It could involve a chairman-to-chairman discussion or the chief executives sorting it.

Q: Could we now move our focus to the contracting process, the information required, including the all-important costings upon which contracting depends?

HOW THE INTERNAL MARKET WORKS AT THE UNIT LEVEL

The contracting process

Q: Do you have what we might call a contracting strategy, a set of policies about contracting?

A: No, not if you mean a contracting strategy that drives other things. It is the other way about; these other things drive the strategy. You start with a determination of the business you want to be in, then an analysis of what you are doing at the moment against market conditions. From this comes the contracting strategy.

Let me elaborate as the process can be quite complex. We adopted a 'star-chamber approach' to review all our clinical specialties. An outside assessor, a senior academic, came in and chaired the group conducting the evaluation.

That SWOT (strengths, weaknesses, opportunities, threats) evaluation, specialty by specialty, was a fairly formal examination of how each medical specialism rated in terms of such things as academic excellence, ability to attract contracts, the demand in the community, the view of GPs, the ability to attract and retain staff of the highest calibre and the like.

Q: Can you give me some examples of the high and low scorers, as it were?

A: The review indicated strengths in liver disease (fairly obviously as we are a national centre) and neonatology, diabetes and dermatology. Our weaknesses include rheumatology, where we have a service which is struggling because it's small and underdeveloped and there is a stronger department close to our shores at Guy's.

Q: Would you think of running down such a specialism?

A: Not necessarily. We moved from the internal SWOT analysis to a review of strengths and weaknesses in market terms.

The internal analysis of ophthalmology, for instance, suggested there was no need to have it on an in-patient basis at King's. It's a very small specialty and possibly could be combined with a new Unit nearby as has often been the case in other centres.

However, when we came to test that against the market, it rapidly became apparent that the ophthalmology service at King's was highly regarded by SELCA in terms of quality and cost and was in a very good position to attract more income and additional contracts – and that's what has happened. We realized there was an opportunity not only to retain current provision but expand it on a cost-and-volume basis for procedures like cataracts.

The conclusion is clear: purely internal analysis of our services may lead you to one conclusion. Once you start looking at the market opportunities and threats, it can quite often turn things on their head. Clearly all the elements, the external as well as the internal, must be brought to bear before deciding what the future is for a particular speciality.

The information provided for SELCA and other purchasers

Q: What sort of access do purchasers – SELCA, other DHA purchasers, GPFHs – have to King's and its information systems to check contract compliance?

A: We have prided ourselves in being able to give GPFHs what is regular contract monitoring information for their own purposes. We treat them as autonomous customers and give them their own data sets indicating the number of patients that we are treating against the contract levels they agreed with us under our block contracts. We currently have such agreements with three GPFHs. We usually have regular quarterly meetings with each and go through all the issues including quality matters such as access and speed of referral.

Q: And what about District purchasers?

A: Our main purchasers are SELCA. We have formal monitoring meetings every quarter with them where we consider the financial and quality dimensions. Those meetings are minuted and signed off as a correct record of the discussion and really become part of the contract. Thus, contracts contain very specific agreements about the quantity of data required, its completeness and timeliness.

There is a lot of contact between those meetings, including visits by SELCA officers to look at what we are doing on the ground and assure themselves that what we signed off as done has, in fact, been delivered.

Q: What non-price factors are reflected in contracts?

A: Quality. We have generic quality requirements given to us by SELCA. Because they are such a large purchaser, all of our other commissioning DHAs are happy to piggyback on those quality standards.

SELCA's generic standards are gleaned from DoH and Regional initiatives, the Patient's Charter and issues specific to the provider Unit. Observance of their standards would be evidenced by systems of medical and clinical audit; that we are providing decent information to patients in terms of written communication; by what we are doing about survey instruments to find out what patients think about our services; and by issues about fair access and evidence of a coordinated approach to care planning.

Let's take one clinical directorate or, in our terms, care group[10] within the hospital to show the quantity and quality of information produced for our purchasers. This includes information on customer satisfaction, complaints data about waiting times in out-patients, the number of cancelled out-patient clinics, response time to GP referrals, notes' availability, infection control procedures, the length of waiting lists, admission times, cancelled admissions and so on.

Each of these is reported on in detail. Take two areas, complaints and waiting lists. In the complaints sphere we produce flow charts to show how we deal with written complaints and what our complaints procedures are. So, for example, there is a briefing note about accident and emergency (A&E) and what's happening about improving these services, certainly an issue of high public profile. We compile detailed complaints returns showing the number of complaints logged in each area of the hospital, the number that have been dealt with and those still outstanding. In the waiting list area we assemble information on such matters as the length of time it takes in all our clinics to get a routine or urgent case across the institution, and a detailed breakdown by District of residence within SELCA showing the number of patients waiting for each specialty and for how long.

We have been very keen to ensure, however, that all this monitoring does not become a cottage industry for the benefit of SELCA alone; we need this information too to manage effectively.

In addition to such specialist areas, SELCA receive from us routine reports listing such things as the number of patients treated per speciality against each block contract for each District of residence. We are beginning to develop out-patient monitoring and out-patient contracting. This has been a neglected area in the NHS if only because the Körner requirements didn't specify a great deal about out-patient services. Consequently, at present our monitoring only extends to the in-patient and day-case side of things. In the climate of the internal market this omission of detailed information about out-patient services has already proved rather costly.

Specialty costing, cost behaviour and business planning

Q: 'Managed competition' requires other sorts of information to work, in particular, the costing of procedures and specialties. How far do you feel you have got at King's in this very large undertaking?

A: It's an enormous undertaking and we are still at a pretty rudimentary stage, although less so in multi-District specialties like cardiac surgery and renal services where we have in effect had cost-and-volume agreements running with the RHA since before the current Reforms. For these Regional specialties we are certainly further down the track in terms of costing and separating these costs into their fixed and variable components than the rest of our provision.[11] You can't really run cost-and-volume contracts effectively unless you have got a very clear idea not only on each specialty's bottom-line costs but also on how those costs behave for different case loads.

But beyond our Regional specialties we are still running most of our services against block contracts and our goal for this year is the rather limited one of simply ensuring costs to the institution are covered by income.

Q: What do you do, for instance, with indirect costs or overheads? For most NHS hospitals that seems still to be a particularly raggedy area.

A: It certainly is and for the vast majority of our services at King's Healthcare we still have not got a proper separation of our overheads by speciality. It's a very difficult problem to resolve. Let's just take the example of the Government funding we receive because King's is a teaching hospital: the service increment for teaching and research (SIFTR). In this institution out of 1991–2 total income, including capital charging, of £125 million, SIFTR amounts to £14 million. In other words, it is a significant amount of money and it's not unlike capital charging except, of course, SIFTR reduces our cost level whereas capital charging adds to it. None the less, both are supposed to be part of the 'level playing field'; each must be taken into account to arrive at the real costs of service in competitive terms.

But how to distribute it between specialties, that's our problem. King's School of Medicine and Dentistry has probably made more progress on resolving this than a lot of other NHS teaching hospitals, but it is still rudimentary despite having major implications on how costs are distributed internally.

Given the relatively speedy implementation of the Reforms, getting a grip on things so basic and fundamental as how much things actually cost and therefore what we should really be charging for a particular specialty at the particular volume to a particular purchaser is hardly complete at this stage. For the vast majority of our medical and surgical services we are a long way from being able to say to Croydon DHA, for instance, 'Well, if you want 250 general medical cases next year, it will cost you £x. If you want 270 cases, the extra 20 cases are going to cost you £y.' At the moment the only way we can charge for these extra cases is to *pro rata* the costs upwards and charge on this basis, that is, to ignore the behaviour of most of the costs involved, treating them all as if they were variable even when that is patently not the case. We know we shouldn't be doing that. As we have covered our fixed costs with the 250 cases, we should price the 20 cases on a marginal basis and therefore only consider variable costs.

This creates major headaches for NHS managers for which there is no obvious solution in the short run. Block contracts work on an average price per specialty but, given the cost variability for the different procedures within each specialty, they should be scrapped in favour of cost-and-volume and per-case contracts. But for the moment at least we are on the horns of a dilemma. There are real financial risks for us providers if we stay with block contracts but regrettably the move to more sophisticated contracting must wait till we have more detailed knowledge of cost behaviour.

I'll give you a good example of cost variability within a specialty. In general medicine at King's our costs are very much skewed upwards because of the case mix, particularly in clinical haematology. Arising from our expertise here, we happen to have a somewhat unrecognized, but quite lively, clinical haematology department that tends to attract patients with serious blood disorders like leukaemia and lymphomas. They can cost £30,000 per treatment yet what goes in the contract is the average specialty cost for medicine which is a fraction of that. Thus King's is carrying a major financial risk so long as clinical haematology is included in medicine's block contract.

It has been part of our very clear strategy in the contract negotiations during 1992 establishing the 1992-3 contracts to take haematology out of that block contract and to offer it as a separate contract to SELCA. However, SELCA have so far refused to contemplate this. So we are prepared to accept that we don't have a contract for clinical haematology in 1992-3 and we will charge on an ECR basis for these cases. To do otherwise is to have the financial risk all on our side; it's not being shared equitably.

One moral of this particular story is that we have to concentrate more on trying to separate out our variable and fixed costs for all our specialties. Yet this is such a Herculean task in terms of time and cost to us that we are simply not able to do it at this stage. We have had to concentrate on high-cost procedures that are currently hidden within block contracts; to pull them out and offer them as separate ECR-type or per-case agreements. For example, we have done this with spinal surgery, separating it off from orthopaedics. We have a separate tariff for spinal surgery procedures so that we can cover our costs more effectively. But, unfortunately, the problems arising from an inadequate knowledge of our costs aren't resolved by that step alone. At the moment the majority of these per-case agreements are being charged at the average specialty cost. This is crazy as it is the more complex work that tends to be charged on an ECR basis and in the past we haven't been charging enough to cover our costs.

That is forcing us to do more than simply separate out our high-cost procedures in the existing block contracts. The next step is the detailed study and analysis of costs and already this has led to several new cost-and-volume contracts for hip and knee replacements, cataracts, terminations of pregnancy (TOPs) and the like, that we are going to bid for and hopefully run in 1992–3.

Q: The original image, certainly the media image, of the internal market was one of GPFHs looking at their computer screens in, say, London and finding a good deal in, for instance, Aberdeen, and patients going there. In reality virtually every party – patients, GPs, purchasers and providers – has been entirely resistant to such large-scale alterations and uncertainty surrounding referral patterns. Am I right to think that, even in London, the changes in referrals will not be great?

A: There is not wholesale change. No, we are still talking about changes at the edges but, for us at least here in south London, these changes are significant changes at the edges. This year we already know, for instance, we are going to be doing a materially different amount of ophthalmology because we have attracted extra income and extra contracts.[12] We are working hard to see some relatively major shifts in cardiac surgery, again as part of an explicit strategy of expanding the specialty to ensure it survives.

Q: Clearly a very high percentage of your work load comes from SELCA. In time do you see King's winning some extra out-of-London contracts or will most of these commissioners stay with their local provider?

A: At the moment the signs are that it is going the other way. Thus, as money gets taken away from central London authorities, local purchasers are wanting to concentrate more and more on obtaining contracts locally. Furthermore, if there is a squeeze on budgets and you lose 2–3% of your allocation, that 2–3% is going to be withdrawn from your more distant providers. As long as SELCA pursues the same policy, and I think it is beginning to, this will limit the damage.

Q: Given that there are for you at King's 'changes at the edges', but that these can be none the less significant, within SELCA as much as anything else, what do you know about other Units' prices? To what degree are you operating in the dark in this respect?

A: I haven't seen competitors' prices although there is an agreement within SELCA that there should be free exchange of information amongst providers. However, that's not as clear cut as it sounds; the problem is one of being sure you are comparing like with like. For instance, we were confronted with a situation where Guy's quoted a very different order of costs than us for certain

episodes. Subsequently we learnt that Guy's prices excluded out-patients and
ITU (intensive therapy unit) costs which we had included within our prices.

Q: Can we conclude this part of the interview with some questions about
planning? You have talked about your difficulties with costings. Where does
that leave you now in terms of business planning in which case load and
contracts must be key ingredients? On balance will you largely stay with block
contracts at least in the short run till you know more about your costs?

A: From both a provider and a purchaser point of view, I think it has certainly
been the implicit assumption in everybody's mind that we are moving towards
cost-and-volume contracts as a means by which we equalize more effectively
the risks involved. Certainly, from our standpoint, we want to do that.

We've caught a major cold with block contracts this year. We're treating well
over the Camberwell target on the block contract for which we were getting no
extra income. King's has simply had to absorb the cost pressures that produces
together with the other financial pressures we have already discussed. Our
problem with this year's block contracts arose mainly due to the very high
level of emergency work load that we have encountered. Unfortunately, we
really can't do much about the emergency admissions through A&E until we
have the right sort of information system in place that can analyse in more
detail such things as admission criteria.

Overall, therefore, we are keen to move wherever possible to cost-
and-volume contracts. But, as we have just discussed, nobody should
underestimate the difficulty of costing all our contract activity in an organization as large as this.

Q: How do ECRs figure in your planning? Presumably they make life
easier.

A: There is no doubt that the comfort level is increased. However, because
of the problem all NHS hospitals are having in obtaining reliable cost data for
the range of services provided, Units have also found their ECR estimates to
be somewhat wide of the mark in 1991–2, the first year of contracting.

Actually at King's the situation is not nearly as bad as we first feared it
might be. We have come out more or less on the nail, recovering the income
we planned to. We are pleased about the difficulties we have overcome to
achieve this, particularly in setting up a trading system and to get the
internal disciplines right. Essentially this means doctors cooperating and
only admitting patients through prescribed procedures. For most of them to
start with this was something that went against their cultural grain. To stop
so-called 'back-door admissions', treating patients without any agreement as
to who will pay for them, was the main problem. That problem has now been
cleared away.

What nobody can still predict is how much ECR demand will be affordable
by purchasers for next year. It's a fine judgement for commissioners as to how
much they place up front in their main contracts and how much they keep
back for ECR demand. SELCA have adopted an explicit policy of committing
as much as they possibly can to up-front contracts, not keeping much money

back for ECR payments. They consider that to be the responsible approach as it gives providers a more sensible, firmer basis on which to plan the work for their Units.

Q: It occurs to me as we talk about the nuts and bolts of 'managed competition' – contracting, costing, pricing – that private-sector medicine charges on a per day, or *per diem*, basis and, in block contracting and certainly in per-case and cost-and-volume contracting, NHS managers are being asked to do much more than their private-sector counterparts. Have I got that right?

A: The private sector does have more flexibility in how it prices its services. One of the major factors, if not the major factor always, in determining cost is length of stay. The private sector avoids the costing problems we face and is able the more effectively to exert downward pressure on costs by charging, as you say, on a *per diem* basis. We are not allowed to do this; we are required to charge on episode cost.

But there are things we can do in the NHS. We have wide variations between consultants, between firms basically doing the same work, treating the same people for the same diseases. In terms of their patients' lengths of stay, it is in our interests to try and get *that 'per diem* factor' sorted out and reduced as much as possible. Achieving this is going to be a major focus for NHS managers. Stay length is still a key determinant of episode cost if only because our accountants still use length of stay as the basis for allocating overheads.

Q: In theory at least, some would say medical audit might help you there but it seems to be, quite understandably, an area into which you currently don't have much input.

A: Certainly locally the experience at the moment is that the doctors running medical audit aren't actually particularly interested in management issues. To us as managers they often appear to be narrowly focused around the actual outcome of their treatments. Lengths of stay or readmission rates have not really been examined. They see the patient very much in isolation from other organizational issues and that's something I think is going to have to develop over time.

Q: Not suprisingly and for some time now in this interview you and I have been knocking at the door of my next topic: the reaction of consultants, other doctors and other clinical staff, and their importance in making things happen – or not happen – in the Reformed NHS.

THE REACTION OF DOCTORS AND OTHER HEALTH-CARE PROFESSIONALS TO THE CHANGES

Q: Right at the outset you spoke of the internal market providng new incentives for hospitals to improve their performance.[13] To me a key fact about the NHS is its multiprofessional nature, with all the complexity that it brings. Are these new incentives affecting the clinical staff, especially the doctors and consultants, as the latter so directly affect expenditure levels?

A: There are some pretty powerful incentives now forcing us to respond to the actual demand for health-care services the hospital and its departments face and I find that very healthy indeed. Over time this will produce profound changes in clinical practice. A very good example of this at King's is surgery. It poses some of the classic problems faced by NHS teaching hospitals and this really makes it an even more effective illustration for your purposes.

Our surgical service exists more as a series of quite distinct subspecialities than a fully coherent whole. The important point to remember is that the prior system, certainly in teaching hospitals, encouraged this and all the problems it produced. The net result of surgery being organized essentially by subspecialty is that we have a problem with general surgery – the lumps, bumps and hernias, what the majority of our patients present to their GPs and are referred on to hospitals for. In the past this has not produced the long waiting lists it would have otherwise but only because, frankly, we have had such a superfluity of facilities and staff that it was possible to get through both a large amount of major complex work but also all the minor and intermediate work, the latter being largely done by junior medical staff.

Now, because there is a squeeze on resources – which one could argue would have happened anyway irrespective of the Reforms – those facilities have been reduced. The surgeons' reaction to this has been to preserve above and beyond everything else the major complex work. That continues to rotate very quickly off the front end of the waiting list, leaving a rump of work just sitting there.

What we have been trying to say to the surgeons is that they have got to look at things completely the other way round. If they want to continue to attract contracts and cover the fixed costs of their specialty, they are going to have to meet contract performance in terms of case load, throughput and waiting lists. Unless this minor and intermediate work gets done as a priority of its own right, there simply will not be a surgical presence here at all able to conduct the major complex work which is so important to them.

As far as surgeons in a teaching environment are concerned, up to now all the incentives in the system have encouraged a skewed case mix. You become a surgeon and make a name for yourself as a teaching-hospital surgeon not by doing the routine work but by undertaking the interesting surgery and doing more of it than anybody else. You publish your papers; you become known nationally, perhaps internationally. You get your merit awards. Teaching-hospital surgeons do not get these for being work horses, ploughing away day after day on the minor and intermediate, doing their share in the day surgery centre, and so on.

I think it has to be only a matter of time before the stimulants introduced by the internal market and other Reforms begin to change both attitudes and practices. For managers trying to get this across there is currently a problem in convincing them we face real market considerations and they must be meaningfully dealt with. With the Patient's Charter and local purchasing strategies, unless we do something about the surgical situation, we are going to have a real problem sustaining the speciality. I can't believe King's is alone in facing such difficulties. In specialist medical centres throughout the UK similar problems must exist. There are organizational pressures encouraging change. They need to be complemented by a more realistic, hard-headed approach to the personal incentives doctors face. It doesn't seem to be an issue that has been tackled at the moment on a national basis.

Q: Theoretically at least, could RMI be used to encourage changes in doctor/management relations generally, as well as the particular matter you raised?

A: Let's not be naive about RM. Just putting a doctor in a management position doesn't change anything in itself. King's Healthcare has had RMI and clinical directorates since 1987, well before many other hospitals. We were pretty close to Guy's in introducing that.

Organizationally RM at King's has meant the establishment of 19 clinical directorates or care groups as we call them. Many were headed by consultants but it has to be said less so now than a few years ago, mainly because we are having to get much more hard-headed about success criteria; on what has to be achieved to perform satisfactorily and to remain viable. If for whatever reason – lack of interest, commitment to management, etc. – there happens to be no one among the relatively small number of consultants available to lead their colleagues in the way that is essential in the 'New World' in health care, we are prepared to employ other professionals, not infrequently nurses, in full-time clinical management positions. Other King's managers are not clinical at all, having planning or administrative backgrounds. They have proved very effective and, funnily enough, they include those managers whom the doctors have really grown to appreciate.

At our Unit we have also defined different ways in which doctors can become involved in management. We have, for example, a clear distinction between a care group (or clinical) director and a clinical head of service. The latter is responsible for the clinical business management function only, which includes leading the relevant contracting discussions with SELCA and marketing the service to GPs, rather than the full-time management of the service concerned.

We don't need to have doctors managing, in a line management sense, the huge armies of people full-time management would normally be expected to cope with. This day-to-day management function we give to our care group directors. Thus what we have is the doctors in an influential position to purchase that service on behalf of the clinical specialty that they represent. That is the approach we are trying to adopt. It is proving difficult to develop but in time it must come.

These care group directors will not only deal with the detailed management and administration of outside contracts but also will before too long be required to enter into internal contracts with other King's managers. Nobody can really enter into a service agreement with an outside purchasing agency unless they are clear about the supporting systems to back up that agreement.

We need a customer chain with explicit agreements at the different levels. We ought to create a situation where, say, a surgeon will enter into a new external contract with a clear internal agreement of what nurses are going to be doing to support that new work; what the quality standards are going to be; what the throughput arrangements will be; and what all the other effects elsewhere will be.

Q: How have your doctors and other clinical staff reacted to the internal market?

A: Frankly, it's been widely variable. At the leading edge, particularly among those within the multi-District specialties who have been used to the contract environment for some time, they've taken to it very well and are entrepreneurial and actively involved in leading the process.

At the other end of the scale there are people who even now have not bothered to understand what the process is and what it involves. The discussion we had earlier about surgery[14] illustrates the mind set of a group of people whom I suspect are not uncommon in NHS hospitals. They still find it very difficult to understand how the values they have grown up with, in terms of developing their specialties, are being turned on their head by new imperatives in the system that force people to look at things in a different way. They are beginning to change their views but, for them, this is a painful exercise.

Q: Which are the majority, the enthusiasts or the doubters?

A: I would say that there is a significant minority, it could even be a majority, of people working in clinical roles – doctors, nurses and paramedical staff – who are not consciously aware of the changes or of really operating in a market environment.

It is useful to see these in two categories. First, there are those who know about the Reforms including the internal market, and are interested and informed about such things but whose daily work lives have not been affected by the changes. The activities of a physiotherapist or a staff nurse in a ward have not been directly affected by the contracting environment but, none the less, quite often these are people who have always taken seriously initiatives to improve quality, to improve their responsiveness to customers – who see that as important in professional terms, in their own personal view of their job. Now for quite different reasons, market reasons, great emphasis has been put on such matters and so they just continue on. It makes no sense to call such people 'doubters'.

There is, however, a second group of people who don't understand the Reforms, who have either had them explained but haven't made the intellectual jump to get their mind around them or have been alienated at some early stage of the process and since then have switched off, kept away from them deliberately and have taken refuge in their day-to-day work – looking after the patient – consciously switching off whenever anyone comes and talks to them about what needs to be done and why. This is a rapidly diminishing minority.

Q: We have been talking about the internal market for hospital services and the clinical staff reactions to it. Hospitals can lose contracts in this market. This raises the personnel question: what would happen to staff in such a case? Wouldn't you have to retain most of them?

A: You would certainly have to retain the senior people, if only because of the huge severance pay costs.

Q: Technically speaking at least, acquiring Trust status could change that somewhat. But effectively would it make much difference?

A: It would for most staff. But, if you want my candid opinion, Tomlinson or someone has got to sort out senior medical staffing issues in London. Consultants are appointed for 30 years; they have tenure; they are the major determinants of the cost and shape of our clinical services; and, with the Reforms, we have to be able to make rapid changes as and when necessary. The consultant situation does and will continue to hold up the process.

I won't name the specialism but certainly the strong feeling we got from our local purchasers was that one particular change in a clinical specialism that could have taken place this year has not occurred because we are waiting, literally waiting, for the retirement of the consultant concerned. You try and remove a consultant and they simply become a lady or gentleman of leisure, at enormous cost to the taxpayer. As long as those constraints exist, there will be problems.

Q: I want to refocus our discussion now on to our last topic: what sort of organizational changes have you made because of the internal market? What briefly have been some of the main training implications at King's arising from the Reforms? And, to draw the interview to an end, how have the roles of some of the senior participants – let's take those of consultant and your own as head of the acute side – changed as the Reforms are implemented at King's?

THE CHANGE IN ORGANIZATIONAL
STRUCTURE AND TRAINING FOR NEW ROLES

Q: I would like to start by asking for an overview of the changes to the organizational structure.

The main changes in organizational structure

A: We have completely reorganised and reshaped King's Healthcare. The process started some time ago with us asking ourselves how can we best operate in the Reformed NHS of today and tomorrow. The result was spelling out success criteria, both at the operating unit level, the part of King's that actually delivers the service, and the corporate part of the organization.

Having defined explicitly and closely our success criteria, we moved on to the tasks they produced and what people were expected to do. For the first time, evaluation criteria were actually available for use. The final part was organizational redesign: what shape organization will best deliver what is required?

My job as Divisional Manager, General Hospitals Division, illustrates this process. We soon realized it was too big and too wide. We will now have four, roughly equal divisions replacing one huge division (my own), one relatively big division and one tiny division. Support for care group (or clinical) directors has been thinned out and streamlined by rationalizing the number of people in business management and those supporting them. That change has caused some heartache as we will be cutting management posts and actual staff, and thereby making a necessary cost saving. Further, we have decided not to retain the management grade of deputy care group director.

It would be quite wrong to see this as a downgrading of importance of care groups. In fact, they are the key to our success in the internal market and, consistent with this, will receive more specialist support – dedicated financial and business management, HRM (human resource management) and better information. Currently all that type of back-up is organized at divisional level. But to operate successfully in the market, these vital skills are being put right into the front-line of the organization. These experts will be working alongside clinicians in the care groups, not above them or away from them.

In sum, we will be emerging with four divisions and a much enhanced function for care group directorates. The directorates will be the main operating limbs of King's Healthcare; in addition, there will be various corporate aspects reporting direct to the Chief Executive. It will result in a much flatter, slimmer and more agile organization than we currently have, and one suited to functioning under conditions of 'managed competition'.

The training implications

Q: What have been the principal training needs that have arisen to complement the changes you have outlined?

A: Training is being undertaken in a variety of ways. First, 30 of our senior managers will be going through a management development programme. It's being run here but organized by a well-known US college, Pennsylvania State University. The participants on this course will include care group directors and it will run over a full week. The purpose is to do a lot of business simulation work and assist our managers to think coherently in strategic and market terms. It is also important to develop a strong culture among the 30 most senior people in the organization. Region will be helping us pay the costs of this course.

Another larger training area currently being planned is for the middle-management cadre. We have done some work with outside management consultants on competencies and we are developing a training package. In time about 500 middle managers at King's will go through these mandatory training programmes which will cover such areas as recruitment, equal opportunities, and system and procedure development.

The purpose of the entire exercise, all the organizational changes we are in charge of, is to get every member of the staff very clear about what their role is, what the possibilities are, and having some clear systems against which they are monitored. Currently we are slightly behind some other hospitals in as much as, for large tracts of the organization, people just get on and do things against an unwritten specification, and with no system of monitoring what they are doing. The impetus for our organizational changes is mainly financial but also to improve efficiency.

The changing roles of some senior participants

Q: Finally, to end this interview and as an effective way of distilling something of the essence of the change process, I would like to hear briefly how the hospital consultants' role and that of the top managers, as exemplified by your own, are altering as a result of the current Reforms? Can we start with the doctors' role?

A: To give a brief answer I will concentrate on one issue, flexibility. Clinicians are going to have to get used to shifting around their usage of operating theatres, sessions and timetables on a much more flexible basis than hitherto. Gone are the days when a surgeon can be appointed and, for the next 30 years, always do his NHS operating session on a Friday morning, his out-patient clinic on a Wednesday morning, because that is always the way it's been done and so the rest of his life gets carved out in stone around that. Doctors are going to have to get used to the idea that they are going to have to 'Box and Cox' much more to accommodate fluctuations in work load as contracts are won and lost.

Q: What about your own role? How has that been affected, particularly by the internal market?

A: The focus of the job has become much more external. Historically, if you want to caricature it somewhat, community UGMs have been concerned centrally with the interface between their organizations and the community but acute UGMs have been more concerned with the internal workings of their hospitals to the exclusion of almost everything else. The Reforms are forcing everyone to look outwards – managers, doctors and other clinical workers. There is now a need to find out what patients and purchasers think and want from the Service much more than previously.

NOTES

1 The next chapter is an examination of this Trust by one of its doctor managers.
2 The Tomlinson Report recommends the merging of Guy's and St Thomas's Hospitals. At this stage it is unclear whether this will happen or in what form.
3 For more details on this important change refer to p. 65.
4 Refer to Chapter 3 which dwells at length on these regulated *vs* free-market aspects of the changes in the NHS.
5 For a similar view see p. 116.

6 See p. 192 for a similar view but coming from a purchasing standpoint.
7 Again the similar view is held by the author of Chapter 12 who is a DHA commissioner. Cf. pp. 190–1.
8 See p. 209.
9 Tomlinson could, of course, reduce this considerably if it is acted upon.
10 See pp. 223–4 for some more details about King's care groups.
11 For a clarification of this distinction see p. 149.
12 For a more detailed discussion of this see p. 215.
13 Refer to p. 210.
14 See pp. 222–3.

15

Everyone a Trust?: Trust Status in the Experience of the Guy's and Lewisham NHS Trust

Robin Stott

This chapter offers a personal assessment of the role of NHS Trusts in the light of my experience as a doctor and manager at the Guy's and Lewisham NHS Trust. In making such an assessment I am reminded of the words of Chou en Lai, one of my political mentors. He was on one occasion asked by a French journalist what he thought to be the main impact of the French Revolution. He replied without hesitation that it was still too early to tell. If a judgement after 200 years is difficult, to make any pronouncement so soon after the creation of NHS Trusts about their social significance is clearly foolhardy. So whilst I can be eloquent in my support for the theory of Trusts, any of the apparent practical benefits have to be viewed in this light.

In this chapter I will cover the following areas:

(1) I will suggest that even though NHSTs have not realized all their proclaimed advantages, they make possible one over-arching achievement – the 'impositional' management style of the old system can yield to more focused, devolved management.

(2) I will endeavour to demonstrate that such devolved management is both practical and effective by considering 1991–2, the first year of the Guy's and Lewisham Trust, and sketch out how such devolved, participative management enabled us to tap the requisite knowledge of many staff members and effectively position our Trust in the somewhat over crowded internal market in the London area.

(3) Some of the fears voiced about the true meaning of Trusts both inside and outside of the Service will be scrutinized in view of our experience at the Guy's and Lewisham Trust.

(4) By way of conclusion, I will point to both the dangers and penalties of any 'regressions' to the older, impositional managerial style in NHS hospitals when all of them were run by the DHA.

THE CHIEF VIRTUE OF NHS TRUST STATUS

The key to the health Reforms is the successful and cooperative management of the purchaser/provider split. Further, the focused and devolved managerial responsibility inherent in Trust status affords the best opportunity for a provider Unit to work closely with its main purchaser to achieve this end. I intend in this article to elaborate on the benefits of Trust status, and show how we in the Guy's and Lewisham Trust are attempting to capitalize on these, in conjuction with our main purchasing authority, the South East London Commissioning Agency (SELCA), to advance the cause of health in our corner of London.

I am always heartened when tendering arguments in favour of Trust status or 'opting out' because, as a Schumacher devotee and a Green Party member, I support the emancipating role of local, devolved management. Defending the move to local management of hospitals is not a problem for me. Trusts have made real the notion that accountability, responsible authority and finance have come to rest at the same local level, and we should resist a move back to the cumbersome bureaucracy of the old system. In that old system, trickle-down nourished the tip of the multilayered edifice of health provision; trickle-up nourished the base. The middle remained an arid waste. Or put in rather more graphic medical terms, the health system had both oesophageal atresia and Hirschsprung's disease, a punishing combination. The formation of NHSTs is merely a device which enables nourishment to reach all the parts – the essence of good management, as well as an advertisement for Heineken.

Trust status is therefore no more than a management tool, enabling a provider Unit to respond in a focused way to the changes in health care which are upon us, whether related to the present health Reforms or not. Other aspects of the Reforms, which I discuss briefly below, will determine what ultimate health-care benefit can be derived from using this management tool.

The other ostensible advantages of Trusts over direct managed status are two-edged. Even those of us who think that the Nikkei Index is a form of exotic Japanese martial art recognize that the concept of capital freedom has turned out to be illusory, and the move to abandon central wage negotiations is gathering pace throughout the system anyway.[1] Trusts may nudge this process along, as exemplified by the increase in pay for over 1,000 low-paid workers in the Guy's and Lewisham Trust but this is a marginal benefit as compared with that of local management.

POSITIONING THE GUY'S AND LEWISHAM
TRUST IN LONDON'S INTERNAL MARKET

Using the Guy's and Lewisham NHS Trust as an exemplar I will attempt to show how the devolved management of Trust status has enabled this Trust to respond most effectively to the demands of the new Health Reforms.

The Guy's and Lewisham Trust usually communicates via the press, both popular and unpopular, and also uses the media to spread our news across the length and breadth of the land. This news has not always been either accurate or complimentary. I can understand this as there are a number of mixed metaphors around which tend to confuse people. Our Trust has been likened to a 'flagship' and it has been suggested that the Health Service Reforms should have a smooth take-off. It is truly difficult to conceive of a flagship having a smooth take-off. More importantly, it seems to me that this concept could only emanate from the Ministry of Defence, an institution not renowned for its health promotional activities. As the Medical Director of the Trust, I am glad to be able to write about some of the positive initiatives we have been taking, initiatives which I hope will promote good health, and persuade you that Trusts really do promote enabling, participatory management.

As I have indicated, our initiatives have to be put into the context of the purchaser/provider split. This separation means that purchasers have the responsibility for assessing health needs, as well as having most of the available money to pay for these. They are thus able to exert considerable leverage on all parts of the health-care system, and help us all move toward more responsive and sensitive health care. We have recognized the necessity for this kind of change for years, but have never had the collective will to initiate it. Benefits we might derive from other aspects of the health Reforms are more contentious, and, in my view, do not alter the benefits of Trust status. However, I myself doubt whether the GPFHs should be purchasers; have considerable misgivings about the internal market as 'the motor' of the purchaser/provider separation; deplore the fact that debate over the Reforms has clouded the central issue of underfunding of the Health Service; and I feel that there should be a more open and democratic way of selecting the various health authority management boards. Fortunately none of these detract from the benefits that Trust status confers. So I can turn again to the positive, and look to see how the purchaser/provider split has energized us all to begin changing the pattern of health-care delivery, and how Trusts with their devolved management style have been leading the thinking about what and how we might change.

I will touch briefly on the well-known problems which our Trust faced when it was first set up, if only to show that they are not Trust specific. We started the year with a £6.8 million deficit (5% of our revenue), had troubled negotiations over our capital allocation, and difficult negotiations over what was and wasn't the responsibility of the old District. In common with most other provider organizations,[2] we have had difficulties with ECRs. Apart from this last issue, these are depressingly old difficulties, and have occurred not only in our hospitals, but also in most other inner-city hospitals, in each of the 5 years I have been involved in management. These problems in large part relate to chronic Health Service underfunding, finessed in London by RAWP and now capitation funding.[3]

The Trust dealt with these in the all too familiar way, but at least did so promptly, and with a directness which, although not comfortable, was honourable. The devolved management allowed us to come to grips with these issues in a more decisive and ultimately less destabilizing way than the usual death by one thousand cuts of the old regime. As a consequence of this, we are going to break-even in 1991–2, have treated 6,000 more in-patients, spread our fixed costs further, and so have achieved a unit cost reduction of

8% and have reinvested £2 million in delivering the promises we set out in our Trust charter. Perhaps the most important of these was the increase in wages to 1,000 low-paid workers in the Trust. But in addition to all that, we have embarked on another initiative: creating the mission for the Trust in a new and participative manner. This epitomizes the liberating effects of local management, and, in positioning the Trust in a difficult market, is a tangible benefit of Trust status. It is one that is widely 'owned' and therefore affects how we actually function.

Shortly after forming the Trust, we recognized that we would need to find an effective way of defining how we could respond to the changes which were likely to come about in both the manner and content of health-care provision. We believed the most important of these are:

- **the need for care closer to home** with hospital care closer to primary care; also an increase in day-, out-patient and programmed-investigation care;
- **the need for clearer information** to enable patients to make informed decisions about their care, and to make it easier for patients to use our services;
- **the need to research and evaluate** the role not only of what we do now, but of changes which will occur with the introduction of new technology;
- **the need to reorientate teaching** at both under- and postgraduates levels, to ensure that medical education supported the desired changes;
- **the need to link service teaching and research** into a Trust-wide evaluation ethic;
- **the need to improve the quality and effectiveness** of all our services, all of which should be in the top 10% of clinical and cost indicators.

We also recognized that our response would be constrained by a number of important issues. Some of these related to the health Reforms, namely:

- **A loss of money** from our three main local purchasers (SELCA – responsible for 70% of our contracted income plus Greenwich and Bromley DHAs) because 'capitation funding' means that over 5 years between £20 million and £30 million are moving from these three purchasers to other purchasing authorities further away from London.
- **Paying very high interest and depreciation charges** is significantly pushing up our cost per case. So in the financially competitive environment of the internal market in London, the increases in capital investment have to be coupled the Trust management wishes to make **an increase in income**.
- We could increase income either by **reducing the unit cost** of treatment, **or by increasing the number of funded patients** coming into the hospital.
- The present reality, whatever the Government said about money following patients, is that money follows contracts, and so **the getting and fulfilling of contracts becomes vital to us**.

- Contracts come from the 'patient advocates' (GPs and the DHA commissioners), whose views would be of increasing importance. We must assume that **it is GPs**, and possibly some of the tertiary referral agencies, **who exert the main influence on their DHAs, and work with them accordingly**.
- Particularly when multi-District specialities were contracted for at District level, **SELCA would be the purchaser for around 80% of our work**. Therefore, quite apart from the obvious need for us to work together to develop new ideas for health care, we also had compelling financial reasons to work closely with them.
- The recognition, dating from DHA days before the Trust was established, that the two Units in our Trust, Guy's and Lewisham Hospitals, were in many areas of their work and practice **not in the top range of NHS performance indicators**.

The position of the Trust in the NHS internal market and our way of dealing with the challenges and opportunities this poses is only one part of the equation. The other part relates to wider, national issues:

- **Demographic changes, with the expected shortage of manpower, which creates the need to look at new ways of doing things**. The need to improve the working conditions of those in the Health Service, particularly junior doctors, hence becomes a crucial part of looking for new ways of doing things.
- **London has**, in the view of most people, **too many hospitals and an inadequate community-based health network**. On the presumption that no government will wish to put more money into the hospital service of London, **money will be transferred from the hospital sector**,[4] making change in the numbers and functions of hospitals inevitable.

All these issues we felt were common to most inner-city teaching hospitals in the developed world and, in our visionary moments, we hoped that the Guy's and Lewisham Trust could pioneer a satisfactory solution to them.

In the era of unfocused management similar analyses were made but nothing was then done with them. Nowadays and in cooperation with SELCA, we intend to explore not only how we can adapt to these pressures but also how we can create new ways of responding to them which would be of benefit to our patients.

In designing our policy response to all the environmental pressures, we designed a matrix which enabled us to get a sense of the adequacy of what we did now, of how well we did it, and, more importantly, what we should be doing. We involved around 200 people, including clinical directors, GPs, commissioners, health experts and managerial and technical staff in the construction and filling in of the matrix. Following that, the results were discussed with them; indeed, 50 of us spent two weekends together reviewing our findings.

We used the information we had developed to draw up a vision, or mission statement, of where we hoped our hospitals would be in 5–10 years' time. This statement reflected possible solutions to both the aspirations and problems faced. We included benchmarks which we would hope to achieve in a defined and much shorter time scale.

The extensive consultation we have engaged in during this process ensured that we have the support and commitment of a substantial number of senior people within our local health nexus to reconfigure our services within the framework of the vision. This we are now proceeding to do. There will clearly be difficulties as we progress our vision, but again the focused, uncluttered managerial framework of the Trust will allow us rapidly to come to grips with such problems.

THE FEARS AROUSED BY NHS TRUSTS: AN APPRAISAL

Some observers have worried that Trusts might be the secret weapons of privatization of the Health Service. There are practical reasons why this cannot be so, in that the main source of money coming into Trust is from the publically funded commissioning authorities. Given the difficulty the already constituted private hospitals have in generating sufficient income to enable them to run effective, it is unthinkable that a Trust with a contract income of some £160 million would be able to survive on private patients. Again, the effective running of Trusts is entirely dependent upon the involvement of large numbers of Health Service staff, most of whom are opposed to the privatization of health care. NHSTs can compete much more effectively with the private sector than DMUs. Given the resources and talent in the Health Service, Trusts are more likely to erode rather than advance private care.

Some have asked if Trusts will wish to continue their involvement in teaching and research. There are several issues here. First, without an effective research and development base, no major institution will be able to survive the impact of increasing demand and continuing need for evaluation. Any short-term gain will rapidly be eroded, and enlightened commissioners are anyway requiring that evaluation and research structures are in place in the Units with which they deal. Second, the service increment for teaching and research (SIFTR) the income that hospitals (particularly large teaching hospitals) receive to fund their medical training and research roles, will in the future only be related to clearly defined teaching and research initiatives. Third, the presence of junior staff, which requires college accreditation, will be in part based on the availability of high-quality continuing education.

The crucial role of the commissioning authorities also belies the possibility of Trusts turning away from treating those people with 'less profitable' illness, another fear sometimes expressed about NHSTs. If a trust were unilaterally to stop treating the elderly, or mentally ill, it would of course lose the contract income covering these groups, and the commissioners would be in a very strong position to translate their displeasure into financial penalties.[5]

CONCLUSION: AVOIDING REVERSIONS TO THE PREVIOUS MANAGEMENT STYLE

Looking at what our Trust has achieved in 1991–2, we should ask the obvious question, 'Why haven't we done all this before?' I believe the pressure for change has come from the purchaser/provider split. The capacity to respond in an effective manner to the internal market in an over-provided London market for health-care services stems from the fact that we are an organization which has enthusiastically embraced the advantages of devolved management that our Trust status has given us. And NHSTs generally seem to be creating a good track record. For instance, I asked several senior members of the DoH and also Barbara Stocking – Director of the King's Fund Centre and author of an excellent paper on the future of acute services – where most of the major innovations directed to improving health care were coming from. All have said that whilst it is difficult to be certain, they don't know of any non-Trust hospitals which are pushing as vigorously as Trusts for new patterns of care.

What I have tried to do in this chapter is to identify the key virtues of Trust status, and show how we in the Guy's and Lewisham NHS Trust have taken advantage of these. Of course, one of the strengths of devolved management is that we can more readily learn from our mistakes. Not all our decisions have been enabling and participatory. Some have been frankly impositional, and have not lived up to the high standards we have chosen to measure the benefits of devolved management against. These standards are best characterized by a beautiful Taoist poem written in the sixth century BC:

Go to the people
Live amongst them
Start with what they know
Build on what they have
And when the task is done, the mission completed,
Of the best leaders
The people will say
We have done it ourselves.

I will therefore finish with two examples which show how perilous it is to revert to impositional management, one pre- and one post-Trust. As we are known as 'the flagship', I draw the first example from nautical history. In 1628 Gustav Adolphus of Sweden launched his new warship, the *Vassa*. It sailed for 1,500 metres from its launch in Stockholm harbour, capsized in a gust of wind and sank. The *Vassa* was long, narrow, and had a very tall main mast. This would have been fine but Gustav, anxious to have a ship which would out-gun any of his rivals, had unilaterally instructed the master builder to provide an extra layer of 20 one-ton brass cannons. The builder had to acquiesce, but made the prediction that the ship, its centre of gravity radically altered by the brass cannons, would sink on its maiden voyage. It was brought to the surface 350 years later, and with it surfaced this sorry testimony to the inadequacy of impositional management.

I share responsibility for a similar episode of bad management in our Trust.

Eager to communicate our aims we produced the *Trust News*, a paper which rained down on all employees of the Trust. We hoped it would be seen as confetti, but it proved to be more like the biblical plague of locusts. We, experienced managers though we were, had not prepared the way. We had used a cheap, old-fashioned and somewhat impositional method of imparting highly charged information. George Bernard Shaw said the major mistake in communication is to assume that it has happened. We wished on this occasion that he was right but I hope that in this short chapter I have succeeded in communicating the benefits of Trust status to you.

NOTES

1 Refer to Chapter 11 for a full account of the changes to national collective bargaining and NHS industrial relations generally.
2 See also pp. 220–1.
3 The change in the funding formula is the crucial dimension to King's Healthcare as well. Refer to pp. 213–4.
4 The 'Tomlinson factor', including the closing down or merging of London hospitals, was, at the time contributors were writing their chapters, regarded by most as a significant factor. See, for instance, pp. 128–9, 135 and 225.
5 Cf. Chapters 17–18.

REFERENCE

King's Fund Commission on the Future of London's Acute Health Services (1992) *London Health Care 2010: Changing the Future of Services in the Capital*. London: King's Fund.

16
Mainstream Specialisms and the NHS Market: The Case of Surgery

Simon P. Frostick and W. Angus Wallace

The NHS has seen several 'reforms' since its inception in 1948. Such reforms have been aimed at improving the efficiency with which resources are used. The most recent Reform programme propounded in the White Paper *Working for Patients* and subsequently embodied in the National Health Service and Community Care Act 1990 (DoH 1989, 1990) are no exception. The government of the day initiated a review of the NHS with particular reference to management of resources and formulated a report within 1 year. The recommendations were far-reaching and generated much political comment. Within the medical profession clinicians polarized into two opposing forces, for and against. The result of the 1992 general election has ensured that the major changes introduced by the Thatcher government will be confirmed and significantly extended.

The central feature of the Reforms was to separate the purchase of health care from its provision. The purchasers were to be the DHAs and general practices large enough to be allowed to manage their own budgets. The flagships of the provider side were to be the NHSTs. These latter would be independent of interference from the DHAs; be given privileges for obtaining and managing finances when compared with the DMUs; and be allowed to develop their own strategy for health care, as long as a number of specific specialties (originally referred to as 'core specialties' in the White Paper) were provided by each Trust hospital.

For the doctors the so-called 'internal market' (renamed the 'quasi market' by Le Grand 1991) has emphasized the fact that the funding of health care is not a bottomless pit into which governments are willing to pour ever increasing amounts of money. Doctors are forced to consider the need to prioritize health-care needs for the public. The Reforms have also meant a devolution of financial responsibility in hospitals to the level of groups of consultants, the 'clinical directorates'.[1]

The NHS Reforms need to be viewed in the light of changes that are occurring in other Western countries. Many other European nations are finding that the demand for health care is outstripping the resources that can be invested in the system. Canada is experiencing similar problems. In the USA adequate health care only reaches a proportion of the population who either fall into defined groups covered by the State or have health insurance cover. Recently US clinicians are expected to justify every cent spent even for those patients covered by private insurance. The Annual Abstract of Statistics (Central Statistical Office 1992) shows that in 1990 the UK health spent 5.6% of the gross national product (GNP) on health care. Taking similar factors for GNP into account the figure for the USA was 11.6%. In Canada the figure stands around 10% but is falling.

Further, the expectations of the general public have increased in recent years. No longer will patients and relatives tolerate long waiting times for out-patient appointments and in-patient treatment. No longer will the general public accept poor levels of care. Moreover, the public expects there to be increasing care at consultant level and improvement in the standard of information given to them.

We write this chapter as a review of the internal market as it is perceived by the two of us who are orthopaedic surgeons working and researching in a large NHS teaching hospital. Our review covers this market viewed against the backdrop of those other NHS Reforms that are internally related to it. Drawing extensively on illustrations and examples from our own clinical specialism we consider especially the following matters:

(1)   What sort of market is this internal market for health-care services?
(2)   How do the DHAs and GPFHs, the purchasers of these services, enter the picture?
(3)   What is the impact of the market on the acute provider?
(4)   Taking the example of hip replacements, we demonstrate the degree of imbalance between what the providers can supply and what their patients demand.
(5)   We examine the vexed question of classifying and costing contracts and the information problems that exist.
(6)   We consider another set of information problems and their implications, around new technology and new treatments, an area of particular interest to surgery generally.
(7)   What are the respective roles of managers and clinicians in RM?
(8)   We consider outcome and quality control measures, another area where the links between managers and clinical staff are central.

Two leading themes run through the chapter: first, that to do with resourcing the Service and its specialisms; and, second, the nature of the doctor–manager relation in an NHS where both groups accept patient care as the leading criterion – and together derive a working definition of what it means in particular contexts.

WHAT IS AN INTERNAL MARKET?

A free market is one in which the consumer has a choice when obtaining commodities and where there is competition between the producers to provide the best commodity at the best price. In the industrial setting the application of quality measures to ensure an adequate standard of product is well established and easy to achieve. If there is a provider monopoly, that is, one producer or provider, a free market cannot be said to exist; similarly if there is a monopsony, that is one purchaser or consumer, free-market conditions do not exist.[2] In the pre-Reforms NHS something even more restrictive than that prevailed: the purchaser and provider were one and the same. The concept of the internal market was designed to introduce some competition to the health-care system by breaking these monopoly conditions in health-care provision and health-care purchasing. A question that needs to be asked at this stage is, 'Who is the consumer?'

In monetary terms the consumers are the DHAs and the GPFHs but where do the patients fit in with this? Are they simply pawns to be manipulated depending upon the funding available or are they also to be regarded as consumers with a mechanism to choose and the right to expect particular standards? The DHAs and GPFHs cannot be regarded as free agents for the patients, able to negotiate the best deal, if only because in the case of DHAs at least they are controlled financially by higher authorities such as the RHAs[3] and, ultimately, the DoH.

The provision of freely available health care for all patients with no constraints is now recognized as being an impossible aim. In a private system the consumers (in this case the health insurers and, to a lesser extent, individual patients) can invoke market forces to ensure that there is competition between the providers of health care, that is, the consultants and private hospitals. In this situation, either the patients will have to travel to the most cost-effective hospital or there will need to be a proliferation of hospitals within a given geographical locality as occurs in the USA. Within the British health-care system the private hospitals have, on the whole, been built to serve a specific population without requiring significant movements of patients for most procedures.

The health insurers have negotiated tight bands of payment eliminating the possibility of competition on the basis of price. For the NHS large-scale funding is never likely to be available to create new hospitals in order to introduce competition between institutions locally.[4] The Government has developed plans for funding to 'follow the patients', indicating an expectation that competition should be generated by patients moving from one DHA to another.[5] What does the internal market mean to the managers and hospitals doctors? The answer to this seems reasonably simple, in the theory of the Reforms at least: the generation of contracts based upon the real cost of delivery of the health-care needs of the population. The providers would negotiate appropriate contracts with the purchasers to deliver a cost-effective service. Implicit in this is the need for quality assurance.

The most central problems that health authorities have had to face are the ability to generate contracts based on real costs and defining quality measures that are appropriate and acceptable. For the doctors the most critical problems relate, first, to the time spent away from treating patients when involved in managerial work and, second, to a lack of expertise when dealing with financial issues. The latter problem has been eased by the appointment of business managers to clinical directorates under RM. Doctors are then only required to make strategic policy decisions and can then leave the detailed application of that policy to a more appropriately trained individual with business skills.[6]

The first problem, that of time spent away from patients, is almost insoluble but is a source of frustration, particularly when the same hospital managers are telling consultants to reduce long waiting lists whilst at the same time expecting a large increase in the involvement of that consultant in the management structure. Ultimately all this means clinicians face the dilemma of prioritization of care provided for the patients. This is an alien concept to most individuals who have decided to become doctors and who have been educated to believe that all patients are equal and should be equally treated.

PURCHASERS OF HEALTH CARE

The DHAs and the GPFHs are the purchasers of health on behalf of the population they serve. They do not have a free hand in determining which services are purchased. Their funding is controlled completely by central government and, because the funding is limited, the purchasers inevitably have to prioritize the activities they wish to support. For DHAs whose hospitals have remained DMUs there has been little change in the way in which the overall delivery of health care has occurred since the start of the internal market. The main effects have been as a result of issues such as the Patient's Charter outlining some quality measures that the Government expects to be implemented. During 1991–2, Year One of the internal market, the DHAs have tended to negotiate block contracts for the entire work performed by a hospital based upon the volume of work complete the previous year and the previous year's resource allocation. These contracts have often been negotiated with very inaccurate data both in terms of the volume of work being performed and, more particularly, most hospitals have been unable to calculate the true cost breakdown for treating individual conditions. As a consequence major inaccuracies have occurred resulting in huge discrepancies, sometimes up to 300%, in the difference of costs for the same procedure.[7] During the financial year 1992–3 and beyond there will be an increasing emphasis on generating income on a cost-and-volume basis for each procedure performed and possibly eventually on the basis of individual invoicing for each patient treated.[8]

The DHA relationship with NHSTs has, during the 1991–2 financial year, been on the same basis as for the DMUs, that is, block contracting. However, the Trusts were encouraged to calculate their costs from professionally pro-duced business plans. As the business consultants employed for this purpose required accurate data that the Trusts could not provide, it is self-evident that the business plans were less than accurate and, in their efforts to compete in the market-place, a number of Trust hospitals under-costed their services.

The GPFHs have been a small proportion of the overall numbers of GPs in any given District. Following the Conservative Party success in the 1992 general election it is likely there will be a rapid expansion of the number of Fundholding practices. The GPFHs have controlled a small but significant percentage of the funds. As a result many hospitals have been forced to negotiate contracts favourable to the GPFHs resulting in preferential treatment to the patients from these practices. For the surgical specialties this is an unacceptable situation as it means there has been queue jumping for operations.

The percentage of the funding that the GPFHs control (only 5–7% in 1991–2) would appear to be sufficient to cause a significant decrease in overall activity for an individual hospital if that money were to be withdrawn. The financial margins within which hospitals currently work would appear to be very narrow. GPFHs have, in addition, been able to purchase care directly from the private sector and this too has resulted in an unfair advantage to patients treated in these practices. Although there is a belief by Government ministers that GPFHs are provided with the same funding levels as DHAs, the discrepancies between patient treatment levels would imply this cannot be the case.

THE PROVIDERS

DMUs and NHSTs are allowed to generate income from three sources: from the DHAs from whom the patients have traditionally been referred, from the GPFHs and from remote DHAs in the form of ECRs. The Trust hospitals also have limited and controlled access to borrowing money. However, neither DMUs nor the NHSTs are allowed to make a profit in the way that would be expected in a free market.[9] Some activities can be regarded as net income generators (e.g. cardiothoracic surgery) and others net income users (e.g. acute services such as trauma). The income generators are those that allow hospitals the leeway to improve their service to the community. A major source of net income generators are the ECRs but these are unpredictable and usually cannot be regarded as a regular source of income.[10] In exceptional circumstances, however, such as the provision of a supra-Regional tumour or spinal surgery service, a more predictable level of demand, and of income, is likely but cannot be guaranteed. Thus, even here planning can be difficult. Some types of hospital, especially those that are providing entirely elective services such as the specialist orthopaedic hospitals, can exert some control over throughput and hence manage resources advantageously as unpredictable acute services are eliminated.

Theoretically, all provider hospitals have the chance of generating extra income from ECRs. If there is sufficient spare capacity in the system patients, together with their funding, could be attracted from far and wide. In reality, it is unlikely that for most routine work in busy specialties – plastic and vascular surgery, ENT (ear, nose and throat), gynaecology and orthopaedics – there is much spare capacity. For some specialized work, for example, scoliosis and acetabular fracture surgery, cardiothoracic and transplant surgery, where there are few specialists, the opportunity for income from ECRs is highly possible but the demand for such procedures is restricted. Patients expect to travel for highly specialized treatment but should they be expected to do so for routine work such as a total hip replacement? It is reasonable to assume that patients recover better in familiar surroundings and can be discharged from hospital more quickly when family and friends are nearby which would not be the case if they have had to travel. Further, it would appear that towards the end of the financial year some DHAs have had difficulty funding ECRs because of a financial shortfall.[11]

As mentioned above,[12] very few hospitals have been able or seem likely to be able to generate accurate data upon which to develop contracts. Hospital management information systems depend upon data being transferred in an accurate fashion from individual departments, coded by clerks and entered into the computers. In many specialties (orthopaedic and traumatic surgery being a prime example) the number of coding inaccuracies is very high (Smith *et al.* 1991) and the coding systems available are inappropriate for modern practice (Radford and Wallace 1990). Moreover, it has proved very difficult for NHS hospitals to cost procedures. As with any labour-intensive industry, a very large proportion of the income generated is used to pay employees needed to run the service. Unlike industry, where labour levels can be manipulated quite significantly in the short term to cope with wage increases and the effects of economic recession, a minimum safe level of labour is required to maintain the NHS. The hospitals are not in a position to control the demand for services particularly for the acute or emergency services where an 'open-door' policy exists but also in the elective services where long waiting times are becoming increasingly unacceptable. Further, pay awards are not agreed at a local level so that hospitals are bound by national pay agreements for which they may not have fully budgeted. Theoretically, NHS Trusts are able to negotiate pay awards locally but, at present, would find it very difficult to make an award that is less than the national figure. The Government has also acted to prevent Trusts awarding junior doctors anything other than nationally negotiated pay rates and conditions.[13]

SUPPLY AND DEMAND

Within any national health service the demand will inevitably always outstrip supply if financial constraints exist. As doctors practically involved in planning activity within a surgical department, we have found the lack of knowledge about the true demand is extremely worrying. For instance, the specialty of orthopaedics has changed dramatically over the last 20 years. Total joint replacements, joint arthroscopy, major spinal surgery, microsurgery and so forth have placed unpredictable burdens on orthopaedic services. The only prediction that can be made is that in many instances the demand for this type of care will continue to increase for the foreseeable future. Total hip replacement surgery can be used to model the problem. The recommended level of hip replacement (*not total* hip replacement) suggested by the DoH is 1,050 per million population. This figure *includes* operations for fracture of the proximal femur treated by hemiarthroplasty. We know from our own figures that hip fractures will continue to increase well into the next century as the age of population of the UK continues to increase. Thorngren (1992) states that the total hip replacement rate in Sweden is 10,000 per year for a population of 8 million (approximately 1,250 per million population per year) and approximately 17,000 hip fractures occur per year. This is based upon a national audit with fully validated data. Keller (1991) from the USA has stated that the rate of total hip replacement is 2,300 to 2,700 per million population. In the USA the waiting time is minimal so that this figure probably reflects the true demand for this type of surgery *but*, as all individuals do not have access to elective health care in the USA, this too is an underestimate. Therefore, in the UK not only is the estimated figure for this single operation likely to be low but it is not possible to estimate the demand for the future.

In the brave new world of the internal market the planning of resource management cannot occur without a massive improvement in information. To date, in our experience, few orthopaedic departments are able to provide validated data about clinical activity and those data which are available, are often very inaccurate and incomplete. The general surgeons have a somewhat better database as a significant proportion of them have had a computer-based clinical system available for several years (Emberton *et al.* 1991). Some general surgeons have also extended their computer systems to generate useful resource data (Ellis 1991).

On the supply side increased demands are being made upon clinicians, especially in the surgical specialties, to increase supply and so reduce the waiting times for both out- and in-patient care. The fact that patients should not wait for 2 years for treatment is accepted by all clinicians and even 1 year is often regarded as too long a wait. Effectively many patients will have been waiting many years for some types of surgery because the GPs have not referred them to a hospital specialist (Foster *et al.* 1991). There has been very little evidence that surgeons abuse their privileges and do not provide an adequate service for NHS patients. On the contrary most consultants work considerably more hours than they are officially contracted for by the NHS.

The fundamental question that doctors are now asking is how the increased demand (determined by population, disease and referral patterns) is going to be provided for and how are the quality measures, such as short waiting times similarly going to be achieved, unless there is a major increase in all resources? In the UK there is one consultant orthopaedic surgeon per 63,000 of the population. There is a marked regional variation. Similarly, there is a marked variation in the waiting times for major joint replacement surgery ranging from a few months to a supposed maximum of 2 years. In other European countries there is one consultant for 30,000–40,000 population; the USA has a ratio of 1:15,000. Direct comparisons are impossible, because of differences in work practices for example, but it is self-evident that there are insufficient orthopaedic surgeons available in the UK. Similar problems exist in other surgical specialties.

The 1989 White Paper (DoH 1989) recommended the appointment of 100 *new* consultants over 3 years. This is but a drop in the ocean when one realizes there are over 1,600 consultants in the NHS and these 100 new consultants represent an overall increase of only 6%. However, simply to increase the number of consultant posts across the board is not the solution. New consultant posts must be properly resourced in every other aspect. Practical problems emerge from such an expansion as, at present, the control over training of surgeons is such that there would not be enough candidates for the new posts which are clearly required to provide the service.

THE BASIS OF COSTS IN CONTRACTS

How should costs be derived? In the USA the Medicare system introduced the concept of diagnostic-related groups (DRGs) which have banded a number of procedures into a set number of groups which pay the hospitals a specified fee. There is a move to introduce a similar set of DRGs into the UK. There are major defects with this system which will result in major errors in remuneration for services if the system is universally adopted in the UK. Munoz *et al.* (1990), Cotler *et al.* (1990) and Smith *et al.* (1991) have all shown there are defects in using DRGs in orthopaedics and trauma. The private health-care companies in the UK also band procedures into a small number of groups: minor, intermediate, major and complex major. Reference then needs to be made to a list of procedures which will allocate the operation to one of these categories. The private companies then add hotel costs to the bill.

This system may be applicable to the NHS but an improvement in the calculation of costs needs to occur. There will be variations in the cost of the same procedure in different hospitals. This will depend upon the size of the hospital, the facilities available, whether or not the hospital has to support core services and probably upon the skill of the clinical team. Low-volume surgeons cost more than high-volume surgeons and their outcomes are worse (Cotler *et al.* 1990). It will be necessary for an accurate list of surgical procedures to be formulated which can then be allocated to the best cost band. Information about lengths of stay and other hotel costs will need to be calculated. Once again, banding of length of stay may be necessary.

Whereas under most circumstances most patients will spend roughly the same time in hospital for a given procedure, some will inevitably stay much longer. If the median length of stay is used to calculate the cost, this will reduce some of the effects of variation for most patients. It must be remembered that cost should include items such as the need for capital equipment and buildings and labour changes. As all hospitals should make allowance for frequent major capital expense, equipment needs to be replaced and upgraded and those costs must be included in contract prices.[14] It has been disturbing to find that the current rules only make it possible to do this if equipment is fairly new and a realistic depreciation cost can be calculated. It seems replacement costs cannot easily be brought into the equation.

NEW TECHNOLOGY AND NEW DEVELOPMENTS

During recent years many new developments in both investigation and treatment have occurred. These are thought to be cost-effective but have not been subjected to formal analysis.[15] The UK usually lags behind other Western nations in implementing new technologies in the clinical setting. This is due to a historical lack of investment. In the era of the internal market and cost accounting a proper cost–benefit analysis of these should be undertaken but this requires investment in a potential risk area until the benefit is demonstrated.

Amongst doctors there is little comprehension of economic concepts such as cost-effectiveness and cost–benefit analysis and once again there is the need to return to the assertion that the information is not available upon which to carry out these analyses. Maynard (1991) states that 'There is an absence of data about inputs, activities and outcomes as well as ignorance about the relationships between these variables.' Maynard goes on to say that 'Public health care systems such as the British National Health Service have no cost data. Furthermore, the expenditure data that are available are related to functions and it is not possible to identify the opportunity cost of a hospital episode.' Therefore, there is little hard evidence available to confirm that new technologies are worthwhile and indeed cost-effective.

Many of those forms of investigation that have been shown to reduce morbidity and improve the overall diagnostic capabilities of a hospital have not had funding routinely made available for capital purchase from either central or local sources but have tended to depend on public donation. To complete this issue, funds for maintenance and replacement of donated equipment have to be found from existing funding.

The major worry for practising surgeons is that the restriction of funds available for the NHS will result in an inability to introduce new methods of treatment. In orthopaedics expensive implants are frequently used. Sometimes there is a tendency by the surgeons to use the flavour of the month which is often the least well tested and the most expensive. Surgeons must show restraint when introducing new technology but management must also appreciate many advances do result in benefit to patients despite being more expensive. The results of the effect of using a new system of total hip replacement, for example, may not be available for many years (similarly disasters may not become apparent for prolonged periods) and a risk must be taken in the introduction of changes to practice.

CLINICAL DIRECTORS

A 'key change' suggested in the White Paper *Working for Patients* (DoH 1989) is 'to make the health service more responsive to the needs of patients, as much power and responsibility as possible will be delegated to local level'. Although RMI started before *Working for Patients* emerged, analytically it can be seen as an important part of the current NHS Reforms.

This initiative means that the day-to-day management of resources for each specialty is being devolved to the clinician level, the clinical directorate. The head of a directorate is usually a consultant chosen by his or her colleagues. Directorates also exist in the paramedical services and are led by an appropriate individual. The clinical directors are assisted by a nurse manager and a business manager.

Within different hospitals the make-up of the directorates varies. In the smaller hospitals there will probably be a surgical directorate taking in many, if not all, surgical specialties. This may be a source of friction among some specialties who might see their independence being eroded. The unity of the directorate will depend, first, on the need to prevent domination by one group and, second, by a regular rotation of the clinical director. In larger hospitals the different surgical specialties may operate as independent directorates. The central role, within the internal market, for the directorates is to manage their own resources and eventually develop contracts for the delivery of their services. The directorates need to develop the strategy for the specialty (or specialties) they represent and it is the role of the clinical director to coordinate this activity and to 'put the case' to the hospital management board for the appropriate level of finance.

It has to be remembered that the clinical director is a consultant. Some clinicians may have the interest and knowledge to fulfil the role with ease; others are appointed because of their degree of seniority and the respect colleagues have for them but lack any particular skill in the management process. The business manager and nurse manager play a fundamental role in providing much of the necessary expertise for the directorate to function. It is obvious that the consultant is in a unique position in being able to discuss strategy with clinical colleagues and determine the activities of the Unit in the future.

The clinical director, therefore, has two roles (Bradford and Dinsmore 1992): first, as the director of clinical services and, second, as a member of the hospital management board which determines the 'corporate management' of the hospital. The director of clinical services is expected to be responsible for the management of the Unit budget, develop contracts, be responsible for the overall management of the services in the Unit and develop quality measures and medical audit.

This requires a tremendous commitment by the individual concerned. The DoH has suggested that one or two sessions per week will be required. It is the experience of many of the clinical directors that this is a gross underestimate of the time required even if all the necessary back-up is available. Moreover, it is not only the clinical director who is involved in this process, all the consultants will be spending some time in the management area. Some consultant contracts do mention that a session is allocated to management and audit activities. There is considerable unease from many consultants about the time spent on these activities especially when at the same time hospital management complain about waiting lists. Presumably one of the basic principles behind the clinical directorates is that the resources can be used more effectively by the clinicians directly involved in the delivery of health care. This is not very useful when there is a long-standing legacy of patients waiting for treatment and very severe controls over the level of resources available.

CLINICAL AUDIT, OUTCOME MEASURES AND QUALITY CONTROL

'To ensure that all concerned with delivering services to the patient make the best use of the resources available to them, quality of service and value of money will be rigorously audited' (DoH 1989). During the last few years there has been a considerable amount of activity concerned with setting up and developing medical audit strategies (Devlin 1990). These discussions have been concerned with audit of clinical activity and have ignored the 'key change' quoted above from the White Paper. It is obvious that the Government reason for encouraging medical audit was to improve information about resource requirements and utilization. Many clinicians have actively refused to be involved in this area of audit. However, it is self-evident that the link between medical audit and resource management is such that they cannot be separated. The aim of audit is to improve the quality of care delivered to patients. The most effective use of resources is embodied in this need. Frostick *et al.* (1992) have suggested that in order to distinguish the concepts of purely medical audit from audit linked to resource management, a further definition of audit was required. They have suggested that a form of audit called patient care audit, defined as a review of all activity within the Health Service having a direct effect on patient care, should be considered and analysed. This analysis is already being undertaken but in a piecemeal fashion. It can only be successful (that is, result in improved patient care) if all individuals involved in the care of the patients being considered, discuss their areas of concern together.

For the implementation of audit, extra central funding has been made available in the short term. The level of funding has been insufficient to properly install and develop the necessary high technology strategies and, in future years, further implementation will have to be financed from Unit funds. Unless further funding is made available, the very basis upon which the internal market is founded, that is, accurate data from which contracts can be formulated, will not exist.

The Patient's Charter (DoH 1991) has stated a number of quality measures that *must* be introduced in order to improve the patients' access to health care. Within any contracts resulting from the Patient's Charter both 'managerial' quality measures and 'medical' quality assurance now have to be included. In many specialties an accurate assessment of outcome is both difficult to undertake with any degree of accuracy and expensive to carry out. Elements such as patient satisfaction are either ignored or are reduced to estimating a single item such as pain.

Many of the quality measures put forward in the Patient's Charter are easy to measure (but much harder to achieve). But other areas, such as assessing the success or otherwise of a surgical operation, require outcome measures that look at short- medium- and long-term outcomes, and few objective measures of outcome are currently available.[16] Some contracts will state the acceptable levels of complications following particular procedures. This is again an almost impossible task because of the complex factors involved in diagnosing and determining the effects of adverse events (Frostick and Hunter 1992).

It is very easy to be negative about the introduction of quality assurance in health care. However, the patients do require reassurance that they are being treated to the highest possible level and do expect that waiting times will be kept to a minimum. The Government needs to know that the resources are being used in a cost-effective fashion. Individual clinicians should be interested in ensuring that their delivery of health care is to an expected level. It must be stressed that, unlike manufacturing industry, objectivity is substantially impossible and that quality measures will take time to develop and will continue to evolve.

CLINICAL FREEDOM AND PRIORITIZATION OF CARE

There are not enough resources available to the Health Service to fulfil all the health requirements of all the population. Some surgical procedures (minor in nature at present) are already not available on the NHS. Other patients effectively have their care rationed or do not receive any at all because of the long waiting times. Frequently a validation of a surgical waiting list will find a number of patients who have died or cannot benefit from the proposed procedure for other reasons.

It has become necessary for clinicians to justify clinical decisions and sometimes the options for treatment are limited because of a limitation on the resources available. It is, therefore, increasingly necessary for clinicians to prioritize patient care. The economists would like us to allocate care on the basis of useful or healthy life gained from a procedure. The most popular 'measure' at present is the quality adjusted life year (QALY). Measures of quality of life examine the effects of disability and distress in particular illnesses and calculate the amount of quality life that the procedure will give to a patient.

There is much argument as to the value of the assessments. There are complications, however. For instance Avorn (1984) has suggested that some measures of quality of life have been based on questionnaires given to well people. When the same questions are asked of the real patients, a totally different view is given. The situation is further confused when cost data are combined with quality-of-life measures. Unfortunately there is clearly a tendency towards using these types of data to prioritize resource allocations. It is reasonable to assess the cost-effectiveness of particular procedures and, subsequently, influence the way clinicians approach groups of patients but, in some instances, it may only be the least cost-effective treatment that is available and thus ethically it cannot be withheld.

CONCLUSIONS

In this chapter we offer two orthopaedic surgeons' views of the internal market, with this market discussed in terms of the wider Reform context within which it functions. To begin with, the internal market is here to stay. There is always going to be a restriction on the level of resources available to the NHS. The need to reduce waiting times and improve the quality of care is almost incompatible with this financial restriction. In orthopaedics there is a need for increased resources as the system is already working close to full capacity with the prospect of further major increases in demand. It is likely that similar problems are occurring in the other surgical specialties. In order that funds are being used efficiently a substantial improvement in the type and level of data is urgently required. Outcome measures need to be developed. There may be a place for measures of quality of life to help to decide on priorities. Finally, management and clinicians must work together in a cooperative, not adversarial, fashion as both should have the aim of treating patients properly as their first and foremost criterion. All other considerations must be secondary to this.

Le Grand (1991) concludes his review of the NHS quasi market:

> Many of the ideas are directly amenable to economic analysis. . . . It has provided a set of quasi-market 'experiments' against which to test those theories. Properly monitored, these should be able to provide economists and other analysts of social policy with evidence whether, suitably adapted and extended, quasi-markets constitute the way forward for social policy – or whether they are a retrograde development that will need reversing as soon as politically and practically feasible.

NOTES

1 RMI predates the White Paper. However, viewed analytically it can be seen as an important part of the current Reform package. Refer pp. 38–40.
2 See Chapter 5 above on different ways of conceptualizing markets.
3 See pp. 192 and 211 for more on the lack of clarity surrounding the role of RHAs today.
4 Cf. pp. 109–12 on the degree of competition actually spawned by the current health initiatives.
5 The rhetoric, perhaps only the early media presentation of the internal market, spoke in such terms. The reality can be very different. For example, the internal market can allow local providers and purchasers to build up a specialty at the DGH and stem the flow of patients to a more specialist provider.
6 Cf. pp. 223–4.
7 Cf pp. 147–9 on price variability.
8 Cost-and-volume and per-case contracting depends on an even more accurate knowledge of cost behaviour than than required for block contracting. See pp. 218–9 where this is explored. Refer also to Chapter 10 from which it is clear that, although costing in the NHS will have to improve, management accounting can never produce the accurate, real costs that some still naively hope for.
9 Their return is fixed by Government. See p. 61.
10 Cf. pp. 196–7 and 220–1 for more on ECRs from a purchaser and provider manager.
11 Opit sees this as a serious problem. Refer to p. 185.
12 Refer to p. 239.
13 The NHS industrial relations sphere is reviewed in Chapter 11.
14 Cf. pp. 197–9 for additional reasons for pricing variability.
15 The need for comprehensive evaluation of procedures is something that the

purchaser/provider split heightens. As pp. 194–5 indicate, very few hospital treatments have been evaluated in the way required.
16 Refer also to pp. 64–5.

REFERENCES

Avorn, J. (1984) Benefit and cost analysis in geriatric care: turning age discrimination into health policy, *New England Journal of Medicine*, 1294–301.

Bradford, A. and Dinsmore, M. (1992) Resource management and budget holding, in S.P. Frostick *et al*. (eds.) *Medical Audit: Rationale and Practicalities*. Cambridge: Cambridge University Press.

Central Statistical Office (1992) *Annual Abstract of Statistics*. London: HMSO.

Cotler, H.B. *et al*. (1990) The medical and economic impact of closed cervical spine dislocations, *Spine*, 448–52.

DoH (Department of Health) (1989) *Working for Patients*. London: HMSO.

DoH (Department of Health) (1990) *National Health Service and Community Care Act*. London: HMSO.

DoH (Department of Health) (1991) *The Patient's Charter: Raising the Standard*. London: HMSO.

Devlin, H.B. (1990) Audit and the quality of care, *Annals of the Royal College of Surgeons of England (Supplement)*, 3–14.

Ellis, B. (1991) Management importance of common treatments: contribution of top 20 procedures to surgical workload and cost, *British Medical Journal*, 882–4.

Emberton, M. *et al*. (1991) Comparative audit: a new method of delivery audit, *Annals of the Royal College of Surgeons of England (Supplement)*, 117–20.

Foster, H.E. *et al*. (1991) Provision of medical and community services to people with severe arthritis: an audit, *British Journal of Rheumatology*, 356–60.

Frostick, S.P. and Hunter, J.B. (1992) Complications and outcome measures, in J.C. Fairbank *et al*. (eds.) *Outcome Measures in Trauma and Orthopaedics*. London: Butterworth Heinemann.

Frostick, S.P. *et al*. (1992) Introduction, in S.P. Frostick *et al*. (eds) *Medical Audit: Rationale and Practicalities*. Cambridge: Cambridge University Press.

Keller, R. (1991) Personal communication.

Le Grand, J. (1991) Quasi-markets and social policy, *The Economic Journal*, 1256–67.

Maynard, A. (1991) Developing the health-care market, *The Economic Journal*, 1277–86.

Munoz, E. *et al*. (1990) Economies of scale, physician volume for orthopedic surgical patients and the DRG prospective payment system, *Orthopedics*, 39–44.

Radford, P.J. and Wallace, W.A. (1990) The code war, *British Journal of Healthcare Computing*, 22–4.

Smith, S.H. *et al*. (1991) PIS and DRGs: coding and their consequences for resource management, *Journal of Public Health Medicine*, 40–1.

Thorngren, K.G. (1992) Medical audit: experience from Sweden, in S.P. Frostick *et al*. (eds.) *Medical Audit: Rationale and Practicalities*. Cambridge: Cambridge University Press.

17

Psychiatry and the Purchaser/Provider Divide

Stuart Turner and Nigel Fisher

Mental health services, even before the NHS Reforms, were organized differently from other hospital services. Specifically they:

(1) were essentially local services for tightly defined catchment areas;
(2) operated within fixed budgets to provide a defined range of services;
(3) spanned, to a greater or lesser extent, the hospital–community interface;
(4) were accustomed to working with private-sector institutions (e.g. secure hospital care).

In other words, they were, even if only loosely, defined in quality, quantity and cost in a fixed relationship between service and a DHA. The impact of the current Reforms has been less marked than in some of the other acute specialties precisely because these prior (contracting) relationships existed.

The aim of this chapter is to consider the new framework created by the internal market and related Reforms (for example, changes in the method of funding that express themselves eventually by which service agreements are entered into) and consider what opportunities and threats this creates and is likely to create for psychiatric services, especially in view of their differences from other acute services.

To this end we will consider the ramifications of 'managed competition' for our profession under the following themes:

(1) in the light of the key issues facing mental health services today and in relation to the acute and community provision;
(2) how, to date, the work load for psychiatric services is being affected by the new contracting process;
(3) what new information on cost and quality might emerge under the new arrangements;
(4) the likely effects of an explicit process of needs assessment by DHA purchasers;
(5) the insensitivity of the new weighted capitation formula for NHS funding to social deprivation including homelessness, one crucial social background often underlying mental health problems;

(6) whether preventive medicine is likely to benefit from the internal market;

(7) the future of psychiatric teaching and research under their new funding arrangements;

(8) finally, and growing out of the foregoing, where psychiatric services are best located in terms of the organizational structures for providers under the Reforms: specifically, will our services flourish more in an acute- or community-based NHST?

Let's begin our review by indicating the most important issues mental health currently faces.

THE NATURE OF THE MENTAL HEALTH SERVICE

Over the last two decades increasing attention has been directed to the need to make adequate community and local hospital provision for the closure of the Victorian asylums. Failure to meet all these needs, particularly in inner cities such as London, has led to increasing pressures on users and their families. Although, in general, long-stay residents of the large hospitals have been offered good-quality community re-provision, there are many new chronic patients who have not been able to access longer-stay services. Some of these vulnerable people have fallen out of care into homelessness and worse.

Hospital and community-outreach mental health services are currently able to contact only a proportion of people with psychological difficulties. They have the potential to meet ever more diverse needs but this can easily be seen as a 'threat' because of the implications for costs. Because they operate as emergency-led services, usually without waiting lists, they are hard to control except by limiting resource. Society has declared that there is a statutory responsibility to detain some individuals – currently under the Mental Health Act 1983 (DHSS 1983) – and demands that the service is capable of response. Often the only effective method of control is seen to be financial and cash limits have been routinely applied.

In the pre-Reform NHS, mental health was forced to compete with more 'glamorous' high-technology specialties. Both opportunities for development and quality standards were significantly restricted. The competition for funding has been especially difficult because DHAs, especially teaching authorities, have had the dual responsibilities of maintaining local services and providing a range of specialist facilities for use by students and people from other communities. There has been a lack of clarity about how to balance these competing claims (community versus specialty service) on the local DHA budget.

The complexity of psychiatric services is often not appreciated. They include, for example, work in child and family psychiatry; out-patient psychotherapy; support for community services; hospital treatment and continuing care; secure treatment of mentally ill offenders; liaison work with general hospital doctors and GPs; and work with drug and alcohol dependencies and psychiatry of older people. They stand to have an important impact on many aspects of health and social care. To take just one of many examples, about a fifth of people admitted to general hospital beds have significant problems with alcohol misuse; simple psychiatric interventions can reduce readmission rates. Despite more recent work carried out by the Royal College of Psychiatrists, for long periods there has been a lack of consensus on appropriate balances and methods of service delivery.

Mental health services also require close cooperation between primary health-care and specialist services, between health professionals, social work and voluntary agencies, in other words, between a range of hospital and community services. The boundaries between social and medical care are blurred and for good practical as well as theoretical reasons. There are interacting forces in operation: the homeless man might be in crisis because he has no accommodation but the reason for this might be to do with his chronic schizophrenic disorder and the effect of this on ability to work or access social support.

PSYCHIATRY AND THE PURCHASER/PROVIDER SPLIT

Competition is not new to the NHS. Rather, the Reforms have clarified and modified the system. They have opened up many areas where previously there were ambiguities. For example, the DHA managing a large London teaching hospital which had to decide between the relative merits of a service for local people and the wider benefits of a high-technology acute hospital development, now has a mechanism for resolving this dilemma. Similarly the competing interests of teaching and research, on the one hand, and clinical service, on the other, were often hard to resolve but are now explicitly covered in the SIFTR[1] and Working Paper No.10 funding allocation (DoH 1989).

Drawing a distinction between purchasers and providers has provided a useful framework in which to resolve some of these difficulties. The task of maintaining large medical institutions now falls increasingly to the acute provider Units, both DMUs and NHSTs, which have to attract patient referrals (and hence resources) from a range of purchasers. On the other hand, the responsibility for defining and prioritizing the medical needs of local people lies with the local DHA as purchaser. Locality-based services, such as mental health, should therefore be able to compete equally on the basis of need within the same defined population as other specialties.

Because psychiatric services have traditionally been based on catchment areas coterminous with local DHA boundaries, the baseline contracts of the first year of the internal market are largely with single home-purchaser health authorities. This is in stark contrast, for example, to other London acute services which depend heavily on contracts with a multitude of Districts to maintain revenue. The 'market forces' affecting these other acute services have not yet had much impact on psychiatry. The process of withdrawing contracts from remote centres in favour of developing local services, which is affecting some of the general hospital flows, is unnecessary.[2]

The initial opportunity under the internal market is to define a common interest with the home purchaser in providing an appropriate service to meet the needs of the local residents. Because the services have long been based on this relationship, the first steps should be more to do with refining quality and cost standards than with changing contracting flows. Although there are still relatively few GPFHs in London, it seems to be particularly important both for providers and for purchasers to ensure that local GPs, whether or not Fundholding, have an effective voice in determining the pattern of services.[3]

COST AND QUALITY OF SERVICES

At this stage quality standards are often rather basic but the more these can be made explicit as part of the contract between provider and purchaser, the more the debate about style and method of service delivery can be opened out to include users and other interest groups. In the short term this may be uncomfortable for service providers and there are risks that anti-psychiatry pressure groups will replace the older medical advice structures. However, as long as any developments are based on best available evidence rather than anecdote or prejudice, and are thoroughly evaluated, in the long term this wider debate is likely to be beneficial for the Service. It is essential that the potential for an open market in health care is moderated by quality criteria. Only the future will show whether the quality rhetoric assumes real value in determining competition or whether financial argument – as in the past – simply dominates everything else.

There is scope for considerably more sophistication in resource management. The identification of realistic costs for parts of a service, including capital charges and proportion of medical, management and support services, should allow much more realistic judgements about relative standards of efficiency and effectiveness. Again it is vital to take an informed view of data but the contracting imperative to hold valid information provides an opportunity to examine prejudices. In one recent exercise examining a range of ward sizes, one of the smaller wards, which was able to maintain an intensive treatment approach and an associated high turnover, was (predictably) relatively expensive in terms of cost per bed-day but was the cheapest option when the cost per completed episode was calculated.

There are exceptions to this account of a simple relationship between home purchaser and locality service. Although in-patient services have been heavily restricted to catchment area even within teaching hospitals, there has been some opportunity to specialize at an out-patient level. In this way, teaching hospital psychotherapy services tend to be better developed and often include more variety than in other Units. There are some immediate opportunities and threats, therefore, to specific elements of service which need to be confronted.

There are other hidden complexities. Liaison (general hospital) psychiatry in which the mental health service provides consultation to people admitted into medical and surgical beds, from the whole range of geographical areas which those services cover will also involve a relationship with other purchasers. This is particularly important to clarify where the general hospital itself receives a substantial flow of distant patients; failure to consider this will lead to these costs being carried by the home purchaser and will divert money away from other psychiatric services for local residents.

NEEDS ASSESSMENT

Fundamental to the rational implementation of the Reforms is the obligation on purchasers to determine more systematically than hereto the needs of local people. A substantial criticism of all health services is that they are led by demands of individual patients. Although, because of the nature of the catchment area and community service, this is much less true in mental health than some other specialties, there are no grounds for complacency.

Difficulty in gaining access to appropriate health care by black and other minority groups has frequently been raised. For as long as services were working to high levels of activity, within geographical and cash limits, there was little motivation for the Service as a whole to seek additional work. There has been no systematic development of statutory services for refugees and asylum seekers in this country in contrast to many other developed host countries.

Similarly, the clinical and moral case for providing psychiatric sessions to local courts is obvious. It would mean that large numbers of people facing minor charges could avoid being remanded in custody for long periods simply to obtain an assessment. Now it is possible to use the tension between purchaser and provider to achieve shifts in attitudes and priorities. It remains to be seen how far this will happen and whether any financial assistance will be available to start these projects.

The Jarman Index (Jarman 1983), a measure of social deprivation, has been used to allocate resources at both primary and secondary levels of health care. Although the subject of criticism (Davey-Smith 1991), the Jarman Index has the advantage of being calculable from existing data and of combining a range of measures of social deprivation into a single figure. Significantly for mental health services, homelessness is not one of the measures. Indeed, the Jarman Index and other similar indices (Scott-Samuel 1984; Townsend *et al.* 1985) measure the deprivation only of households, by definition omitting the effects of the homeless on demands for health-care resources. The numbers and health-care problems of the homeless have been thoroughly investigated in other communities (for reviews see Tessler and Dennis 1989; Morrissey and Levine 1987). This work indicates that there are many people with serious mental health problems who are not identified by service providers.

It is essential that this process of needs assessment takes place carefully and yet quickly. The risk is that the planning process will become dominated by different, but no more accurate, anecdote and stereotype.[4] No service is more at risk of these political pressures than psychiatry. Service providers, for all their undeniable limitations, do have a good knowledge of many of the local issues. To distance them from the commissioning process may serve to shift the balance of opinion too far away from professional clinical advice. There are lessons to be learnt from other countries where the balance of decision-making has become too remote from professional knowledge. In some parts of the world people are denied access to one of the most effective forms of treatment for the most serious form of depression, evaluated using properly controlled scientific experiments. The decision to ban electroconvulsive therapy (ECT) is a tragedy for the small group of people for whom it may, quite literally, be a lifesaver.

A balance must be introduced into needs assessment. People with severe mental disorders who present with disturbed and dangerous behaviour constitute only a small minority of the total patient population. None the less, small numbers of people each year need to be cared for in secure accommodation. These are people who would pose a considerable threat if allowed to leave hospital or cared for in a hospital environment which was inadequately supported. Danger does not just apply in the streets; it also applies in hospital wards, both to staff and patients where the environment and the staffing ratio are inappropriate. The needs of people in this category are obvious and, in general, no District would be able to resist an appropriate request to find a safe level of care for dangerous patients. The risk is that others, whose own needs may be just as great but who are quiet or isolated, may not achieve such a high profile and will therefore continue to suffer in the competition for resources.

PURCHASER PRESSURE ARISING FROM THE NEW NHS FUNDING FORMULA

There are some particular difficulties facing the purchasers of mental-health services. Needs vary from District to District and, if standards are to be maintained, this needs to be reflected in resource allocation. In the new NHS funding formula, needs variability is less sensitively provided for by social deprivation indices than previously.

There are, for example, frequent problems in resourcing adequately the health care of homeless people (Fisher *et al.* 1991). Estimates of the numbers of homeless people in London vary widely (for a review see Oldman 1990). However, the number accepted as homeless, by local authorities, has increased by over 117% in inner London since 1979, although changing thresholds and patterns of acceptance must qualify these data. In a hospital survey, about 1 in 9 psychiatric in-patients in an inner London acute service was unable to give any indication of a place which they would describe as home (Fisher *et al.* 1990).

Given that schizophrenia is characterized not just by the 'positive' symptoms of hallucinations (e.g. hearing voices) and delusions (e.g. a belief in a conspiracy to observe the individual through television screens) but also the 'negative' symptoms such as isolation, withdrawal, loss of drive, loss of feeling and loss of concentration, it is hardly surprising that people with chronic schizophrenias are particularly vulnerable to failure in social and community care. Many may find themselves becoming homeless, partly as a consequence of this special vulnerability. Indeed, it has been suggested that up to 40% of single homeless people in London have major mental disorders (Weller *et al.* 1989), although this estimate rests on assumptions about the definition of homelessness and sampling techniques.

In one London District it has been estimated that a third of all acute psychiatry beds are occupied by homeless people (Fisher *et al.* 1990). This implies that local residents can only occupy two-thirds of the provision, equivalent to adding half as much again to the effective size of the catchment area. This has not yet been adequately addressed in any of the weighted capitation formulae. Simply to estimate numbers of homeless people in a District and add these numbers to the total population is quite inadequate. There are two main reasons for this. First, surveys always underestimate the numbers of people who preferentially migrate to inner-city areas and to Districts with hostel provision. Second, this calculation fails to take account of the prevalence of serious morbidity in this group; this is an additional factor over and above the social deprivation factor.

Needs-assessment methodology is important, therefore, not only in aiding purchasers to prioritize the allocation of resource within a purchasing budget, it also stands to be helpful in dividing resources appropriately between purchasers. The problem of care is made more complex by the historical and theoretical overlap between social care, for example social work or housing assistance, and medical care for people in difficulty. There is scope for pointless argument about the boundaries between social and health care. In the same London District one of the local authorities has experienced a prolonged social work strike. Failure to work as effectively as usual inevitably leads to increased pressures on the Health Service and, more importantly, on its users. The current funding formula makes no provision for damaging effects such as this.

PREVENTIVE MEASURES AND CONTRACTING

Preventive measures in psychiatry often feature in planning documents as no more than a pious hope or, alternatively, as a panacea to take the role of all treatment services. Both extremes miss the point that there are certain situations where prevention is possible; these include considerable elements of the work in community care. However, none of these measures is likely to produce significant lower costs and therefore the fate of preventive medicine in the internal market is perhaps uncertain.

To take two specific examples: first, there is now a substantial research basis for the assertion that family intervention, where one member has schizophrenia, can assist in relapse prevention (e.g. Leff and Vaughn 1981). Second, there is some evidence that early (within 1 or 2 days) critical incident debriefing (CIDB) can prevent late psychological sequelae of major traumas such as natural disasters or combat (Dyregrov 1989). Either of these manoeuvres, if widely introduced, would improve the quality of life of many people. To listen to the self-styled 'forgotten people' who returned from detention as the 'human shield' in the Gulf following the 1991 invasion of Kuwait only underlines the importance of providing an appropriate response following these incidents (Easton and Turner 1991). The risk is that, although a needs assessment might indicate the value of these techniques, unless they can be shown to reduce cost, the effect of market forces might be to stand against their introduction.

EDUCATION AND RESEARCH IN THE INTERNAL MARKET

Another of the potential advantages of the Reforms is the separation of health purchaser from medical education purchaser. Identifiable budgets for undergraduate teaching are available to teaching Units in the form of the Service Increment for Teaching and Research (SIFTR). In some cases this will reduce the costs of services below DGH levels; students may be a benefit as well as a cost. In other cases, it will help to clarify the cross-subsidization of teaching and research by clinical service funds. In either situation, it will help both teaching and clinical purchasers to examine the quality and quantity of the service for which they are contracting.

In psychiatry, because the service has been restricted by catchment area and budget, there has often been a conflict between teaching, service and research. An academic with an interest in an esoteric disorder stood the risk of being criticized by colleagues working under pressure with local people. The purchaser/provider divide may improve this situation by allowing more easy access of such patients to specialist Units, providing that appropriate health purchasers can see the merit in a distant referral and there is also adequate support for the research and teaching element.

CONFIGURATION OF TRUSTS IN RELATION TO PSYCHIATRY

One of the main advantages for psychiatry as a community service is the separation of responsibility for local services from specialist high-technology acute hospital services. There would appear to be a case for psychiatry entering into a community-based Trust rather than merging with these specialist services in a compound hospital-based Trust.[5] Although theoretically it should be the case that budgets for psychiatric services will be determined by contracts independent of the condition of the rest of the Trust, inevitably there will be a focus of management time and resource into some areas at the expense of others. Psychiatric services have too often been the poor relation in these arrangements.[6]

There are probably more natural relationships with other community specialties and with the services provided by the FHSA. Bearing in mind the vulnerability of the large teaching-hospital Trusts in inner London,[7] there are sound reasons of finance and stability for psychiatric services to consider actively joining a community-based rather than an acute hospital-based Trust.

CONCLUSION

In this chapter some of the differences between psychiatry and other hospital services have been examined in the light of the new purchaser/provider divide. The nature of the pre-existing arrangements may account for the lesser impact of the changes on psychiatric than other acute specialties, perhaps nowhere more obviously than in London teaching hospitals subjected to significant changes in distant patient-flows.

So far,[8] the main impact of the reform for psychiatry appears to be in determining that the purchaser has the primary responsibility for carrying out a needs assessment of the local population and commissioning appropriate services. In the future there will be more opportunity for market competition. Unless this is based on rational assumptions about local needs, the whole system will remain flawed. Indeed, the simple capitation approach, if it fails to give sufficient weight both to deprivation factors and homelessness, may lead to a poor quality (because under-resourced) service being purchased by inner-city authorities in contrast to more affluent districts.

The complex relationship with local voluntary and social services agencies, the need to operate within the other NHS Reforms (namely care in the community) and strong historical precedents mean that competition on a large scale is less likely. However, these relationships will probably need further attention as funding arrangements become more clearly understood. The implications of moving service pressures from one agency to another will increasingly be seen in terms not just of quality but also of cost. It is to be hoped that a sophisticated view of the interacting social and medical forces is taken to avoid unnecessary and clinically meaningless conflict between carers.

Psychiatry needs to meet the challenges of the new Reforms by defining its services more clearly, demonstrating effectiveness wherever possible, listening to users of the service – especially those detained – and tackling some of the issues of prevention where this is achievable. The Reforms will not, in themselves, solve any of the long-standing difficulties in this service, but they do provide a different framework in which to argue for change. As with any development, it is essential that we take up as many of the opportunities as possible without being blind to the threats to the quality of care.

NOTES

1 SIFTR is the Service Increment for Teaching and Research. Refer p.217 for the difficulties in spreading SIFTR across the specialties for costing purposes.
2 Refer to the mini case studies in Chapter 8 where this problem, feared (SLTH) or realized (ILT and LDH) is a significant factor in the overall strategic response for acute services.

3 The enhanced status and the courting of GPs is a major change produced by the Reforms, especially the internal market. Refer Chapter 13.
4 Cf. Chapter 6 on the many technical and other problems needs assessment must face. At this stage the process is rudimentary in nature. See pp. 192–5.
5 New combined Trusts are no longer favoured by the DoH. See p. 124.
6 Refer to pp. 193–4 for a commissioner's view of the place of the so-called Cinderella specialties like psychiatry in the overall contracting plan.
7 Refer to Chapter 8.
8 In the first year of contracting, the so-called 'steady-state' period.

REFERENCES

Davey-Smith, G. (1991) Second thoughts on the Jarman Index, *British Medical Journal*, 359–60.

DHSS (Department of Health and Social Security) (1983) *Mental Health Act*. London: HMSO.

DoH (Department of Health) (1989) *Education and Training. Working for Patients, Working Paper No. 10*. London: HMSO.

Dyregrov, A. (1989) Caring for helpers in disaster situations: psychological debriefing, *Disaster Management*, 25–30.

Easton, J.A. and Turner, S.W. (1991) Detention of British citizens in the Gulf: health, psychological and family consequences, *British Medical Journal*, 1231–4.

Fisher, N.R. *et al*. (1990) Homeless and mentally ill, *Lancet*, 14 April.

Fisher, N.R. *et al*. (1991) Working for patients: will it work in practice?, *The Psychiatric Bulletin*, 73–5.

Jarman, B. (1983) Identification of underprivileged areas, *British Medical Journal*, 1705–8.

Leff, J. and Vaughn, C. (1981) The role of maintenance therapy and relative expressed emotion in relapse of schizophrenia: a two-year follow-up, *British Journal of Psychiatry*, 102–4.

Morrissey, J.P. and Levine, I.S. (1987) Researchers discuss latest findings: examine needs of homeless mentally-ill persons, *Hospital and Community Psychiatry*, 811–12.

Oldman, J. (1990) *Who Says There's No Housing Problem? Facts and Figures on Housing and Homelessness*. London: Shelter.

Scott-Samuel, A. (1984) Need for primary health care: an objective indicator, *British Medical Journal*, 457–8.

Tessler, R. and Dennis, D.A. (1989) *A Synthesis of NIMH-Funded Research concerning Persons who are Mentally Ill*. Washington, DC: National Institute of Mental Health.

Townsend, P. *et al*. (1985) Inequalities in health in the city of Bristol: a preliminary review of statistical evidence, *International Journal of Health Services*, 637–63.

Weller, M. *et al*. (1989) Destitution at the festive season, *Lancet*, 220.

18

Health Care of the Elderly and the Internal Market

Shah Ebrahim

Health care of the elderly came into its own as a recognized specialty after the birth of the NHS, although the need for a medical approach to the care of the aged and the chronically sick was recognized long before this. The National Assistance Act (Ministry of Health 1948) delegated responsibility for frail old people to local authorities (under Part 3 of the Act) rather than the NHS, much against the advice of Lord Amulree, a pioneer of health care of the elderly working at the Ministry of Health (Bennett and Ebrahim 1992).

Health care of the elderly wrestles with this dichotomy between medical and social views of the nature of problems and their solutions. Over the last century a consensus has emerged which places the responsibility for frail elderly people with *both* medical and social agencies. Attempting to solve chronic problems (such as confusion or incontinence) or acute crises simply by a medical *or* a social intervention is usually inadequate (Campion *et al.* 1983; Rubin and Beckard 1972). Communication and joint working between social and Health Service agencies has been of great benefit to patients and has led to joint planning of a wide range of new services for elderly people and training programmes for staff and carers.[1]

This chapter will endeavour to give a comprehensive account of medical care of the elderly and how it has been affected by the Government's health policy with particular reference to the internal market. The chapter will therefore cover:

(1) the nature of our hospital-based service and some indication of how it developed;
(2) the major policy objectives behind the internal market seen in relation to elderly patients and a comparison of the rhetoric of 'managed competition' with its reality;
(3) how the market challenges the three distinctive elements of health care of the elderly plus the strengths and complications in health-care-of-the-elderly catchment areas and how the latter are exacerbated by the internal market;

(4) the lessons we have already learnt from the large market in private-sector institutional care for the elderly;

(5) a demonstration of how extensive the detailed ramifications of the internal market are for this specialty in particular:

- the case for high-tech acute provision for the elderly and how this is being fundamentally challenged by the Reforms;
- the impact of GPFHs on the primary-care side of working with elderly patients;
- the ripple effects of health-care-of-the-elderly's difficulties on its complementary paramedical professions;
- how health care of the elderly is disadvantaged by existing economic evaluations of treatments and procedures.
- questions of spare capacity and real choice in the provision of our services;
- complexities around costs for this specialty;
- common ownership of the Reforms as the key challenge that management must take up;

(6) finally, some thoughts on the profound funding problems created by an ageing population.

HOSPITAL CARE OF THE ELDERLY

Throughout the development of health care of the elderly there has been a misunderstanding of its role in hospital and a concern that it has 'medicalized' old age and is just concerned with keeping old people alive for longer. The aims of health care of the elderly in hospital are many and include the acute management of disease, the rehabilitation and resettlement of elderly people suffering from chronic diseases and the long-term institutional care of those frail elderly people who are unable to live in their own homes. Over the last 40 years elderly people have consistently been housed in some of the worst buildings, with some of the worst levels of staffing and at lower cost than other groups of patients, although new building and an awakening of interest in this hospital specialty have done much to improve these circumstances in much of the country.

More recently health care of the elderly has been seen by some as a means of ensuring that elderly people do not 'block' beds, particularly in acute specialities. The efficiency produced by adequately resourced multidisciplinary teams working in designated wards has been self-evident and has led to a rapid expansion of the specialty. However, health care of the elderly is more than just a 'take-away' service. Sick elderly people often require the skills provided by teamwork from the very beginning of a hospital admission and various forms of age-related and integrated admission policies have evolved to ensure that the majority of elderly patients find themselves in the right bed at the right time and with the care of the right team (Hall 1988).

Many health-care-of-the-elderly services are justifiably proud of what has been achieved in a short space of time: new wards; day hospitals; linked working with psychiatry, orthopaedics, internal medicine; close relationships with local social service departments; input into local residential and nursing homes; emphasis on preventive health care; development of chiropody, dentistry, hearing aid services, communication therapies, continence-nurse advisers, liaison nurses. The morale, enthusiasm and expertise that has been built up is remarkable compared with even a decade ago.

Against this background of development and achievement the NHS Reforms have come as a tremendous blow to many who work with elderly people. The need for appropriate reform was most evident in surgical specialities where investment had been low for a decade, waiting lists for cold surgery had risen, and crises in the availability of expensive areas of acute care, particularly intensive care, had reached the point where the case for an immediate increase in resources appeared self-evident to most of the professions involved (Perrin 1992). To the Conservative Government the need was rather to ensure that the service was better managed and would therefore be more efficient. Given what I have said earlier about the efficiency and confidence of the health-care-of-the-elderly services, the need for further efficiency was not a particularly clear one.

THE AIMS OF THE INTERNAL MARKET

A major aim of the internal market was to ensure that 'cash should follow patients' thus avoiding the busiest hospitals outstripping their budget allocations: the more work done under contract, the more income to the hospital. Further aims were to avoid scandals related to underprovision of health care and to pass the accountability for rationing to the Health Service itself rather than the Government.

Central to the market philosophy has been the idea of choice which assumes that consumers are aware of the value of the commodity being bought or sold. Consumers of health care of the elderly are not discerning customers. Most do not know what they want or need and are not in a position to make rational choices, neither are their relatives or even, in many cases, are GPs. Many elderly consumers of health care do not want to be associated with geriatric medicine even if it is what they need most to ensure the best outcome. Late referral for a 'long-stay bed' of elderly patients who might have benefited from rehabilitation and respite care is commonplace among so-called 'good' GPs. In a market, demand for a commodity is related to supply by price. Given that all health services in the world, including the British NHS, practise differing methods of cost containment, their chief characteristic is rationing of services which automatically removes choice from the consumer.

THE REALITY OF THE INTERNAL MARKET

The accountability of purchasers to the general public is extremely weak[2] and cannot be seen as an enhancement of the rights of consumers to get what they want out of the services they buy through taxation. The internal market has empowered directors of public health medicine and general managers (but not patients) so not surprisingly these directors and managers have few complaints. It is difficult to see how purchasers will be responsive to local need as no efficient means of measuring need has been developed,[3] nor is there a direct relationship between Health Service provision and the burden of illness in a community. Hence services that may be effective in a limited sense of improving the outcomes for individual patients cannot hope to compete with the wider and stronger forces of unemployment, ignorance and poverty as major determinants of the community burden of illness (Townsend and Davidson 1982).

As of March 1992, the market has not yet started operation in anything other than a token sense (NHSME 1992). There has been a toning down of the language of the market-place. The market is heavily controlled and it now appears unlikely that any real competition (with winners and losers) will result.[4] It is also becoming clear that the internal market is limiting choice for some patients. Resources for ECRs are extremely limited and much time is currently spent on assessing requests in departments of public health medicine. An option that is used in London is simply to say no to all requests and let the provider make the decision of carrying out treatment without payment or take the blame for callously discharging the patient. Consequently, the idea that cash will follow patients remains a forlorn hope and could have been achieved more easily by simply paying hospitals for the volume of work done without introducing the purchaser/provider split (Perrin 1992).

The political rhetoric that the internal market, rather than increases in funding, will lead to greater efficiency and quality of care remains unsupported by clear evidence even in the best-documented areas of waiting lists for cold surgery (Beecham 1992a). In the majority of the hospital sector's activities – acute admissions – the internal market appears to be an irrelevance at best and at worst will divert resources from patient care into setting up the detailed accounting machinery. The bulk of health care of the elderly does not lend itself to market forces as it consists of unregulated presentations of acute illness that have to be dealt with immediately and at unforeseeable cost. The model of the market might be appropriate for a small proportion of cold surgery where costs can be more readily defined and choices made ahead of time. It is remarkable that the entire system of health care is subverted by an internal market that makes marginal sense for only a small proportion of the work.

A potential benefit of an internal market is the opportunity to iron out inconsistencies in the amount or quality of health services. This will require purchasers to be knowledgeable and shrewd in their negotiations. Time will tell whether this opportunity is realized.

REQUIREMENTS OF HEALTH CARE OF THE ELDERLY

Effective patterns of working require three main elements: comprehensiveness of care, continuity of care and cooperation between health- and social-service sectors. The workings of the internal market seem set to challenge these requirements and dismantle the patterns of care that have served elderly people well. I will discuss how each of these three elements is likely to be adversely affected by 'managed competition'.

Comprehensive care ensures that, regardless of where an elderly person enters the 'system', her subsequent management will be determined by her needs. This involves often very complex – and unpredictable – liaison with other hospital specialists, with home-care services, with primary-care teams, with relatives and friends, and even with the cats' home! Follow-up work may range from informal telephone calls to check all is well to the patient attending a day hospital 3 days a week. Comprehensive care implies that the patient cannot be viewed as a pre-planned, income-generating episode of care. The costs involved in such management are difficult to quantify and depend more on the willingness of staff to communicate well and a shared sense of purpose, namely, the good of the patient.

Continuity of care is vital for elderly people and their relatives. It is the knowledge built up over time that guides decisions and reassures carers that help will be forthcoming when needed. The uncertainty associated with the internal market has caused relatives to question the motives of consultants and GPs as never before: 'You are sending her out to save money' and 'I'm afraid I'm going to be too expensive to look after soon' are commonplace comments these days. The general public are assuming that the elderly will get the cheapest possible care and will miss out on care that they might need but that cannot be afforded.

The cooperation between local authorities and hospitals seems destined to die as both parties attempt to save money. Already in 1991–2 the exercise of joint planning between authorities has achieved very little as hospitals have effectively opted out of the scheme, claiming to have no resources for such liaison work as they have had to balance the books in the last 2 years. The innovation that joint planning was capable of introducing seems unlikely to be resurrected as it becomes clear that some hospital managers want to play a different sort of game, and one in which elderly people are a local authority, not a Health Service responsibility.

MARKETS AND CATCHMENT AREAS

Health-care-of-the-elderly services have traditionally worked with defined catchment areas and resources have been allocated on the basis of population served.[5] This arrangement makes communication easier between different sectors within the same geographical area and ensures that a shared philosophy of care can be developed. Work with elderly people usually requires a high level of advocacy which is eased if professionals know each other well. Contracts are often held by purchasers with several Health Service providers which are not coterminous with the patient's local authority services. This leads to major difficulties of communication, of prior assessment by community staff on discharge and unwillingness to offer appropriate follow-up.

A further dilemma is that patients who are admitted to an out-of-catchment hospital may fail to be accepted by the local health-care-of-the-elderly service because they are not the responsibility of that service and no extra resources will flow to the service for the extra work. In essence, two systems are working in parallel; staff understand the old system and are unwilling to embrace the new, particularly as no extra beds or staff are available to cope with the extra work.

EFFECTS OF MARKET FORCES: THE LESSONS LEARNT TO DATE

Health care of the elderly has already been substantially privatized with the dramatic increase in private-sector institutional care over the last decade (Laing 1988). Indeed, this unprecedented change in the NHS occurred with minimal public debate and has had unexpected consequences, not least the £2 billion of taxpayers' money now spent each year on income support to residents in the private and voluntary sector.

The private institutional care sector is indeed a proper market. There is a ready supply of the commodity. The consumer is free to choose which home to use, and has direct access to the necessary money to make her choice. If she doesn't like the services on offer, she can leave the home, taking her money with her. This free market in private institutional care has demonstrated that not everyone who self-selects for a nursing home needs that level of care; thorough multidisciplinary assessment and treatment prior to resettlement is not available; homes vary in quality; inspection systems are not capable of ensuring good standards; the homes that do go out of business are not necessarily the worst ones; and closing a private home leaves frail elderly people on the streets.

Hospital departments of health care of the elderly have been asked to provide beds to avoid the scandal when things go seriously wrong at a particular private-sector home. This private-sector market has also demonstrated that making money out of institutional care is easy in areas where property is cheap but difficult in the south east and London. Consequently, very wide differences in the availability and cost of private homes exist because of market forces. In general, moving the patient to where the homes are does not help relatives to visit and may be associated with increased morbidity and even death.

Markets are protective of their interests and in the hospital sector the main concern is to ensure that budgets are not exceeded, particularly this year. This has led to some questionable decisions. In one psychogeriatric service some 40 demented elderly people were moved *en masse* from NHS facilities to a private-sector home some 200 miles away. This was done because their hospital was considered inadequate; the patients were too demented to know where they were; and none had any relatives to speak up for their interests. From the purchaser point of view this was an excellent decision because care costs would no longer come from their budget but from centrally funded income support grants to individual patients. From the provider point of view it was a good decision because it permitted two wards to be shut thus saving around £500,000 a year. From the patients' point of view it was a scandalous decision as the care provided in the private nursing home was so poor (but cheap and within the income support limits) that the home was the subject of a television exposé and was quickly shut down.

This story is dramatic but every day individual patients are discharged to the private sector for institutional care, not because it is better or cheaper, but simply because the hospital's budget is protected. This self-interest is about to be checked. In April 1993 the community care legislation (DoH 1990) will come into effect, transferring the current centrally funded income-support payments for institutional care to local social services departments. Some social services departments may be unwilling to consider hospital patients as their responsibility, particularly if they need nursing care. The results for hospitals may be profound with a rapid increase in length of stay and a reduction in efficiency unless local solutions to this problem are found.

A consequence of the local authority social services department having the key responsibility for care of elderly people is a need to define the responsibilities of health and local authorities: for example, is bathing a social or a nursing responsibility? This route is strewn with elderly people who have come to grief because of social or medical definitions of their problems. The central lesson of health care of the elderly is that no one discipline has supremacy but that multidisciplinary teamwork and blurring of roles benefits elderly people by ensuring that disease is treated, appropriate rehabilitation found, aids for living and home-care services are provided, and that social engagement and housing problems are dealt with as well. Considerable vigilance will be required to ensure that community care plans recognize the importance of multidisciplinary teamwork, use the available expertise of existing hospital departments of health care of the elderly and built in mechanisms for auditing the quality of service from both a service and consumer perspective.

HIGH-TECH AND LOW-TECH HOSPITALS

The development of income-producing surgical specialties,[6] 'glamour' services such as laser angioplasty and acute services will leave little room for health care of the elderly in acute DGHs. One of the hardest battles of the last 20 years has been the establishment of acute units for elderly people within DGHs and the closure of many peripheral, small hospitals with inadequate staff and facilities for the safe management of sick, elderly people.

This battle is being refought with some hospital managers who wish to define health care of the elderly as 'low tech' and thus something that can be done anywhere, but not on an acute hospital site. Elderly people are capable of benefitting from high-tech medicine, particularly minimally invasive surgery, joint replacement and modern imaging techniques. Often high tech for elderly people is the safest, quickest and most effective way of dealing with their problems. It is, however, expensive and age has always been a popular yardstick for rationing in the UK.

One way of avoiding the costs of maintaining health-care-of-the-elderly beds on a DGH site is to 'rationalize' provision and simply offer all elderly services as part of general internal medicine, a solution proposed by a London teaching-hospital Trust. Such a solution could be good for elderly patients if medical wards were places where elderly patients would get the time and type of care they need. Only limited progress has been made in improving standards of care of elderly patients in internal medicine so, for the present, the main beneficiary of such a strategy would be the hospital budget.

The probability of two-tier services is one of the most frequent criticisms of the internal market; some hospitals will get worse and worse until they close. Since the political nerve to shut hospitals frequently fails Secretaries of State for Health, the alternative 'death by a thousand cuts' method is used. After a period of financial attrition and one or two scandals of inadequate care, the local view then becomes very positive towards closure.

The internal market appears to lead inevitably to popular and unpopular hospitals being labelled as 'good' and 'bad' without evidence that their outcomes or standards are any different. The raw material they work with – the patients – and the fabric of the buildings are likely to be the chief differences in the popularity stakes. Given the choice of attending a dilapidated hospital in the poorest part of the east end of London or a modern hospital in the richest part of London which would the 'discerning customer' choose?

GENERAL PRACTICE AND BUDGET HOLDING

Health care of the elderly is a two-way street: it requires responsibility and action from GPs as well as from the hospital; both parties are direct providers of care. For the hospital team to do a good job, it is essential that the GP and primary-care team do a good job and do not simply wash their hands of elderly patients. Reciprocal contracts between hospital and primary care providers are needed in most disciplines, particularly health care of the elderly, psychiatry and child health. The hospital task is made possible by high standards of primary care which includes careful monitoring of frail elderly people in the community, rapid response to acute problems, willingness to deal with social crises. Without good-quality primary care, hospital services get overloaded with the community's work that they are not capable of doing well.

GPs are being encouraged to take up budgets as this is a way of making hospital providers more responsive to their (and hopefully their patients') needs. The concept of budget holding has been strongly criticized because it threatens to distort the provision of services in a maverick way with cost being the overwhelming consideration in referral choice. It is also thought to be inequitable as the access of patients to health care will depend on whether their GPs are budget holders. The administrative burdens of placing contracts for individual patients, particularly in smaller practices, is likely to be considerable, let alone the knowledge base required to evaluate constantly whether hospital A is cheaper,[7] quicker and as good at the job as hospital B.

Most of the new software available to GPs gives listings of the most expensive and highest consulting patients on the list. Most are elderly and presumably, if times get much harder, it will be in the practices' interests to remove such patients from their lists. Already it is hard for private-sector nursing homes to find GPs willing to take on new residents. FHSAs will have to ensure that GPFHs are acting in their patients' interests.[8] Referral, investigation and treatment audits may be useful in examining the ways in which budget holding affects health care. Removal and refusal to accept elderly patients should result in a review of the circumstances with a patient advocate if necessary.

SCARCE SERVICES

Elderly people depend on teamwork provided by a wide range of people, particularly in the hospital sector. With increasing interest in controlling and passing costs on to other sectors it is possible that some services, for example occupational therapy (OT), clinical psychology or social work,[9] may disappear from many hospitals. Social work is paid for by local authorities and, following the Seebohm Report (Home Office 1968), the good sense of close relationships between social services and hospitals was cemented into practice. OT is widely used in health care of the elderly but not by other hospital departments. Without widespread demand for OT and other similar services they are in danger of disappearing from hospitals.

The solution to ensuring that elderly (and other disabled) patients have ready access to the right skills is to ensure that the standards of practice common on health-care-of-the-elderly wards spread throughout the acute and elective wards of hospitals. The use of systematic team assessments, goal setting and consultant-led team meetings are already part of the best internal medicine with elderly people and need to be extended to the rest. The danger is that under the Reforms things will go in the opposite direction.

EXPLICIT RATIONING

The most obvious benefit of internal markets is that they have the potential to provide explicit criteria for rationing of health-care resources. It remains to be seen whether managers will be bold enough to be explicit in their decisions and whether such decisions will receive any public discussion or have any general currency. In general, elderly people do not do well in resource arguments because they evoke so little interest and the costs of their care are high. It is therefore possible that the elderly will suffer as decisions about spending are determined more by public opinion than the potential for benefit for their health care arising from canvassing opinions on such a wide scale.[10]

It must always be remembered that pensioners are an important part of the electorate and until recently have accepted a position of social gratitude for the welfare state's handouts. Pensioners are likely to have much stronger public voices in future and to expect greater rights, access to health care among them. The available means of economic valuation of the benefits of treatment will inevitably place old people at a disadvantage, as they will tend to represent a bad trade-off between cost of treatment and years of survival resulting, whether adjusted or not. In some preventive health care, by contrast, older people are better targets than younger people as they are at greater risk of many preventable diseases (Gray 1985). For example, treating elderly people with high blood pressure to prevent stroke requires half as many patients to be treated to avoid one stroke than if younger patients are the target group (Beard *et al.* 1992). Thus it is essential that economic appraisal, as an aid to rationing, develops and uses more equitable measures of outcome and that evaluations of service impact always consider elderly people.

CHOICE IN PROVISION OF CARE

The idea of purchasers bullying providers into doing what the purchasers want is fine if there is a choice of providers. Only in the big conurbations is this choice available and most professional (as opposed to manager) providers do not relish the prospect of competing with colleagues. Furthermore, it is very unlikely that any health-care-of-the-elderly service would want to take on the contract of another purchaser even if extra resources were provided. There is little slack in the hospital elderly service unlike some of the cold-surgery specialities which seem able to take on extra work at short notice and without staff increases. For elderly patients who do need cold surgery, the internal market might speed things up although on current evidence it appears that any reduction in waiting times is better attributed to the waiting list initiatives (i.e. more money) than the internal market (Beecham 1992a).

Choice assumes a supply excess exists. The majority of elderly people are simply not players in such a market. The services available are often extremely resource limited so any element of choice becomes take it (with gratitude) or leave it. The emphasis on *choice* in the promotion of the NHS Reforms is likely to become extremely embarrassing as it becomes obvious to the general public that rationing and choice cannot coexist in a rational world (Allen *et al.* 1992). A more viable approach would be to limit individual choice (a political heresy) with a view to achieving the greatest good for the greatest number. Clearly the public need to have a voice in deciding where such limits to choice would fall although at present such decisions are taken by local purchaser groups.

ALLOCATION OF COSTS OF CARE

As the internal market begins to work it is likely that costs will be passed on to the 'appropriate' sector. For elderly people this will be the immediate family and less frequently the local authority. Given the organizational problems of providing and maintaining good-quality community care, it is likely that hospitals will remain the safety net for many of the community's crises. Cross-charging of local authorities for time spent in hospital for non-medical reasons may be the spur required to ensure that hospital beds are not simply used as an expedient solution to deficiencies in community care.

Economic analysis of the effects of different Health Service strategies will become much more complex with the need to account for costs, such as those of caring, which are hard to measure and value. Such analysis may have to be organized at a Regional or central level to ensure that appropriately trained Health Service researchers do a competent job and to avoid any charge of local self-interest in the way in which costs and benefits are appraised.[11]

MANAGING CHANGE IN THE NHS

Health services all over the world are subject to increasingly intense pressures to change (Ham 1992). The management of change emphasizes the need to develop human resources, to ensure that the goals of an industry are known and valued (by all employees) and that all employees 'own' the strategies by which goals will be achieved. A major challenge for NHS management will be to ensure that a more common ownership of the Reforms is reached.

One of the most depressing aspects of the NHS Reforms has been the way in which the most precious resource – staff morale – has been squandered. Despite the well-known opposition of virtually all staff working in hospitals (with the exception of small numbers of self-interested consultants), decisions were made by a variety of managements to go for Trust status. Since the changes in status of hospitals little work or money has been put into winning back staff opinion. There is even a complacent and unsubstantiated view that morale has not fallen and that the management of change has been a 'remarkable success' (Klein 1992). The NHSME appears to ignore staff anxieties and insecurities associated with change (Warden 1992). In academic medicine a survey of attitudes and morale has been conducted recently which showed that morale has declined as the Reforms were implemented (Beecham 1992b).

NHS management must grasp that change and its effective management have been, and will be in the future, central to any organization that hopes to be successful into the next century. The need for a major investment in staff development programmes and common ownership of the means of achieving change are the major challenges for Health Service managers over the next 5 years.

FUTURE PATTERNS OF CARE

In a true market elderly people are the best patients as they generate so much work. In the internal market – a quasi market – they are the worst as they are complicated, do not fit into clear diagnostic categories, do not get better quickly, and have problems that cross professional and sector boundaries.

Purchasers

Purchasers are likely to be perplexed by their difficulty in measuring whether providers come 'up to spec' and in knowing whether the extra cost to achieve target levels of performance or quality represent money well spent. They may find themselves unable to negotiate better deals as no alternative and acceptable providers exist. The arguments with local social service departments over who is responsible for what, will continue with minor skirmishes into no-man's land. Finally, they will come to realize that they lack and need adequate indicators of outcome for making purchasing plans relate what is bought with what is obtained.

Purchasers will have to set standards of practice for elderly people that are applicable to the varied places in which old people are treated: general medicine, surgery, ophthalmology, etc., to ensure that their specific needs are not neglected. It is likely that voluntary sector agencies such as Age Concern will have a long-term job reminding purchasers of the need to consider elderly people in their decisions.

Providers

Providers of health care of the elderly should find themselves in great demand as their skills in assessment, case management and rehabilitation are needed by the increasing number of the oldest old. They will have to be nimble to avoid being caught in a stranglehold of hospital-oriented services and will have to demonstrate their worth to primary care, local authorities and the independent sector.

British geriatricians are in danger of being used solely as bed clearers for the rest of the hospital. While this work needs to be done, this burden should be shared by hospital consultants rather than falling so disproportionately to my specialty. Training for hospital medicine requires a substantial input of health care of the elderly to ensure that consultants who will inevitably carry out the bulk of their work with older people know what they are doing.

Geriatricians and psychogeriatricians have a big task on their hands: they will have to develop community networks, modify their traditional power base of the in-patient ward and redefine themselves as a speciality working at the interface between hospital and community, with a strong role in leading primary and secondary prevention, and in providing ready access from local social services and private sectors to hospital and community rehabilitation and acute-treatment resources.

Consumers

The consumers of health care of the elderly have probably seen little change in services since the start of the internal market. What can they hope for? While it may not be possible to change negative attitudes to old people, it is essential that the NHS itself documents problems of access and the process of service delivery and that such problems are resolved. They may find that trust in their doctor and the system is difficult during the testing early years of the Reforms when inter-sector rivalry and competitiveness have not yet exhausted themselves and they will need strong advocacy which will always be found in the voluntary-sector agencies.

If the NHS Reforms mean anything at all, it is about the transfer of power from professions/providers to consumers. This change in the traditional balance could potentially improve health care for older people by ensuring that their, and not the providers', priorities are tackled first. Improved rights – perhaps as a 'charter for elderly people' – could help but inevitably it would bring responsibilities. Many elderly people gladly take on the task of looking after other elderly people more frail than themselves and are therefore committed to their half of a new social contract already. Elderly people and their advocates may find it hard to adjust during a transitional phase but it seems inevitable that part of the cost of obtaining rights will be an increased financial obligation for some health and social care placed on the elderly people themselves. This may mean that the right to pass on property to children is forgone as the means of paying for care in later life. Talk of an internal market in health care generates powerful expectations about choice. This may encourage a consumerism that is expensive. If the State does not put in enough resource, there must be extra costs to the end user.

NOTES

1 See p.195 for an example of such joint care planning.
2 This is a major problem, certainly for DHA purchasers but also in a different way for GPFHs. Directly or indirectly it is raised in both pieces in this collection on purchasing. Refer to pp.83–5 and pp.192–5.
3 Our psychiatric authors (pp.255–6) are also anxious about how effective needs assessment might be, as is Professor Opit (pp.88–91) who none the less endeavours to suggest ways of improving it. Finally Chapter 12 indicates what one DHA is doing in this area.
4 Cf. the mini case studies in Chapter 8, where competition and protectionism are shown to be relative standpoints and see also Chapter 3 which looks at regulation.
5 Refer to pp.253–4 for an account of the psychiatric service and its traditional organizational basis of catchment areas, and what this means under the internal market.
6 See pp.241–2 for a surgeon's assessment of their specialty and its income-producing potential.
7 The costing and pricing data generated by providers are, and to a significant extent are likely to remain, a difficult, even insecure base for purchasing decisions. Refer to Chapters 10 and 12–14 in particular on these matters.
8 Whether they have effective sanctions at present is unclear. Refer to Chapter 13 and p.185 on the relative lack of accountability of GPFHs.
9 Cf. p.194.
10 Perhaps the reply to this is that the canvassing of local opinions about health priorities would be but one dimension to the assessment. National and Regional prioritizing could provide the framework in which such local opinions would be sought. Refer also to pp.194–5.
11 Refer to pp.64–5 on the difficulty of such appraisals.

REFERENCES

Allen, I. *et al.* (1992) *Elderly People: Choice, Participation and Satisfaction*. London: Policy Studies Institute.

Beard, K. *et al.* (1992) Management of elderly people with sustained hypertension, *British Medical Journal*, 412–16.

Beecham, L. (1992a) Government's drive on waiting lists, *British Medical Journal*, 403.

Beecham, L. (1992b) Medical academics' falling morale despite job satisfaction, *British Medical Journal*, 73.

Bennett, G. and Ebrahim, S. (1992) *Essentials of Health Care of the Elderly*. London: Edward Arnold.

Campion, E. *et al.* (1983) An inter-disciplinary consultation service: a controlled trial, *Journal of the American Geriatrics Society*, 792–6.

DoH (Department of Health) (1990) *National Health Service and Community Care Act 1990*. London: HMSO.

Gray, J.A.M. (ed.) (1985) *Prevention of Disease in the Elderly*. London: Churchill Livingstone.

Hall, M. (1988) Geriatric medicine today, in N. Wells and C. Freer (eds.) *The Ageing Population: Burden or Challenge?* London: Macmillan, 65–86.

Ham, C. (1992) Paying for Health Services, *British Medical Journal*, 328.

Home Office (1968) *Report of the Committee on Local Authority and Allied Personal Social Services* (Seebohm Report). London: HMSO.

Klein, R. (1992) NHS Reforms: the first six months, *British Medical Journal*, 199–200.

Laing, W. (1988) Living environments for the elderly: the mixed economy in long-term care, in N. Wells and C. Freer (eds.) *The Ageing Population: Burden or Challenge*. London: Macmillan, 235–48.

Ministry of health (1948) *National Assistance Act*. London: HMSO.

NHSME (National Health Service Management Executive) (1992) *NHS Reforms: The First Six Months*. London: DoH.

Perrin, J. (1992) Administration and financial management of health-care services, in E. Beck *et al.* (eds.) *In the Best of Health: The Status and Future of Health Care in the UK*. London: Chapman & Hall, 251–72.

Rubin, I.M. and Beckard, R. (1972) Factors influencing the effectiveness of health teams, *Milbank Quarterly*, 317–35.

Townsend, P. and Davidson, N. (1982) *Inequalities in Health*. Harmondsworth: Penguin.

Warden, J. (1992) Fear or facts on Trusts, *British Medical Journal*, 276.

19
Can Nurses Learn to Dance?
Nursing and 'Managed Competition'

Stephanie Stanwick

If the new game of business is indeed like Alice-in-Wonderland croquet, then winning it requires faster action, more creative manoeuvring, more flexibility, and closer partnerships with employees and customers than was typical in the traditional corporate bureaucracy. It requires more agile, limber management that pursues opportunity without being bogged down by cumbersome structures or weighty procedures that impede action. Corporate giants, in short, must learn how to dance.

(Kanter, 1989)

There remains probably only one consistent factor about the NHS that is as true today as it was in 1948 with its inception, and that is that the needs of people are at its centre. There have undoubtedly been enormous changes since then, but the fact remains that even with the latest NHS Reforms, meeting the needs of people has featured high on the agenda. However, the NHS Reforms of the 1990s are more fundamental than any experienced since its beginning.

The Reforms stem from the three White Papers: *Promoting Better Health, Working for Patients* and *Caring for People* (DoH 1987, 1989a and 1989b), and were designed to tackle the underlying problems of management and funding. The most important of the Reforms introduced:

- a system of contractual funding;
- proposals to strengthen management at all levels;
- new arrangements for allocating resources;
- measures to manage clinical activity;
- measures to improve the quality and efficiency of services;
- ways of reinforcing the importance of the community as the focus for the provision of services.

Ham (1991) describes the idea of there being a clearer purchasing role within the NHS as being at the heart of the Reforms. This places hospitals and other provider units under competitive pressure to improve the quality and efficiency of their services, and contractual funding brings about 'managed competition', or an 'internal market' between provider units.

For some time the NHS has been trying to get to grips with the fact that the potential for increased demand and costs for health care is unlimited. Inevitably this results in the need to examine priorities for health services which are articulated in Government policy and DoH service objectives. Issues which the 'purchasers' or 'commissioners' of health care, in the purchaser/provider split, have to deal with.

Heginbotham (1992) describes rationing and priority setting as the central isssue to purchasing dilemmas; the issue of acute versus community care; of what he calls 'horizontal or vertical equity', that is equity across all care groups, versus priorities within those care groups; the issue of quality of life versus that of saving life; and the issue of looking at health 'conditions' versus the importance of specific health gain or outcome.

WHAT IMPACT HAS ALL THIS HAD ON NURSES AND NURSING?

It must be said that at one level, the level of practice and patient care, the impact to date has been minimal. The issues about efficiency and value for money remain the same. There are still complaints about insufficient numbers of beds, inadequate and out-of-date equipment, shortages of staff, all reported in the papers and journals almost daily. Patients frequently have operations cancelled, wait in accident and emergency departments a long time both to be seen by a doctor and then to be admitted to a bed; they miss their meals because of the scheduling of departmental investigations, and are discharged home from hospital with very little or no warning, and with minimal back-up care and support; they wait a long time in out-patient departments and then do not understand the information that is subsequently given to them about their condition by professionals.

To nurses and midwives working on a day-to-day basis with these patients in all care settings, nothing changes and all remains the same. Any improvements in nursing and midwifery practice itself have occurred despite and not because of the Reforms.

At another level, the level of the organization, much can be seen to have changed. Managers and employers are different, many have lost their traditional nurse managers or are managed by non-nurses, and are employed by Trust Hospitals or Units and not health authorities. Similarly wards, departments and community are organized into care groups or directorates with their own managers, accountants, budgets and resources. In many situations ward sisters or charge nurses find themselves managing their own budgets, and generally the accountability for the use of resources is at a much lower level of the organization, closer in fact to where patient care decisions are being made. In the community the Family Practitioner Committee has been replaced by the the FHSA; GPs and dentists work to contracts; and since 1991 GPFHs have come into being[1] and, like NHS Trusts, will increase in numbers every year with each further implementation 'wave'. The size and composition of staff working in general practice has also changed and continues to change. The numbers of practice nurses has increased substantially, nurse practitioners are beginning to be appointed and community nursing services will soon be purchased directly by practices from community health services.

MARKET – MYTH OR REALITY?

Undoubtedly the NHS Reforms have introduced an underlying 'market' philosophy to health care, but is this market myth or reality, and how will this market philosophy of itself impact upon nurses and nursing? Salter (1991) maintains that the internal market set out to control demand by prioritizing and rationing the supply of health care by means of the commissioning process. In a pure market situation the relationship between supply and demand is determined by price, but in the internal market of the NHS there is more than one type of demand, and only one is sensitive to price. In the main, patients follow commissioners' money, and money does not follow the patient. It may well be the case that the demand for health-care services expressed by consumers may be different to the demand actioned by commissioners of services.[2] Providers may well find themselves under pressure from two different directions.

This could mean that in the future nurses or midwives, by acting as patients' advocates and thus enabling patients to choose care or to articulate choice, may bring about conflict between that choice and the security of the business. So, for example, helping patients or carers to choose the kind of service they want, may mean that they opt out of the services offered by one provider Unit to use the services offered by another.

Paton (1991) argues that markets require competition to provide efficiency, and where there are unnecessary investments or failures, and closures are not permitted, then there will be and can be no competitive market. If, on the other hand, closures are allowed, this would undoubtedly mean that nurses would find their continued long-term employment to be vulnerable, and the issues of redundancy and unemployment more of a reality for them as a professional group than has ever been the case before. A true market would demand flexibility from nurses and midwives not only in where they work, but in the way they practise.

The certainty is just in any scenario patients will continue to need nurses and midwives; the uncertainty lies perhaps in individual specialist versus generalist skills. In describing the most recent NHS market simulation exercise, Rubber Windmill three, Liddell and Parston (1992) describe how the market 'froze', GPFHs wanting to move paediatric care from the hospital setting to the community and putting pressure on the acute services to release resources. Similarly purchasers cut back on their contracts with acute providers. If this were a real example, it is questionable whether the nurses involved would be facilitated in moving between what could be different employers. The new employers would not necessarily want to maintain current employment conditions, or even protect wholesale the grades and skills of staff.[3]

CHANGING PATTERNS OF SERVICE

The King's Fund Commission (1992) report *London Health Care 2010* examines the implications and issues of health-care services in the capital.[4] Millar (1992), reviewing the report, highlights the following:

- Health care will look substantialy different as the social and demographic contexts alter.
- Medical technology will blur the distinctions between primary and secondary care, and between professional roles and specialties.
- Secondary and tertiary care should be organized so as to enhance and support the capacity of primary health care.
- There should be a 25% reduction in beds over an 8-year period – a loss of 5,000 beds.

The report went on to say that major developments in community care would be clinically dependent on a programme of closures, and that 30 of the 41 acute hospitals only would be retained.

Butler and Millar (1992), reporting on the problems facing the University College and Middlesex Hospitals in London, surmised that once the brakes had been taken off the internal market no one expected the market to 'scuttle away with the speed it has'. These London hospitals expected a 15–20% reduction in activity from distant purchasing authorities, but in reality some purchasing authorities decreased referals by as much as 71% in 1 year.

There is a view that the new independent hospitals will attempt to differentiate their products, and will eventually corner discrete areas of specialist health care. This inevitably makes some of the London hospital specialties, and by implication the staff who work within them, vulnerable. It may mean that the labour market for some nursing specialist skills may shift from London to the provider Units outside. Alternatively, local providers who are developing these so called specialties may want to develop the skills and expertise of their own staff. For instance the South East Thames Nursing and Midwifery Strategy, *A Quantum Leap* (SETRHA 1992a), identifies key issues for the future development of nursing and midwifery policy and practice: 'the management of nursing through devolved accountability; responsive and effective practice; the adoption of a corporate approach; and consumer responsiveness. This reinforces the need for nursing to respond to health service needs at a local level.'

GENERAL PRACTITIONER FUNDHOLDERS

Discussions about the changing patterns of service would not be complete without some examination of the implications around GPFH and the impact that the initiative has on the health-services market. Willis (1992) argues that, although GPFH was introduced with a view to kick-starting the market, it is not the main instrument of the market itself. He argues that there is a duplication of effort between GPFH and commissioners and that only in the mature market will the proper coordination and liasion occur between all parties. However, a recent report of a study into GPFH undertaken by the London School of Economics, reported by Robinson *et al.* (1992), describes how Fundholders have begun to 'exercise exits'. These have occurred where problems identified have not been addressed, where patients have indicated a preference or where waiting lists are too long. GPFHs have also begun to look at alternatives, for example a private contract agreed with medical consultants to provide local services, or negotiating with private clinics to provide cut-price deals.

South East Thames Regional Health Authority's recently published document, *Primary Care in South East Thames – An Agenda for Debate* (SETRHA 1992b) identifies the following shifts in service as examples of good practice: the increasing number of GPs involved in minor surgical procedures; the increasing number of practice nurses employed and the recognition being made of the potential role of nurse practitioners; and protocols for shared care between hospital and community. The document urges the development of a variety of primary care facilities and services, for example: health shops, poly clinics, and outreach into the community where the local population are particularly disadvantaged.

The outcome from a recent consensus conference on community nursing (SETRHA 1991) identified the following characteristics of the future of community nursing services: flexibility, imagination, responsiveness, a respect for patients and colleagues, and opportunism – all key issues if nursing is to respond to local changes in service.

The results of the proposals for GPFH to purchase community nursing are as yet unknown, but there is no guarantee at all that GPs will want to perpetuate the status quo; indeed they are likely to challenge current thinking and rationales for practice.

CAN NURSES LEARN TO DANCE?

Whether all the changes mentioned in this chapter occur as a result of the internal market, the Reforms as a whole, or from developing services that are led by demographics, is almost immaterial. The results will be the same, but the pace of the changes themselves may vary as a result. Nurses and midwives will need to develop new roles in new settings both in the hospital and the community[5]. They will need to be led by a new kind of manager, who thrives in a changing and challenging environment; they will need to lead innovation and demonstrate imagination in meeting patients' needs; they will need not to feel threatened by issues relating to role overlap and professional boundary changes. To prepare them to work in this new world there will have to be new programmes of education designed to be flexible and cost-effective. In short, like the corporate giants referred to at the opening of this chapter, the nursing profession must learn how to dance.

NOTES

1 For more on the new GP contract and GP Fundholding see pp.204–5.
2 Cf. pp.83–5 for more on this issue of consumer choice and commissioning.
3 Refer to pp.173–4 for a discussion of competitive tendering and business objectives which ultimately impel employees to move to different employers resulting often in lowered pay and conditions.
4 Refer also to Tomlinson (1992) for recommendations concerning health-care provision in London.
5 See pp.223–4 for more on the reactions of clinical staff within a provider Unit to the internal market and the Reforms.

REFERENCES

Butler, P. and Millar, B. (1992) No gain without pain, *Health Service Journal*, 25 June, 10–11.
DoH (Department of Health) (1987) *Promoting Better Health*. London: HMSO.
DoH (Department of Health) (1989a) *Caring for People*. London: HMSO.
DoH (Department of Health) (1989b) *Working for Patients*. London: HMSO.
Ham, C. (1991) *The New National Health Service: Organization and Management*. Oxford: Radcliffe Medical Press.
Heginbotham, C. (1992) Jam tomorrow, *Health Service Journal*, 5 March, 24–5.
Kanter, R.M. (1989) *When the Giants Learn to Dance*. London: Unwin.
King's Fund Commission on the Future of London's Acute Health Services (1992) *London Health Care 2010: Changing the Future of Services in the Capital*. London: King's Fund.
Liddell, A. and Parston, G. (1992) Frozen assets, *Health Service Journal*, 28 May, 18–20.
Paton, C. (1991) Myths of competition, *Health Service Journal*, 30 May, 22–3.
Robinson, R. *et al.* (1992) A foothold in Fundholding, *Health Service Journal*, 13 February, 18–20.
Salter, B. (1991) Demand and fallacy, *Health Service Journal*, 5 December, 19.
SETRHA (South East Thames Regional Health Authority) (1991) *Nursing in the Community*. A Consensus Conference in South East Thames Region, 5–6 July. Nursing and Quality Directorate, SETRHA.
SETRHA (South East Thames Regional Health Authority) (1992a) *A Quantum Leap: The Future of Nursing and Midwifery in South East Thames*. Nursing and Quality Directorate, SETRHA.
SETRHA (South East Thames Regional Health Authority) (1992b) *Primary Care in South East Thames: An Agenda for Debate*. SETRHA.
Tomlinson, B. (1992) *Report on the Inquiry into London's Health Service, Medical Education and Research*. London: HMSO.
Willis, A. (1992) Who needs fundholding?, *Health Service Journal*, 30 April, 24.

20

Concluding Remarks: The Value of an Enhanced 'Organizational R&D' Function in a Rapidly Changing NHS

Ian Tilley

Managing the Internal Market inquires into the management and operation of the key institutions of the NHS market in acute services into the second year of commissioning. It does so in the form of a readings book whose contributors are both academic health commentators and practitioners, two worlds not frequently brought together in a single text. As the academics come from a variety of different disciplinary backgrounds and the practitioners from management, medicine and nursing, the three dominant professional groups in NHS hospitals, this book not only has a multiple authorship but also deploys a range of approaches; is based on different intellectual traditions grounded in a variety of academic subjects; considers different aspects of internal market implementation; and, finally, reflects varied opinions and value judgements about the issues raised.

If this chapter is to respect and value this diversity around an agreed subject, it is encumbent upon me as editor to avoid the temptation of ending this book with a chapter that endeavours to push everything neatly and tidily together. The reality of NHS organization and management, in the midst of yet more years of ever increasing change, is one in which such an appearance of tidiness and order could only be largely imposed.

All change, from that at the personal level through to large-scale organizational change as exemplified by the NHS – not that the two can really be separated – is a rather messy process. Moreover, prediction must be a particularly hazardous business to engage in at a time when many uncertain, complex and contradictory forces, both 'inner' and 'outer', are at work.

Consequently, this concluding chapter will neither attempt to force the necessarily somewhat tangled and still unfolding story of the implementation of the NHS acute-sector market into tidy, reassuring boxes nor launch into bold predictions. Rather it will attempt the following:

(1) To enumerate the seven themes (see Table 20.1) that emerge for me from reading the preceding chapters.
(2) To take the first and broadest of these themes and explore it in somewhat more detail. The purpose of this is to begin to illustrate

what is the thread running through the chapter: that there is a real need for an enhanced, diverse and innovative 'organizational R&D' to support NHS managers and clinicians at this time of significant, prolonged change.

(3) To suggest that, viewing the Reforms and NHS market analytically as simply another management change project, the most neglected part of the whole exercise is evaluation.

(4) To indicate that these Reforms generally, but particularly 'managed competition', not infrequently evoke, as much inside the Health Service as outside it, oversimplified responses expressing either complete approval or utter rejection.

(5) To show that one response to both (3) and (4) above is to upgrade and profoundly change the nature of the traditionally rather neglected research function as it relates to NHS organization, management and control. Thence sections (3) and (4) of the chapter lend weight to (2). This is also likely to occur if readers think about the preceding chapters in terms of their explicit and more often implicit research implications, again using the term in the new and broadened way I am endeavouring to capture with the expression 'organizational R&D'.

SOME THEMES AND THEIR LINKS WITH PREVIOUS CHAPTERS

My first task is simply to list some of what I regarded as significant themes as I too worked through the foregoing chapters in my editorial role. Hopefully at minimum this listing of themes may stimulate readers to reflect and construct their own list of themes. If the links between my themes and the preceding chapters are also indicated, readers might also want to use the themes as a part of the process of selecting the particular chapters most relevant to their interests. This list and the links between themes and chapters are precisely what Table 20.1 provides.

Theme 1 elaborated

Seeing how Theme 1 works is, in effect, the task of the whole book. The institutions of the internal market were first discussed in the Introduction of this book and, in their different ways, all subsequent chapters have been concerned with elaborating and refining that initial review. Therefore in terms of the material covered in *Managing the Internal Market*, Theme 1 is by far the broadest of the seven offered in Table 20.1. For that reason it is well suited for further examination, and an examination designed to illustrate the need for an enhanced 'organizational R&D' function in the Reformed NHS.

The elaboration of Theme 1, being illustrative not comprehensive, simply focuses on two of the many possible areas that might have been discussed.

(a) GP relations under 'managed competition'

Let's start by looking at 'the fly in the NHS ointment', the GPFHs. Initially their small numbers in most Districts meant that their 'bogeyman' status in

Table 20.1 Seven themes on 'managed competition' and their links with earlier chapters

Theme number	Theme	Associated earlier chapters
1	The purchasing and providing institutions of the internal market	6, (7)*, (8), 12, 13, 14, 15
2	Priorities and accountability in commissioning	4, (6), 12, 13
3	The non-price aspects of contracting, in particular quality	(4), 9, 12, (18)
4	The professional, both clinical and managerial, response to the internal market implementation in the provider Units	2, (8), 11, 16, 17, 18, 19
5	Resource allocation and rationing health care in the Reformed NHS acute sector	4, (8), 14
6	Regulation versus a 'free market' in hospital services	3, (4), 5
7	The London factor, Tomlinson and the quasi health-care market	(3), (7), 8, (12), 14, 15

* Associated earlier chapter numbers in parenthesis have only an indirect or minor link to their theme.

the minds of many a hospital and health authority manager and consultant was perhaps simply an outlet for pent-up feelings about the Reforms more generally rather than a measured response to the threat, say, the first wave of GPFHs could really represent for NHS managers and doctors.

Their continued expansion and increased 'clustering' boosted their influence over hospitals and as purchasers (Dearden 1991: 173). Thus, the forebodings now might have more substance to them. In most NHS Districts they certainly will in time. In fact, GPFHs have already proved far more popular with GPs than the DoH imagined or the British Medical Association (BMA) feared. They continue to be 'running far ahead of the Government on ideas' to extend the compass of GPFH (Little 1992: 41). As their influence grows, one reason they will continue to evoke the ire of many an NHS manager is because of the perceived unfairness of relatively unequal treatment of DHAs compared with GPFHs; the latter seem to function 'under different rules' (Galloway 1991: 8). GPFHs have even been accused of being likely to be promoting the spread of private health insurance:

> GPFHs with a limited budget will have an incentive to promote private health insurance to their patients in order to reduce their outgoings. It is likely that GPs in the Thames Regions who have a high proportion of patients investing in private health insurance will find it much easier to remain within their budgets. They will therefore be entitled to plough back any savings into making their practices more efficient.
>
> (Turner 1989: 68)

Furthermore, the GPFHs are a reasonably cohesive group as evidenced, for instance, by claims by the leaders of the National Association of Fundholding Practices to have signed up 75% of the 306 first-wave GPFHs (Pulse 1992a: 4). There is still evidence of conflict between GPFHs and hospital consultants (Pulse 1992b: 24). As the minimum patient list size required by GPFH applicants lowers, some non-Fundholding GPs remain concerned about what their DHAs are doing. For example the handling of ECRs in such a way that the GP might regard this as effectively restricting their right to refer patients to the consultant of choice. The counter-reaction always available to such GPs, even if lacking any ideological commitment to Fundholding, will be to apply for their own practice budget (Bowling *et al.* 1991: 294).

How these and other trends about GPFH will work out in the medium to long term is extremely difficult to predict. One thing, however, is clear: not only will DHAs and the managers and consultants in provider hospitals all have to continue working on their relations with GPFHs but there are important developments among the non-Fundholding GPs as well. As Chapter 13 among others makes clear, most of these GPs too are enjoying their enhanced status and are also becoming more cohesive. Even such occasions as GPs' continuing postgraduate education are being used as a 'forum for discussing, agreeing and implementing clinical management guidelines with the members of the appropriate specialist-GP liaison group' (Willis 1992: 26).

The need for GPs and hospitals to be more effectively linked information-wise has been recognized for some time (Jones and Kerr 1986: 71). Recently some commentators have called for new links that at first sight might seem unlikely to really take off. For instance, Nicklin *et al.* (1991: 17) have argued that there is a genuine need for all GPs, including Fundholders, to share information with DHAs.

Perhaps this may surprise some but the more general point is that there has been so little systematic investigation of GP relations in the Reformed NHS, yet both GPFHs and non-Fundholding GPs are taking on new and significant roles that need to be much more fully understood if only because of the high costs to NHS managers of not understanding such important matters more fully.

(b) Current challenges for health authorities

The NHS purchasers have been told by the policy-makers that they 'hold the key to the future' (Moore 1991; MacLachlin *et al.* 1991). The tasks they face are quite daunting: 'to focus on the health of the population, to create opportunities for greater user choice, to reshape the boundaries between primary and secondary care and between prevention and cure, and to create new alliances with other agencies in caring for people in the community' (Spry 1991: 8).

Other events have hardly been supportive of health authorities in adequately discharging these responsibilities, at least in the short term. Quite a few lost 'top managerial talent' to the 'more exciting' NHSTs where salary levels were thought to be more fluid (Light 1991: 570). Beyond that depletion, the Districts are expected to have to shed more management posts (Ham 1990: 5) as the number of NHSTs (over which the District has no managerial responsibilities) and GPFHs (who erode their budget) continue to rise – and new managerial opportunities are less apparent now in many of the NHSTs who themselves are shedding posts (see, for instance, Chapter 14). In the well-known Rubber Windmill market simulations of the internal market DHAs were identified as:

'the players with the weak hands . . . while the strong men were the Trusts and GPFHs. The "new boys" seemed to have a better hold on events. The FHSA did not seem to have a hand at all' (Dickson 1991: 22).

In early 1991 the then new Deputy Chief Executive of the NHSME, Andrew Foster, accepted the centre had by then done little to guide the commissioning side (Thompson and Flanagan 1991: 24) because, as was discussed in Chapter 1, the initial stress was on the newly established institutions of the Government's health policy, the NHSTs and GPFHs.

The effective discharging of the DHA's new and novel responsibilities suggests the need for research – broadly conceived – that is both immense in terms of what is needed and urgent with respect to the need for it beginning to come on-stream. Forging local health strategies; involving the patients in the choice process with a framework, as yet largely to be created, of national, perhaps even Regional (especially if RHAs acquire an explicit, formal regulatory role in the internal market) needs assessments and evaluation of treatments and procedures; and the complex process of endeavouring to move towards a preventive and promotive health policy which lays more stress on primary and community care and less on secondary health in hospitals all need such 'R & D'. Much of it will be novel in nature. For instance, needs assessment requires collaborative effort involving epidemiologists, health economists, and social and organizational researchers as well as academically based and practising doctors.

Thus, needs assessment and the evaluation of different treatments require a new and novel type of multidisciplinary research that clearly can be no respecter of the current academic division of labour. This poses real difficulties as, for instance, the career structures of potential researchers are still well and truly focused on existing academic disciplines. The only way through such problems is for NHS managers to see the need for such work and thence ensure that it is adequately promoted and funded.

Of course, realistically the overall endeavour must be seen as a long-term one. But if that is used to induce complacency and inaction, adverse consequences will flow. For instance, the current information gap could well work to the detriment of improving the traditionally 'poor services' often received by the most vulnerable NHS patient groups – the mentally ill, the mentally handicapped, the elderly – who, despite being 'bulk users' of the Service, lack 'consumer clout' (Murphy 1990: 78; Cunningham 1990: 18).

Another area of concern, organization restructuring, as DHAs, FHSAs and social service departments become more closely associated, raises 'R&D' issues of quite a different order. None the less, they still require the Health Service to become more concerned about and involved in systematically understanding itself as it engages in yet other reorganization. This is not, however, a plea for passive investigations governed more by academic norms than Service requirements.

In a variety of ways the NHS has long been a major sponsor of medical and scientific research. It has a much less enviable reputation as a sponsor of 'organizational R&D' into itself. Yet in the midst of the current upheavals, more 'self-knowledge' of the detailed institutional workings of the Service are urgently required and on a widespread basis. It ought to go without saying that such 'R&D' can only be one strategy, not a cure-all for the complicated situations created by the Reforms. Still less can such 'R&D' of itself be relied upon to resolve conflicting views or assessments. It might do this in some of the simpler, more clear-cut cases. Beyond this it may only clarify the issues at stake and some of their implications rather than end the disputed views.

Put more boldly, responding adequately to the increasing rate of organizational uncertainty and change in the NHS calls for, first, informed 'environmental scanning' within the Health Service and at its many different organizational levels, and, second, an understanding of how this wider picture interacts with internal processes and structures. Finally, the foregoing will itself help operating managers deciding on appropriate organizational interventions in response to such scanning which could well lead to more evaluation and so on.

What is being described as appropriate in quite a few situations is action research as well as more traditionally based research which endeavours much more to stand apart from the organizational behaviour it is studying. Action research is likely to involve both specialist NHS personnel and outsiders. Interestingly enough, one British variant of action research received much of its pioneering development on work in the NHS (Revans 1982; Cope 1981). There are, however, a variety of conceptually and practically different approaches to action research, including such classic and underpinning work as Miller and Rice (1967) as well as more recent work like that of Whyte (1991) and Klein and Eason (1991) to name some of the more distinctive ones.

To understand something of how action research is likely to have a role to play in the restructuring faced by health authorities, it is useful to look a little more closely at these reorganizations themselves and some of the tensions they are already producing.

If the increased collaborative efforts of health authorities and local government social service departments is in anticipation of the implementation of care in the community in April 1993, the new links and mergers already being created between different health authorities are the result of such pressures as the need to increase the bargaining power of purchasers and help ensure good value even when facing strong providers. In many parts of the UK providers have effective monopoly powers in one District but these might be eroded if several DHAs join together. The net result of these mergers and associations between health authorities is to create what some have seen as an effective 'return' to the old health Areas or 'mini Regions' (Paton 1992: 85–6).

Beyond this, DHAs and FHSAs are also forming closer associations. Whilst some speak confidently of such joint commissioning as 'an important staging post on the route to greater integration of primary and secondary care' (Huntington 1991: 17), others talk of the 'days of the independent FHSA look[ing] numbered' (Meldrum 1992: 41). Certainly, at this stage of the process, some of the FHSA managers are anxious and making such points as that the 'merger mania' between the two types of health authority is often proceeding without being fully debated (Eminson 1991: 8). There is certainly a fear in FHSAs of being taken over by DHAs, and that FHSAs' distinctive priorities, history and traditions will be lost within resultant 'unitary' purchasing authorities dominated by DHAs whose own history is much more hospital based (Ruddy 1991: 8).

All this is occurring before the even more complex, agitating and emotionally laden step of health authorities being led in care in the community by social service departments who will hold the budget. In terms of party politics this is a bipartisan policy supported by both the Conservatives and Labour. The Labour Party (1992: 7) even speak of renaming the DoH as the Department of Health and Community Care to underline its commitment in this direction. Although questions to do with the level of funding, ring-fenced budgets (Paton 1992: 83) and the like underlie much of the current concern, the prior history of collaboration between the different health, local government and voluntary agencies has not been a 'spectacular success' (Wright 1990: 214) for cultural, historical and professional, as well as economic, reasons.

Given the degree of upheaval in the UK public sector generally, research, action research and consultancy-based work on the problems, pain and ways through such inter-agency mergers and associations is just beginning to emerge (Shapiro and Carr 1991; Woodhouse and Pengelly 1991) in addition to the mainstream management literature on managing health-care change (for example, Margulies and Adams 1982; Spurgeon and Barwell 1991; Stewart 1989; Boss 1989) or more general change literature (for example, McCalman and Paton 1992; Buchanan and Boddy 1992; Boddy and Buchanan 1992).

More conventional research on inter-organization relations is also required and a famous US social researcher has laid down rather concisely and effectively something of what is involved, its complexity and how research and action research have different, but interacting, agendas:

> Every organisation requires other organisations to implement its projects, programs and even routine activities: to get itself services, perhaps to get itself financially or politically off the ground, to swap technology and ideas, to have others purchase its products or services, perhaps to fight against common enemies. It is also highly competitive or in conflict with some of those other organisations, so it may have special agreements with them to keep the conflict or competition within manageable bounds. Few, if any, of those inter-organisational arrangements, let alone 'agreements' or formal contracts, could be instituted and maintained without negotiation.
>
> (Strauss 1991: 134)

What broad conclusions can be reached from the brief elaboration of Theme 1 in this section? First, NHS managers and clinicians function in an organizational world of increasing intricacy and uncertainty. Second, 'organizational R&D', even of the broad, diverse and innovative kind put forward in this chapter, cannot magically remove such difficulties. Third, it is, however, a necessary part of the repertoire upon which managers and clinicians with managerial functions must be able increasingly to draw in order to survive, far less thrive, in the ever turbulent world of NHS organization and management.

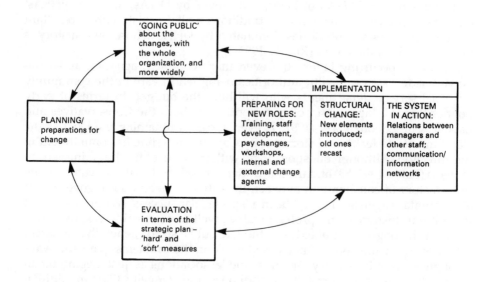

Figure 20.1   A simplified change model

THE NHS REFORMS AND INTERNAL MARKET AS A MANAGEMENT CHANGE PROCESS: LOOKING FOR GAPS

The management of change, if not a glamorous subject in the midst of a prolonged recession, is one of the most popular parts of business studies courses, which says something quite clear about the degree of organizational change and restructuring that is occurring in both the corporate and public-sector worlds in contemporary Britain. One of the first topics considered by students is how to study change. Buchanan and Boddy (1992) summarize the now dominant view in change management theory, if not always its practice, when they say, 'Rational–linear models of change have long since been discredited as descriptions or as explanations of organisational change'.

Figure 20.1 does move some way from these earlier sequential models but has not been brought in here as a description or explanation of organizational change. Those wanting richer frameworks with which better to achieve such tasks could look to such diverse change writers as March and Olsen (1979), Mangham (1979), Quinn (1980), Pettigrew and Whipp (1991) and Pfeffer (1992), all of whom helped establish this move away from the simplistic models of the past with their tendency to depict organizational change in rational, orderly terms. These writers also offer more plausible, alternative ways of coming to grips with complex change processes.

The value of the simplified change model in Figure 20.1 is simply to offer a set of big issues or areas in planned change programmes, originally derived mainly from private-business change, but which can be used here as something of a checklist to help identify any significant gaps in the Government's health Reforms, including the introduction of what Chapter 3 calls the implied market in acute health-care services. This will be carried out by viewing these changes as simply another managerial change process and seeing how thoroughly each issue or area is being covered. To this end, I will review such each area in Figure 20.1, starting with the planning/preparations for change.

It should be clear even from the first chapter that this part of the recent NHS changes is one in which there are plenty of omissions and confusions and that quite a deal of the planning of policy and ways of implementing the changes was undertaken on a purely *ad hoc* basis.

This feature of the NHS planning was detected from the outset (Williams 1990: 237). To some extent this was inevitable in a change programme as large and radical as that which is occurring in the health sphere. Nevertheless, from reading this book alone, it is clear that not all such weaknesses in the planning/preparation area can be so easily accounted for.

The next area, 'going public' throughout the organization and beyond, is clearly a crucial one for the current health Reforms, including 'managed competition'. Again because of its size and novelty, and because of the professional reaction (particularly of the doctors and the BMA) and that of the general public too, there has been considerable change of direction since the Prime Ministerial Review and White Paper (DoH 1989). Two foreign health commentators, Saltman and von Otter, particularly stress this and single out the internal market itself as the key place where policy has softened:

> The central defining of the actual Reform process, once it got underway some ten years into Conservative Party rule, has been a pronounced hesitancy to push announced proposals through to completion. By Spring 1991, a Reform package which had initially emphasised multiple market-style mechanisms, including a mixed public/private market for service provision, had been scaled back to a considerably less radical framework within which most market initiatives will be . . . 'tightly controlled from the centre'.
>
> (Saltman and van Otter 1992: 22)

Apart from the early chapters of *Managing the Internal Market*, there is an increasing number of analyses of recent UK health policy development that touch on the question of policy shifts. These include Klein (1989), Small (1989), Harrison *et al.* (1990, 1992) and Paton (1992). Thus, the 'going public' aspect of the changes is not only much more complex than it is ever likely to be for large-scale private-sector change but also it was much more deeply and publicly canvassed by both the Reforms' promoters and detractors (for instance, the Labour Party (1992) and the Liberal Democratic Party (1992)) and opinion mobilized inside and outside the Service.

The implementation area, being the focus of this book, is the most carefully considered aspect of the Reforms and NHS market in this collection. In broad terms it is clear that the prime focus of attention from the policy-makers and DoH civil servants seems to have altered. In what is evidently very much a top-down change programme and in an organization with a long history of power being placed in the hands of the central bureaucracy, their actions are clearly important. Initially the policy-makers and civil servants focused more on the providing side than anywhere else, and especially on the NHSTs, and also the GPFHs who had an unexpectedly successful impact on GPs – thence their importance from a DoH standpoint has correspondingly risen. But eventually a degree of refocusing on to the DHA commissioning role is occurring, especially in such areas as the District's new responsibilities for a health audit of its residents and for needs appraisal, although it is evident, even from material presented earlier in this chapter, that much remains to be done.

Perhaps the next major focus will be regulation, a move from *ad hoc*, partial and uncertain regulation to a detailed, more public accountability of all purchasers and providers and the development of new agencies to discharge this or, more likely, existing ones to be given powers to examine these institutions, report their findings and bring the erring ones into line.

The last change issue in Figure 20.1 is evaluation, ideally against the organization's strategic plan. There is, however, little evidence of any systematic evaluation of the implementation of the NHS market, certainly not much that has been in any way publicly revealed. Despite injunctions in the change literature reiterating the importance of this part of the change process and of building in clear ways of accomplishing it right from initial planning, the reality of change in action is that surprisingly few organizations, whether in the private or public sector of the British economy, engage in anything close to adequate evaluation.

Perhaps bodies like the NHS have particular problems around assessing change. For instance, the appraisal process could well involve specifying objectives against which a change programme is to be judged (Brazier *et al.* 1990: 223). Whether these are sought inside or outside the Service, one thing is indisputable: there will be scant agreement and more likely considerable discord surrounding such matters. The policy-makers would say, for example, that the main purpose of creating NHSTs is to inaugurate a new system of incentives and freedoms because of which their managements and staff can more efficiently deliver some of the nation's crucially required health services, and retain the fruits of these efficiencies, or at least most of them, thus resourcing even more effective delivery of services and improved facilities in the future. Detractors could see NHSTs as chiefly a way in which the current policy-makers endeavour to distance themselves from the actions of the Trusts, for example by staff redundancies or ward closures, in what they would argue is a significantly underfunded NHS. Besides this, they may claim the hidden agenda for NHSTs is 'privatization by stealth' (refer Labour Party 1992).

Despite such claims and counter-claims, the NHS is the largest public body in the UK and certainly one of the most expensive services provided by the State (Perrin 1992: 221). Given this, sufficient publicly available evaluation is a reasonable expectation for the British public to hold. Some officially generated assessments have emerged (e.g. NHSME 1992). Other examples of evolution include Chapter 7 in this readings book, which details a large-scale study of the Reforms commissioned by the King's Fund and carried out by the

National Association of Health Authorities and Trusts, and 'aiming to track and monitor key features of "managed competition"' (Appleby *et al.* 1990: 31). The existence of such studies would be a real help even if the DoH itself provided a significant number of publicly available evaluation studies. Changes as socially consequential as those intended for the NHS require many evaluations by diverse groups of researchers. Saying this returns one direct to the call in this closing chapter for a considerably upgraded 'organizational R & D' function to be available to NHS decision-makers at all significant levels apart from discharging public accountability through such work.

COMMON RESPONSES TO THE HEALTH REFORMS: ON THE PREVALENCE OF OVER-SIMPLIFIED DICHOTOMIES

Not surprisingly perhaps, the Reforms, in particular the introduction of 'managed competition', continue to arouse considerable debate and disagreement from NHS personnel and more widely. The controversial nature of the changes was first mentioned in Chapter 1 and has featured throughout the entire book.

In Chapter 1 it was suggested that this frequently emerges in the form of somewhat over-simplified dichotomies. Thus it was, for instance, suggested in that chapter that the overall effect of the NHS market is still often assessed as either nil or else that it animates the whole of the NHS Reforms.

Other examples of such thinking processes would include, first, those who regard the private sector (or more likely some mythical private sector with boundless energy, productivity and efficiency) as the source for regenerating a sluggish, resource-hungry public sector dominated by inflexible interest groups, in this case including the strongest, most cohesive and publicly esteemed of interest groups, the medical profession. The opposing image would also see the influence of private-sector practice but would deeply resent this and thence deny any efficacy or value for all the recent health Reforms. Willcocks and Harrow (1992), in a recently released reader on public-sector, including NHS, management refer to the idea of a two-way flow, of the public sector certainly being able to learn valuable lessons from the world of private business but of the converse being true as well – again this is an idea that could stimulate useful research.

Another case of 'binary thinking' concerns GPFHs. Some see GPFHs' chief effect as introducing a 'two-tier' Health Service that disadvantages non-GPFHs' patients and, if the scheme spreads far enough, that unfair advantage will be lost and all that will remain is the increased 'paper chase' and escalating costs of sustaining it.

At the opposite end of this particular spectrum are those who see the same GPFHs in an entirely different light: as having a truly vanguard role in improving hospital practice, its efficiency and quality and domination by hospital consultants, because they believe that these advances GPFHs make for their patients will be rapidly diffused throughout the system as DHAs put similar conditions in their agreements too (Robinson and Scheuer 1992: 20).

Another illustration, and a truly major one, is the tendency for the subject of the Health Service and its reorganization to kindle black-and-white reactions: 'the NHS – underfunded or inefficient?' (Bourn 1989: 173). Two choices are advanced as mutually exclusive sources of all the Services' woes.

The first problem with such formulations is that both raise quite vast, entirely indigestible areas better thought about in terms of the large number of distinct spheres of investigation subsumed within each. While it is certainly clear that funding is an all-pervasive factor in the matters covered by this book, it is not clear that the simple juxtaposition of all the matters involved in properly assessing the level of NHS funding with the alleged inefficiency of the staff and institutions making up the Health Service really helps at all in understanding either the NHS or its much discussed Reforms.

Let us concentrate first on the funding side, albeit briefly. Problems in this area are common to health-care delivery systems everywhere: 'containing the cost of health care has become the aim of virtually all countries in the world' (Abel-Smith 1992: vii). Establishing the appropriate level for resourcing the Health Service is a fraught task (Appleby 1992: Chapter 4). None the less, even in a brief discussion significant points can be made. First, the British NHS's funding 'has been the most successfully protected from economic crises, with almost continuous growth in real terms, even though at rates varying through time, of all the major public services' (Perrin 1992: 221).

Nevertheless, of the around 8% compound growth per annum, about 7% is accounted for by inflation and the 1% left is fully required to keep up with the expenditure rises concomitant upon Britain's ageing population who are high users of the Service. If one adds to this the continuingly rapid technological growth in medicine and pharmaceuticals and the rising expectations of the entire population for its Health Service, it is not hard to see that tight funding or underfunding is the likely outcome. The question of how to deal with this ultimately rests on national decisions about priorities inside the health budget and compared with other areas of state expenditure – the old guns versus butter question of a first-year economics textbook.

The issues are quite basic and hardly comfortable ones with easy solutions. Readers could at this point reflect upon the closing sections of Chapter 18 where Professor Ebrahim suggests a variety of ways – hard to contemplate perhaps – to pay for some of the rapidly rising costs of providing for the health-care needs of the elderly in an adequate and humane manner.

Another frequently encountered dichotomy, and one which certainly can have damaging effects, is between, on the one hand, the general management model initiated in the NHS by the adoption by the Government of the Griffiths Report (1983) in which one manager at each level in the Health Service has, in principle at least, ultimate responsibility and decision-making power over all staff, clinical and non-clinical, contained within that level and, on the other hand, the so-called 'consensus' model of management that in various forms preceded general management. This dichotomy can be easily associated with Theme 6 in Table 20.1 above and the large number of chapters in this book associated with it. In fact, as was pointed out in Chapter 1, the shape of this particular book has been much influenced by, first, the multidisciplinary nature of the Service in all its branches and activities, second by the fact that large numbers of doctors, nurses, paramedics and others, in no way designated as managers, fulfil important managerial functions and, third, not only are the professional managers at an early stage of professionalization but the 'core business' of hospitals is highly technical and still essentially in the hands of the medical profession.

Criticisms of this 'professional dominance' from doctors comes not only from the rising general managers but also from nursing and other clincially based professions. One thing is clear, if NHS general managers, *qua* managers, aspire to impose themselves upon other groups in hospitals, they are likely to have limited success at best and even that could easily turn into a Pyrrhic victory due to the resultant damage to relations between the different professions that do undertake the *primary mission* of hospitals.

Leaving this to one side for the moment, what impact do the Reforms and the quasi market in health have in terms of the strengthening, or otherwise, of the NHS general management position in relation to doctors, nurses and other staff? The influence of the Reforms, including RMI, has been considered at length in the existing literature. Readers could refer to Chapter 2 in this collection, the associated Harrison *et al.* (1990, 1992) and Tilley *et al.* (1991) to name just some accounts.

What of 'managed competition' itself? Might it affect NHS general managers' power and influence over other groupings in their hospitals? In theory it could substantially strengthen such management's hand. In the early days of introducing general management into the Health Service, much was made of administrators metamorphosing into quite different beings, general managers, even if most commentators expected this to be a long journey. The recent Reforms certainly have been aimed at shortening the journey time.

A key difference that could be made between NHS administrators and managers is that the former operate under conditions of relative certainty in outcome terms and, therefore, given their relative weakness in terms of the core technical activities of a hospital, the professions that are dominant in this technical core, will effectively run the hospital, with the administrators servicing senior doctors and nurses.

The internal market might change this relative certainty factor. Chapters 7 and 8 are germane here. From them, it seems clear that even in those parts of the NHS where it is least appropriate to speak of a market in health services, there still is more operating uncertainty for hospitals as, for example, GPFHs both grow in numbers and cluster together to exert greater influence, directly and indirectly, over hospitals. In some parts of London the uncertainty factor derives from many additional and potent sources although if the Tomlinson Report (1992) were implemented this would reduce. But in the circumstances currently encountered by some inner London hospitals, general managers perceived to be competent and successful in the face of adverse and somewhat unpredictable circumstances could emerge as general managers with power and control over their organizations not too dissimilar to that found more frequently in private-sector management. The bulk of NHS managers will be lying between the two poles outlined above, although even if it is present, what use is made of the varying degrees of environmental uncertainty will be influenced by complicated and diverse factors including the past history of the provider and its inter- and intra-professional relations, the personalities and aspirations of key players, etc. The influence of environmental uncertainty on organizational politics in hospitals has also been pointed out by Harrison (1992: 7) and is sufficiently important to warrant closer study.

I would like to close this discussion of NHS general management by thinking briefly about the sort of power and influence that might be won and its costs in terms of organizational effectiveness. In fact, the idea of NHS managers vigorously endeavouring to impose themselves on the rest of their organization is not a model for general management endorsed by the top gurus private-sector managers might well be listening to. In fact, such 'macho' versions of general management are frequently identified by such writers as increasingly dysfunctional in today's business world. I will start with a British guru who points out that 'Paradoxically top [business] managers now mouth the words "our people are our major asset" but do not behave as if this is so' (Garratt 1990: xiv).

Morgan (1988: 55) speaks of 'people as a key resource'. This view is also central to Peters' thinking: he speaks of 'the minimisation of the role of labour' as one of the 'sacred cows of the American economic belief system' that is holding the US economy back relative to its main competitors (Peters 1989: 20). In a similar vein Moss Kanter is concerned to find 'what is it about the structure and culture – the roadblocks erected [in many major US corporations] – . . . that keeps managers and employees from contributing more to productive change' in their working lives when they are often highly adaptive and creative in their non-work lives (Moss Kanter 1985: 71). Tichy and Devanna (1986: x) say that 'the challenge is for transformational leadership [to be sought out and encouraged] at all levels in an organisation' not just at the top. In his well-known study of US general managers in private business, Kotter (1982: 142) speaks of the need to minimize the 'I can do anything' syndrome common in such circles. Schein (1985: 314) offers a telling warning: 'Do not assume that culture can be manipulated like other matters under the control of managers. Culture controls the manager more than the manager controls culture.' And in another of his well-known management studies, this time in the area of career management, he reminds managers that it is an essential requirement of business effectiveness to balance the organizational and individual needs of all employees (Schein 1978: 243).

At first sight it may seem odd to some to be quoting mainly top US management authorities in a book on the British NHS. I adjudged it well worthwhile, first, because of the current enthusiasm for private-sector management ideas and for things American in the present-day NHS and, second, as they provide ample support for the view that, although numerous changes in the relationship between doctors and managers, and between these two groupings and other NHS professional groups, may well be highly desirable, the only realistic conceptions of NHS management today must put high value on the idea of partnership, and this need not end up as the 'consensus management' of the past which is no better suited to the much less certain, faster changing world of the NHS of today and tomorrow. To aim for various types of intersecting managerial partnerships at various levels even in the one hospital requires the active seeking of real partnership all the way along if the aim is to mean anything at all.

This, as with the other dichotomies that limit discussion in and about the NHS, seems to demand extensive research, once again of the broad, flexible, often action-based variety much mentioned in this chapter. The dichotomies often rest on reductionist arguments: 'The problem with the NHS, or this bit of the NHS, is nothing but . . .'. Broad, diverse and innovative 'R&D' can provide knowledge that could, at minimum, help clarify what in its real complexity the situation is. Certainly all the different constituencies the NHS serves, those operating either inside or outside of it, could well benefit from that. One obvious warning that none the less ought to be stated is that although such research helps clarify isssues, this is not to say it can, as if by magic, remove the sometimes deeper disagreements and diverging interests that may have given rise to the polarized views in the first place.

ON THE RESEARCH IMPLICATIONS OF THIS BOOK

A final source upon which to draw to support and elaborate the argument that underscores Chapter 20 – the need to intensify the NHS's 'organizational R&D' function – comes from the collection itself and its research implications, certainly those explicitly identified by contributors but, much more, those implicit in the collection. As this is something individual readers can best do for themselves, I intend to offer only one example of the near endless ones that might have been identified.

Chapters 6 and 12, in particular, identify the huge, quite daunting requirement for local needs assessment within DoH and possibly other (say, Regional) frameworks. Demone and Gibelman (1989) suggest a useful distinction that could help the large, multidisciplinary research effort required. It is between monitoring and evaluation and not unlike the broader distinction in management and organizational literature between programmed and non-programmed decision-making but applied to health commissioning. Monitoring is really about ensuring contract compliance; evaluation is a questioning of the choices behind the contracts. Monitoring may raise some thorny issues around quality, etc., but, when established, has many routine features. Evaluation tends to remain novel, often qualitative in nature and even requiring longitudinal studies. Unlike monitoring, it can be undertaken in-house and/or by third-party researchers. This distinction is useful as it enables the gigantic tasks facing DHA purchasers to be split up and the research effort for the much more difficult evaluation side appropriately shared out.

Where, then, has Chapter 20 taken us? Rather than offer a tidy conclusion forced on rather untidy and multiple realities, it provides some concluding remarks all centred round the now urgent need for the traditionally neglected

NHS research function to be much upgraded as well as being more broadly and, where necessary, experimentally undertaken as the Health Service enters the end of almost two decades of near continuous reorganization and major organizational change. The current Government health Reforms, the latest and largest block of organizational changes, introduce varying degrees of environmental uncertainty and thence one task for this enhanced 'organizational R&D' function is to help managers and clinicians to scan that environment.

The chapter has travelled in a variety of directions, all of which reinforce and amplify this new 'R&D' function. First, the broadest theme from Table 20.1 above was enlarged upon. This discussion included indicating some specific fields where research and action research are required. Second, the whole change programme, including the NHS market, was considered, at the analytical level at least, as simply another management-of-change exercise. Not surprisingly the evaluation area was the most obviously incomplete aspect identified and again broadly based, diverse and innovative 'organizational R&D' could fill some of this gap. Third, more knowledge from research was a way of at least clarifying the many dichotomous reactions to key NHS issues. Fourth, the many explicit and implicit research implications of *Managing the Internal Market* that readers could identify would be likely to provide further support for the idea that a much enlarged, more broadly conceived, diverse and novel 'R&D' function could aid the NHS at this important phase in its history.

Somewhat paradoxically it is by no means clear that a Reformed NHS operating within an internal market will be a more generous patron of this newly conceived research function than the Service was in its past. If this pessimistic conclusion is borne out by events, it is likely to have unfortunate implications. The basic problem is that, though the Reforms were introduced in a simple top-down manner characteristic of the public sector generally and the NHS in particular, complexity immediately takes over as much of the implementation process cannot be controlled (March and Olsen 1989: 65). NHS managers and those clinicians performing a managerial function need detailed, comparative material gathered over significant parts of the Service that the 'new R&D' could, in time, produce. What seems clear is the Reforms and the quasi health market are beginning to produce fairly widespread change: 'the various actors in the health-care game [are] start[ing] to learn how to play by new rules' (Appleby 1992: 25). All NHS stakeholders, certainly Health Service managers and clinicians with management roles, will be hampered in terms of playing this rather important 'game' unless more attention is paid to their intelligence/information-gathering needs relating to both inner and outer circumstance and relevant information is both meaningfully interpreted and acted upon.

REFERENCES

Abel-Smith, B. (1992) *Cost Containment and New Priorities in Health Care*. Aldershot: Avebury.

Appleby, J. (1992) *Financing Health Care in the 1990s*. Buckingham: Open University Press.

Appleby, J. *et al.* (1990) The use of markets in the Health Service: the NHS Reforms and managed competition, *Public Money and Management*, Winter, 27–33.

Boddy, D. and Buchanan, D. (1992) *Take the Lead: Interpersonal Skills for Project Managers*. London: Prentice-Hall.

Boss, R. W. (1989) *Organisation Development in Health Care*. Reading, Mass: Addison-Wesley.

Bourn, M. (1989) Management accounting for recurrent expenditure in the National Health Service, in M. W. Pendlebury (ed.) *Management Accounting in the Public Sector*. London: Heinemann/Chartered Institute of Management Accountants.

Bowling, A. *et al.* (1991) General practitioners' views on quality specifications for outpatient referrals and care contracts, *British Medical Journal*, 3 August, 292–4.

Brazier, J. *et al.* (1990) Evaluating the Reform of the NHS, in A. J. Culyer *et al.* (eds.) *Competition in Health Care: Reforming the NHS*. London: Macmillan, 216–36.

Buchanan, D. and Boddy, D. (1992) *The Expertise of the Change Agent: Public Performance and Backstage Activity*. London: Prentice-Hall.

Cope, D. E. (1981) *Organisational Development and Action Research in Hospitals*. Aldershot: Gower.

Cunningham, D. (1990) Needs assessment, in E. J. Beck and S. A. Adam (eds.) *The White Paper and Beyond*. Oxford: Oxford University Press, 12–22.

Dearden, R. W. (1991) Purchasing with vision, *Health Services Management*, August, 171–3.

Demone, H. W. Jr. and Gibelman, M. (eds.) (1989) *Services for Sale: Purchasing Health and Human Services*. New Brunswick: Rutgers UP.

Dickson, N. (1991) Tilting at those Rubber Windmills, *Health Service Journal*, 6 June, 22–3.

DoH (Department of Health) (1989) *Working for Patients*. London: HMSO.

Eminson, J. (1991) Why small is beautiful, *Health Service Journal*, 22 August, 8.

Galloway, M. (1991) Saying no to two tiers, *Health Service Journal*, 23 May, 8.

Garratt, B. (1990) *Creating a Learning Organisation: A Guide to Leadership, Learning and Development*. Cambridge: Director Books.

Griffiths, R. (1983) *NHS Management Inquiry Report*. London: Department of Health and Social Security.

Ham, C. (1990) *Holding on While Letting Go: A Report on the Relationship between Directly Managed Units and DHAs*. London: King's Fund College.

Harrison, S. *et al.* (1990) *The Dynamics of British Health Policy*. London: Unwin Hyman.

Harrison, S. *et al.* (1992) *Just Managing: Power and Culture in the National Health Service*. London: Macmillan.

Huntington, J. (1991) When two worlds collide, *Health Service Journal*, 10 October, 17.

Jones, T. and Kerr, C. (1986) *Money, Medics and Management: The English and American Systems Compared*. London: Certified Accountants Educational Trust.

Klein, L. and Eason, K. (1991) *Putting Social Science to Work*. Cambridge: Cambridge University Press.

Klein, R. (1989) *The Politics of the National Health Service* (2nd edn). London: Longman.

Kotter, J. P. (1982) *The General Managers*. New York: Free Press.

Labour Party (1992) *Your Good Health: A White Paper for a Labour Government*. London: Labour Party.

Liberal Democratic Party (1992) *Restoring the Nation's Health: Liberal Democrat Policies for Health Care and the National Health Service*. London: Liberal Democrat Publications.

Light, D. W. (1991) Observations on the NHS Reforms: an American perspective, *British Medical Journal*, 7 September, 568–70.

Little, S. (1992) Government funding clampdown forecast, *Pulse*, 9 May, 4.

McCalman, J. and Paton, R.A. (1992) *Change Management: A Guide to Effective Implementation*. London: Paul Chapman.

MacLachlin, R. *et al.* (1991) Illogical, inconsistent and too tight with cash, *Health Service Journal*, 13 June, 14.

Mangham, I. (1979) *The Politics of Organisational Change*. London: Associated Business Press.

March, J. G. and Olsen, J.P. (1979) *Ambiguity and Choice in Organisations*. Bergen: Universitetsforleget.

March, J.G. and Olsen, J.P. (1989) *Rediscovering Institutions: The Organisational Basis of Politics*. New York: Free Press.

Margulies, N. and Adams, J.D. (1982) *Organisational Development in Health-Care Organisations*. Reading, Mass: Addison-Wesley.

Meldrum, H. (1992) Will mergers benefit GPs?, *Pulse*, 18 April, 41.

Miller, E.J. and Rice, A.K. (1967) *Systems of Organisation: The Control of Task and Sentient Boundaries*. London: Tavistock.

Moore, W. (1991) Purchasers move to centre stage, *Health Service Journal*, 23 May, 14.

Morgan, G. (1988) *Riding the Waves of Change: Developing Managerial Competencies for a Turbulent World*. San Francisco: Jossey-Bass.

Moss Kanter, R. (1985) *The Change Masters: Corporate Entrepreneurs at Work*. London: Unwin.

Murphy, E. (1990) Meeting the needs of the most vulnerable, in E.J. Beck and S.A. Adam (eds.) *The White Paper and Beyond: One Year on*. Oxford: Oxford University Press, 78–87.

National Health Service Management Executive (NHSME) (1992) *NHS Reforms: The First Six Months*. London: DoH.

Nicklin, P. *et al.* (1991) Exchange rates, *British Journal of Healthcare Computing*, April, 16–7.

Paton, C. (1992) *Competition and Planning in the National Health Service: The Danger of Unplanned Markets*. London: Chapman & Hall.

Perrin, J. (1992) The National Health Service, in D. Henley *et al.* (eds.) *Public Sector Accounting and Financial Control*. London: Chapman & Hall.

Peters, T. (1989) *Thriving on Chaos: Handbook for a Management Revolution*. London: Pan/Macmillan.

Pettigrew, A. and Whipp, R. (1991) *Managing Change for Competitive Success*. Oxford: Blackwell.

Pfeffer, J. (1992) *Managing with Power: Politics and Influence in Organisations*. Boston, Mass: Harvard Business School Press.

Pulse (1992a) GP split over Fundholding headed off, *Pulse*, 9 May, 4.

Pulse (1992b) GPs back purchaser/provider split, *Pulse*, 4 April, 24.

Quinn, J.B. (1980) *Strategies for Change: Logical Incrementalism*. Homewood, Ill: Irwin.

Revans, R.W. (1982) *The Origins and Growth of Action Learning*. London: Chartwell-Bratt.

Robinson, R. and Scheuer, M.A. (1992) Fishing for Fundholders, *Health Service Journal*, 13 February, 18–20.

Ruddy, B. (1991) A dinosaur in waiting?, *Health Service Journal*, 11 July, 8.

Saltman, R.B. and von Otter, C. (1992) *Planned Markets and Public Competition: Strategic Reform in Northern European Health Systems*. Buckingham: Open University Press.

Schein, E.H. (1978) *Career Dynamics: Matching Individual and Organisational Needs*. Reading, Mass: Addison-Wesley.

Schein, E.H. (1985) *Organisational Culture and Leadership*. San Francisco: Jossey-Bass.

Shapiro, E.R. and Carr, W. (1991) *Lost in Familiar Places: Creating New Connections Between the Individual and Society*. New Haven: Yale University Press.

Small, N. (1989) *Politics and Planning in the National Health Service*. Milton Keynes: Open University Press.

Spry, C. (1991) Oxygen-rich purchasing, *Health Service Journal*, 16 May, 8.

Spurgeon, P. and Barwell, F. (1991) *Implementing Change in the NHS: A Practical Guide for General Managers*. London: Chapman & Hall.

Stewart, R. (1989) *Leading in the NHS: A Practical Guide*. London: Macmillan.

Strauss, A. (1991) Interorganisational negotiation, in K. Plummer (ed.) *Symbolic Interactionism, Vol. II: Contemporary issues*. Aldershot: Edward Elgar, 134–51.

Thompson, D. and Flanagan, H. (1991) Where Darwin meets Beveridge, *Health Service Journal*, 27 June, 24–5.

Tichy, N.M. and Devanna, M.A. (1986) *The Transformational Leader*. New York: Wiley.

Tilley, I. *et al.* (1991) Hospital organisation and intrahospital interest groups: a preliminary look at change perspectives in an NHS hospital. Papers presented to the British Sociological Association annual conference, March, University of Manchester.

Tomlinson, B. (1992) *Report of the Inquiry into London's Health Service, Medical Education and Research*. London: HMSO.

Turner, D. (1989) Insider trading: public funds for private medicine, *Medeconomics*, June, 64–8.

Whyte, W.F. (ed.) (1991) *Participatory Action Research*. New Brunswick, Calif: Sage.

Willcocks, L. and Harrow, J. (eds.) (1992) *Rediscovering Public Services Management*. London: McGraw-Hill.

Williams, A. (1990) Research implications of the NHS review, in A.J. Culyer *et al.* (eds.) *Competition in Health Care: Reforming the NHS*. London: Macmillan, 237–52.

Willis, A. (1992) Who needs Fundholding?, *Health Service Journal*, 30 April, 24–6.

Wright, K.G. (1990) The challenge of community care Reform, in A.J. Culyer *et al.* (eds.) *Competition in Health Care: Reforming the NHS*. London: Macmillan.

Woodhouse, D. and Pengelly, P. (1991) *Anxiety and the Dynamics of Collaboration*. Aberdeen: Aberdeen University Press.

Index